PSYCHOSOCIAL PERSPECTIVES ON AIDS

Etiology, Prevention, and Treatment

PSYCHOSOCIAL PERSPECTIVES ON AIDS

Etiology, Prevention, and Treatment

Edited by

Lydia Temoshok
Henry M. Jackson Foundation
Walter Reed Army Medical Center

Andrew Baum
F. Edward Hébert School of Medicine
Uniformed Services University of the Health Sciences

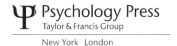
Psychology Press
Taylor & Francis Group

New York London

First Published by
Lawrence Erlbaum Associates, Inc., Publishers
365 Broadway
Hillsdale, New Jersey 07642

Transferred to Digital Printing 2009 by Psychology Press
270 Madison Ave, New York NY 10016
27 Church Road, Hove, East Sussex, BN3 2FA

Library of Congress Cataloging-in-Publication Data

Psychosocial perspectives on AIDS : etiology, prevention, and
  treatment / edited by Lydia Temoshok, Andrew Baum.
      p. cm.
  Includes bibliographical references.
  ISBN 0-8058-0207-X
    1. AIDS (Disease)—Psychological aspects. 2. AIDS (Disease)—
Social aspects. I. Temoshok, Lydia. II. Baum, Andrew.
RC607.A26P7946 1990
362.1'969792—dc20   90-31604
                                       CIP

ISBN 0-8058-0207-X

Publisher's Note
The publisher has gone to great lengths to ensure the quality of this reprint
but points out that some imperfections in the original may be apparent.

This book is dedicated to the people with HIV disease whose courageous contributions to research have made a meaningful difference to all of those touched by the disease.

Contents

Preface

The Acquired Immunodeficiency Syndrome (AIDS) and the virus that causes it (human immunodeficiency virus Type I, HIV-1) have challenged the world's scientists, health care systems, and public health policies as much or more than any medical problem in recorded history. Perhaps this is because AIDS and HIV infection constitute more than a medical problem; they are enmeshed in psychological, social, cultural, political, and economic contexts. Consequently, AIDS/HIV affects — and is affected by — all these contexts. A problem of such massive proportions requires extensive collaborative efforts between biomedical and behavioral scientists at the basic, clinical, and public health levels to inform intervention and prevention efforts.

Although much basic research in virology and immunology can be accomplished within the biomedical domain, biobehavioral disciplines such as behavioral medicine offer more opportunities for the comprehensive approach necessary to confront the AIDS/HIV problem. Behavioral medicine encompasses the entire health-illness spectrum, from basic scientific exploration of brain-body mechanism issues to public health strategies for disease prevention and health promotion at the community level. Applied to the problem of AIDS/HIV, this model suggests that the health and well being of individuals affected by HIV are not solely dependent on the achievements of medicine. Such an assertion is particularly important to reinforce at this time when there is no medical cure for AIDS and the possibility of a vaccine is distant. To the extent that psychosocial and behavioral variables influence risk of exposure to HIV infection, quality of life, and possibly progression of HIV disease and longevity, then these variables become critical to consider in HIV prevention and intervention.

Some of the chapters in this book appeared as more circumscribed, research-based articles in a special issue of *The Journal of Applied Social Psychology* (1987, Volume 17, Number 3). To our knowledge, this was the first collection of research-based articles representing a comprehensive biopsychosocial perspective on the problem of AIDS/HIV. There was a particular need at that time to provide data on the problem, as many assertions and assumptions were being promulgated that were based on little more than opinion and politics. Since then, there has been an explosion of behavioral science research articles in medical, psychological, and public health journals. However, there have been few attempts to combine research and applied aims and efforts. These circumstances have contributed to the present urgency to implement methods and apply research results to HIV/AIDS intervention and prevention efforts in a variety of settings and populations.

In response to this need, we went back to the original authors of the articles in the special issue and asked them to extend their analyses of their findings. In addition, we invited several additional contributions, representing areas not addressed in the 1987 collections. We believe that these areas are critical to an understanding of the multidimensional problems occasioned by HIV/AIDS, and the relative success or failure of their attempted solutions.

This book does not set out to discuss theoretical issues arising from an increasing understanding of factors involved in HIV infection and progression, nor does it discuss in detail ethical or political implications of behavioral science research and application. Rather, the chapters in this book address the need for pragmatic and research-based suggestions on how to address some important psychological, social, and public health problems associated with HIV/AIDS.

It is part of the complexity and frustration of research and intervention efforts regarding the AIDS/HIV problem that we are dealing with a "moving target." It is likely that some of the problems and attempted solutions described in this volume will be of mainly historical interest after its publication. This observation in itself suggests an approach to research and intervention/prevention efforts for AIDS/HIV — an approach that would probably be equally useful applied to other problems. This approach would emphasize flexibility of response to changing knowledge, patterns of the pandemic, new treatments, and shifts in public opinion and behavior. Unfortunately, most funding agencies are ill equipped to respond flexibly and creatively to the changing nature of the AIDS/HIV problem. Further, many agencies are categorical in nature, and again unfortunately, tend to fragment the AIDS/HIV biopsychosocial problem, instead of taking a comprehensive approach. A third major problem is the frequent separation of research and applied efforts. The most efficient way for research to inform practice is for a constant feedback process to exist between research and application within each level of the health care system, and at each step of public health decision and policy making. If changes can be made in these three areas, they will go a long way to allowing behavioral science researchers and practitioners to do the work necessary to anticipate and confront the multifaceted problems of HIV/AIDS in the last decade of the twentieth century.

We are grateful to a number of persons who made this volume possible. Victor Winston, publisher of the *Journal of Applied Social Psychology,* was extraordinarily supportive and facilitated the publication of the special issue on AIDS/HIV in 1987, and his cooperation in allowing us to publish some of the articles from that issue in this book is also greatly appreciated. Several colleagues and friends were important sources of advice and inspiration including George F. Solomon, Don Des Jarlais, Jeffrey Moulton, Susan Tross, Peter Bourne, Leonard Zegans, Harry Holloway, Neil Schneiderman, and Jeff Kelly. We also thank Cheryl Palacios and Martha Gisriel for their great help on these projects.

Lydia Temoshok and Andrew Baum
January 1990

Psychosocial Aspects of Acquired Immunodeficiency Syndrome

1

Andrew Baum
Uniformed Services University of the Health Sciences

Lydia Temoshok
University of California, San Francisco

Since 1980, acquired immunodeficiency syndrome (AIDS) has had, arguably, more impact on the minds and behavior of people throughout the world than any epidemic—or pandemic—in recent history. The urgency of the AIDS problem is undeniable: It is a killer that must be controlled in spite of the fact that we have no vaccine, no cures, and few treatments. It kills fewer people than do heart disease, cancer, and other illnesses common in the U.S., but like other potent diseases throughout history such as influenza, polio, or the plague, it is communicable, lethal, and poorly understood. Unlike heart disease, it does not develop out of a lifetime of unhealthy behavior: One can become infected with the AIDS virus as a result of one careless act. Unlike cancer, which may develop when immunosurveillance breaks down, AIDS is a disorder of the immune system itself and, as such, may short-circuit normal protection against it. As a result, a great deal of effort has been mobilized to better understand AIDS, how it is spread, how it develops once the causal virus (human immunodeficiency virus Type 1, HIV-1, hereafter referred to as HIV) has been unleashed, and, perhaps most importantly, how to stop it.

A common denominator of all the contributions in this book is a biopsychosocial approach to understanding and combating AIDS/HIV. Some chapters will lean more in one direction or another, but all take as a point of departure the necessity of considering the biological, psychological, and social domains *in interaction.* Another common denominator is the extension of research

The opinions or assertions contained herein are the private ones of the authors and are not to be construed as official or reflecting the views of the Department of Defense or the Uniformed Services University of the Health Sciences.

findings into areas of clinical or policy applications. In this chapter, we will launch a discussion of the areas in which most of this research has been done—areas represented by the contributors to this volume—and then consider some of the many issues requiring further investigation. We believe that such issues cannot be addressed in the context of applying the traditional medical model to the multidimensional problems of AIDS and HIV disease.

Behavioral scientists have a great deal to contribute in addressing such multidimensional questions. For example, how do medical status and the increasingly recognized neuropsychological complications of HIV affect a person's coping, well-being, and/or disease progression? AIDS and HIV disease offer a rich arena—perhaps richer than other diseases—in which to examine interactions among biological, psychological, and social levels of functioning (Coates, Temoshok, & Mandel, 1984). Superimposed on the pressing need to apply what we already know to the control of this dreaded disease, the opportunity to observe basic processes is an important by-product of the effort to treat and prevent HIV infection. The traveler down the road of biopsychosocial AIDS/HIV research should be forewarned, however, that the road is unpaved and often precarious (Temoshok & Baum, 1987).

AIDS/HIV itself is a rapidly changing disease phenomenon, particularly in terms of its epidemiology. Because it is a new disease, and one that is being intensely researched by scientists around the world, information about it constantly expands, changes, and becomes obsolete. Since 1982 (when behavioral scientists initiated work on AIDS), the virus that is associated with AIDS was discovered and given at least three different names. The classification of AIDS-spectrum disorders by the Centers for Disease Control in Atlanta was changed several times, and other classification systems were proposed. Numerous tests were developed to detect antibodies to the virus, and a number of biological treatments of AIDS were heralded—most, unfortunately, for a short time—as cures for the disease. Behavioral scientists working in health and medical arenas are accustomed to the need to educate themselves about the health phenomena being studied: heart diseaase, cancer, asthma, and so forth. To stay minimally abreast of scientific developments in HIV research requires hours of dedicated scientific journal reading per week, frequent participation in related conferences and workshops, and active correspondence with researchers worldwide (Temoshok, Zich, & Green, 1987).

It can be cogently argued that the greatest potential contribution of behavioral scientists to the AIDS/HIV problem may be through avenues such as health promotion, health education, and counseling. As there is currently no vaccine against HIV and promising treatments are still experimental, prevention has emerged as our most effective strategy against the disease. Partly because prevention may be achieved by behavioral intervention and because one's risk of infection may be reduced to near zero by eliminating or altering risky behaviors, this is an area in which behavioral scientists have a great deal to offer.

AIDS/HIV also challenges us to look more closely at the social dimension of the biopsychosocial model. It is critical to examine the differences as well as commonalities in response to AIDS or the threat of AIDS across various subgroups of persons whose behaviors put them most at risk: gay men, intravenous drug users (a large percentage of whom are minorities), partners of risk-group members, and sexually active heterosexuals. Different prevention and intervention approaches may be required for black, white, or Hispanic communities; for heterosexuals or homosexuals; for men or women; and for adults or adolescents.

Moreover, biopsychosocial AIDS/HIV researchers must be aware of public-health initiatives, political decisions, and sociocultural events that will have far-reaching repercussions once they are publicized. The widespread availability of testing for the HIV antibody; the announcements of new treatments for AIDS, such as AZT (zidovudine, Retrovir); and new government policies and proposed regulations concerning antibody testing have had unexpected turns and effects on all segments of society. The story of Rock Hudson's struggle and ultimate death from AIDS in late 1985 brought home to millions around the world that AIDS can touch anyone. It is obvious that each of these events had a significant impact on levels of knowledge, fear, optimism, and depression in persons with HIV disease, persons whose behaviors place them at risk for HIV, and the general public.

The AIDS epidemic has generated a tumultuous series of events. Aside from the medical and psychological problems directly posed by the disease, it has sent shock waves through some social groups and is having some effects on behavior at a societal level. The role of sexual behavior in spreading the disease has led to changes in how we view sex, from references to condoms on television shows to renewed emphasis on abstinence and monogamy. It is in this context that the study of various aspects of AIDS/HIV must be studied. We will consider research needs in three general areas: etiology and progression of the disease, patient care, and prevention.

ETIOLOGY AND PROGRESSION

The development of HIV disease, beginning when one is infected and encompassing a number of stages including AIDS, is of crucial importance to our understanding of the disease. It is now clear that the disease progresses at different rates in different people. For some, the initial latency period immediately following infection may be brief; while for others, symptoms of disease progression may not appear for several years. While it has been predicted that nearly all people infected with HIV will eventually develop AIDS (Lui, Darrow, & Rutherford, 1988), the fact that progression occurs at such variable rates suggests that biological and psychosocial variables may influence the manner in which the virus functions and thrives in the body. In this section, we discuss some of these issues, beginning with basic biological aspects of HIV disease and clarification of terminology of AIDS and HIV disease.

Terminology and Basic Biology

People who have been infected by the HIV, who show antibodies for HIV, but who are healthy and exhibit no symptoms of the disease are considered anti-HIV+ or seropositive. Although this means that the possibility of developing AIDS is dramatically increased, it does not tell us very much about when the disease will become evident or what kinds of changes may occur antecedent to the development of AIDS. In this scheme, AIDS refers to the frank and full manifestation of the disease, including profound immunosuppression and certain severe opportunistic infections such as *Pneumocystis carinii* pneumonia, or tumors such as Kaposi's sarcoma. An intermediate stage in which some symptoms are exhibited has been referred to as AIDS-related complex (ARC).

It may be best to refer to the gamut of states of seropositivity through chronic, progressive generalized lymphadenopathy (PGL) and ARC to AIDS as HIV disease. This emphasizes the continuous nature of the illness, rather than a categorization defined by symptoms of the illness. It also raises critical research questions: What kinds of psychological and physiological changes precede, co-occur, or follow changes in disease status? By measuring the basic physiological, cognitive, and emotional changes associated with HIV disease during all phases of the illness, we may be better able to understand and predict its course. Further, as new and more precise staging systems are developed, we will be able to link more closely changes in psychosocial factors and immunologic parameters with clinical status.

Infection with HIV can cause at least two kinds of damage. Best known are its effects on the immune system. The tendency of the virus to attack immune cells and reside in T_4-helper (CD_4) cells has a variety of negative effects on immunosurveillance, allowing opportunistic infections to develop. The targets of HIV are not all known or fully understood, but the resulting immunosuppression leads directly to opportunistic infections, ordinarily the cause of death among persons with AIDS. Neuropsychological deficits have also been observed in asymptomatic seropositive individuals (although there is conflicting evidence), as well as in people with ARC and AIDS. The virus apparently is carried into the central nervous system (CNS) by macrophages, and, once there, it appears to cause a number of cognitive and attentional problems. AIDS Dementia Complex (ADC), the most common neurological complication of AIDS, is characterized by global cognitive deterioration (Navia, Jordan & Price, 1986).

Stress and Immunity

Many studies have suggested that stress is associated with changes in immune system status and incidence of infectious illness, and it is assumed by many that stress and the immune system are linked. "Everyone knows" that stress can make one sick, or at least that one is more likely to get sick during or after dealing with substantial demand or threat. Research tends to support this hypothesis, mostly by documenting relationships between stress and immune system changes or subsequent illness (e.g., Jemmott & Locke, 1984; Kiecolt-Glaser & Glaser, 1987; Rahe, 1975). In the few studies that have investigated stress-induced immunosuppression and subsequent illness, differences in terms of whether the stressor was chronic or acute, severe or mild, or administered early or late in development have made it difficult to generalize about the consequences of stress-related changes in immunity. While much has been learned about how stress may contribute to illness through immune system changes, much remains to be understood about these relationships. In the case of HIV+, ARC, or AIDS patients, questions about the role stress plays in immune changes may be very important.

HIV does not necessarily become active immediately upon entering the body, but may remain latent and not become active or induce clinical symptoms or infections for as long as 7-10 years (Liu et al., 1988). The time between infection and appearance of symptoms of immune deficit is variable. Genetic factors, virus "dose," virus strain, and co-factors such as other sexually transmitted diseases or use of intravenous or other drugs could all affect latency. Research has indicated that stress affects the activation of latent herpes viruses, held in check by immune processes until stress interferes with immunoregulation of the virus (Kiecolt-Glaser & Glaser, 1987). This could apply to activation of HIV (Solomon, Temoshok, O'Leary, & Zich, 1987; Temoshok, Zich, Solomon & Stites, 1987; Temoshok, Solomon, Jenkins, & Sweet, 1989), leading to a number of researchable questions about how stress could affect progression of HIV disease. What are the consequences of stressful life changes associated with and independent of HIV infection? Does stress (or how one reacts) associated with learning that one has tested positive on the HIV antibody test affect the course of the infection? The role of mediators of stress, such as coping and social support, is also crucial as it is in studies of stress and immune function (cf. Kiecolt-Glaser & Glaser, 1987). Does the nature of AIDS cause people to pull away from seropositive and AIDS individuals, depriving them of stress-reducing social support when they need it (Zich & Temoshok, 1987)?

There are several ways to study these issues, ranging from large, correlational, longitudinal studies of high-risk individuals to controlled studies of stress-management or other interventions with HIV seropositives. Although it is perhaps premature to consider stress-management interventions as treatment against progression among individuals with HIV-spectrum disorders, it may be useful to study their effects. Such studies may provide more information about stress and immune function, as have studies of stress reduction and immunity in other populations (e.g., Kiecolt-Glaser et al., 1985). Second, although we do not know that stress reduction will affect immune status and disease state among individuals with HIV-spectrum disorders, the possibility that it may do so is sufficient to justify exploratory studies. Stress also has other effects, including behaviors that affect immunity independently (e.g., cigarette smoking, alcohol use, drug use) and that can affect general physiological status and health (e.g., diet, exercise).

Neuropsychological Problems

Stress may also affect the transport of the HIV into the CNS and/or its consequences once there. The relationships between stress and cognitive functions such as memory are not yet clear. Although stress has been shown to inferfere with performance on a variety of tasks, most of the research on these effects has been conducted in laboratory settings. More critical are the effects of stress on progressive damage by the HIV once it begins to act (Temoshok, Canick, Moulton, Sweet, Zich, Straits, Pivar, Hollander, 1988). Again, studies directed at the *interrelationships* of HIV infection and progression, immunologic changes, stress, performance deficits, and organic brain damage will yield important information (e.g., Temoshok et al., 1989). Ultimately, research directed at evaluating the benefits of stress management with AIDS patients and at the best means of dealing with neurological complications will address survival and quality of life, as well as determine whether intervention among seropositive and high-risk groups produces positive effects on disease progression or on incidence of infection.

A number of questions about the relationship between HIV activity in the periphery and its effects on the CNS can be posed. One of the most significant of these is whether these actions proceed together or occur at different rates governed by different variables. If the latter is the case and CNS effects are more or less independent of consequences for immunity, can evidence of disease be detected before the onset of classic symptoms and the drastic compromising of immunity? Can changes in psychological distress be tied to changes in disease status, and can they be used to predict progression from one disease stage to another? Finally, identification of the pattern or patterns of neuropsychological deficits associated with HIV infection and study of behavioral correlates may ultimately provide important information about how CNS problems affect preventive and treatment behavior, about whether observable behavior changes provide indications of CNS deficits, and about the nature of neuroregulation of behavior.

PATIENT CARE

Closely tied to the issue of progression of HIV disease is the question of how best to care for patients once infection has been documented or symptoms of AIDS have appeared. There are few published empirical studies on treatment or management of distress and other psychological consequences of disease progression, on interventions to slow or stop progression from seropositive status to ARC or AIDS, or on other aspects of patient care. Empirical studies are needed to assess what is effective in reducing psychological distress and promoting adaptive coping to the social stressors associated with HIV-spectrum disorders.

Social Influences

Among the potentially fruitful areas of work with HIV-infected patients are social variables such as support, perceived control, and attributional tendencies. Social support is recognized as an important variable in studies of stress and morbidity and appears to provide some protection from illness or stress effects (e.g., Cohen & Wills, 1985). However, because of fear or other aspects of reaction to victims, it may not be as available to persons with ARC or AIDS as to people with other diseases. Not having social support, losing it, or receiving noncontingent social regard because one is ill are important variables which have not been thoroughly investigated (Coates & Wortman, 1980; Cohen & Wills, 1985). Perceived control is also important. We know that a sense of control can reduce the consequences of stress, and if stress affects HIV disease, it should be important as well. This is particularly true if one recognizes that effects may be bidirectional. Does perceived control change when someone is infected with HIV or as the disease progresses? Do neuropsychological deficits affect perceived control, or does localized brain damage affect these perceptions? What are the effects of control on disease progression?

Clinical Interventions

Clearly, one of the larger issues in patient care is the application of therapeutic techniques and regimens to the care of AIDS patients. Stress management may prove to be important, but other interventions are also of potential significance. How can we modify such motivated misperceptions as immortality or the ability to determine who has AIDS and provide the basis for more accurate risk perception? Are the mental-health needs of persons with ARC or AIDS different from those of seropositive individuals, and do these differ from those of the general population or patients with other illnesses? The identification of techniques and variables that do not help victims of HIV disease, as well as those applications and interventions that are effective in reducing distress, altering risky behavior, ameliorating neuropsychological problems and so on, may tell us a great deal about the process of clinical intervention as well.

At another level, treatments for friends, family, and associates is called for, yet is rarely provided or documented. We know that there are consequences of having a terminally ill spouse or child; bereavement coupled with the unique problems of having a friend or family member become ill with AIDS requires special attention. Much can be learned about family dynamics and multi-target treatments as these issues are addressed. The development of "new" therapies to deal with these and other AIDS-related problems should advance the practice of psychotherapy, as well as help to identify the characteristics of seropositive individuals, the needs of these and other patients, and the psychological sequelae of powerful stigma, prejudice, and discrimination.

PREVENTION

Nowhere are the contributions of behavioral scientists more important than in the prevention of HIV infection. Although information about psychosocial variables and disease progression or data reflecting on the usefulness of supportive patient care will likely prove useful, such efforts will probably have less immediate or widespread impact than will successful education and prevention. Infection with HIV requires contact with the virus through exposure to bodily fluids—most notably through sexual activity, shared drug paraphernalia, exposure to blood products, and so on. These behaviors are generally thought to be modifiable. We presently have no vaccine to prepare the immune system to ward off HIV, and current medical treatments, while showing promise, do not cure patients or eliminate the infection. The only way that we now have to curb the epidemic and reduce the number of victims of HIV disease is to prevent people from coming into contact with the virus. The best ways to achieve this appear to be through screening of blood products, modification of sexual behavior, and alteration of drug-use behaviors.

Knowing what we know, we should be able to take some steps in this direction. We know what causes AIDS and can identify the presence of the virus. We know how it is spread and what behaviors contribute to its spread. Thus, theoretically, we should be able to modify risky behaviors to reduce the likelihood of infection by convincing people to practice safer sex, persuading drug users at least to use clean needles if they are going to continue injecting drugs, and preventing the use of infected blood or blood products. However, people are notoriously poor at assessing risk, at complying with preventive regimens, at dealing with asymptomatic states, and at using contraception. Given the difficulties we have had with preventing sexually transmitted diseases, and convincing people to stop smoking or to wear seat belts, the task appears to be more difficult in reality. There is some evidence that the threat of AIDS has led to risk-reduction behavior in homosexual men, in particular, but also in IV drug users. Little change has been documented, however, among potentially vulnerable adolescents, young adult heterosexuals, or urban black and Hispanic populations (Becker & Joseph, 1988; Fineberg, H.V., 1988).

Sexual Behavior

Sexual activity is one of the two most common routes of HIV transmission, at least at the present time in the U.S. The nature of sexual behavior makes it difficult to study, particularly by direct observation. It is highly personal and intimate, and it is the subject of sufficient societal taboos as to cause embarrassment, reluctance to accurately disclose, and resistance to modification.

Despite these barriers to study of modification of sexual behavior, we have learned a great deal about it over the past decade and must continue this effort. Identification of determinants of sexual behavior and preferences as well as methods of self-control must be evaluated. Information drawn from studies of contraception and sexually transmitted diseases (Brandt, 1988). should be applied in trying to discern ways to instill responsible and protective behaviors. Some of the most commonly used methods of birth control, including the pill, will not protect people from the HIV, so these forms of contraception must be supplemented by condoms and spermicides containing nonoxynol-9 by those who are sexually active.

Development

Special attention should be paid to adolescents, as they typically explore sexual activity and have shown, in past research, that: (a) they are not very reliable users of contraception, and (b) they have a high rate of sexually transmitted diseases, relative to other age groups. The investigation of perceptions of invulnerability among young people is necessary if we are to understand their resistance to preventive behavior. Further, the attitudes and behaviors of parents and older siblings are important to study in order to ascertain how younger people will respond to interventions and educational efforts. It is necessary to learn more about developmental aspects of sexual behavior, as well as the role of such variables as peer pressure in the development of risk-taking behavior. The effects of sex education on promiscuity, attitudes toward sex, contraception, relations with multiple partners, and other behaviors must continue to be evaluated.

Educational Campaigns

Efforts designed to increase people's knowledge about AIDS/HIV have several goals. Educational campaigns seek to provide people with information about AIDS/HIV. By doing this, it is reasoned, people will be better able to assess their risk of infection, the consequences of infection, and how to avoid these consequences by reducing risky behavior. The extent to which educational efforts accomplish these goals is dependent on factors that mediate acceptance and use of information. By increasing information, however, one can also attempt to decrease fear; by providing a clear understanding of the disease and prevention of infection, fear of contact may be moderated. However, it is not known whether information reduces fear, fear affects receptivity, or fear itself has an independent impact on behavior (e.g. Sherr, 1987, Temoshok, Sweet, & Zich, 1987).

The issue of audience is particularly important here in terms of targeting subgroups for particular educational programs. Gay men and IV drug users have constituted the primary risk groups in this country. It makes sense to assume that different groups will respond to different information and that campaigns directed toward one group (e.g., gay men) may not translate well to a second (e.g., teenagers). As we note in the next section, some groups of people may be at risk but not realize it. How one reaches these audiences is an important and difficult issue.

AIDS Education in "Less-at-risk" Groups

Studying the effectiveness of education to prevent infection, particularly in the highest-risk groups, has become a high research priority. Yet, there has been relatively little empirical research on AIDS-related knowledge, attitudes, beliefs, and behaviors of those "less at risk." In terms of AIDS/HIV, relative risk refers to the frequency of behaviors that might expose an individual to the HIV; a gay male is at higher risk than a monogamous heterosexual, and an IV drug user is at higher risk than are people who do not engage in such behavior, all other things being equal.

Studies of those "less at risk" are important for several reasons: Tomorrow's new "high-risk" group will emerge from those who are "less at risk" today. Fears of AIDS spreading beyond the current highest-risk groups into the wider heterosexual community, have, fortunately, not been realized in the U.S. or Europe (Padian, 1987). However, epidemiological evidence suggests that AIDS is a bidirectional, heterosexually transmitted disease in parts of Africa and Haiti (e.g., Melbye et al., 1986; Pape et al., 1985; Van de Perre et al., 1985). By 1990 a sevenfold increase in the number of cases attributed to heterosexual transmission has been predicted (Coolfont Report, 1986). Thus, while a lack of data on the spread of HIV infection into the U.S. general population hampers estimates (Thompson, 1988), there is a strong argument for directing health-education and prevention campaigns toward anyone who is sexually active.

Studies of "less-at-risk" populations have been concerned mainly with high-school and college students (Brown & Fritz, 1988; DiClemente, Zorn, & Temoshok, 1986; Kegeles, Adler, & Irwin, 1988; Price, Desmond, & Kukulka, 1985; Royse, Dhooper, & Hatch, 1987; Simkins & Eberhage, 1984; Simkins & Kushner, 1986; Strunin & Hingson, 1987). Several published studies have addressed AIDS knowledge and attitudes in the wider "general public" (Dawson, Cynamon, & Fitti, 1987; Fink, 1987; Sherr, 1987; Temoshok, Sweet, & Zich, 1987). Most of the work assessing public opinion about AIDS has been in the form of polls by Gallup, Harris, ABC, CBS, NBC, the *Los Angeles Times*, and so forth (Singer & Rogers, 1986; Singer, Rogers, & Corcoran, 1987).

Some studies suggest that there are people who are currently at risk for HIV infection, but who may not consider themselves at risk. Their needs are probably not well addressed by educational and prevention campaigns aimed at those groups of highest risk for acquiring or transmitting HIV. This group of people, at increased but unacknowledged risk, includes the spouses or sexual partners of IV drug users and bisexual men, men who engage in homosexual behavior or who use IV drugs occasionally but who do not identify themselves as homosexuals or IV drug abusers, and sexually active heterosexuals (including prostitutes) who live in high-risk areas. The female partners of infected men face an additional problem: If they are infected and become pregnant, they may transmit the virus to the fetus. Pregnancy can also precipitate overt disease in a mother who is a carrier of HIV (World Health Organization, 1986). Many of these individuals who are currently at increased risk are blacks and Hispanics, and for whom targeted AIDS education is now being urged by the Centers for Disease Control and other experts. Unfortunately, there is some evidence that those at increased risk for HIV are either unaware of this risk or are not doing anything to prevent acquiring the virus (Quinn et al., 1988).

Societal Attitudes and Responses

The issues of societal blame and responsibility are also relevant. It has been argued, for instance, that when an epidemic occurs, primarily in the context of a stigmatized, "legally proscribed" out-group, the tendency will be for society to blame the victims of the disease (Kayal, 1985). The slow response by society to the appearance of AIDS has been contrasted with more timely attempts to isolate and resolve Legionnaire's disease and the toxic-shock syndrome among women using tampons and has been attributed to the fact that the initial victims were marginal or outcast members of society—drug addicts, Haitian refugees, and homosexual men (Cahill, 1984). Some people responded to the advent of the AIDS epidemic with alarm and compassion, while others viewed it as divine retribution on these renegade subcultures, and most were disinterested.

If such attitudes persisted beyond the initial period of public awareness of the epidemic, they may have affected the speed and nature of societal response to it. The misconception that there is something about being gay or a drug user per se that causes or facilitates the onset of AIDS has a number of implications. It suggests that the disease is caused by illegal or "immoral" activities, rather than by a virus and spread by certain behaviors, and that people who do not engage in these behaviors will not be at risk to develop AIDS. At one level, these beliefs can lead to withholding support and resources from persons with HIV-spectrum disorders and can lead to delays in efforts to cure or prevent the disease. At another level, such beliefs may falsely reassure the majority that they are not in danger and may minimize the likelihood that they will behave in ways that reduce their risk of infection.

The links between HIV and morality are complex and extend beyond the realm of homosexual behavior and drug use. During the past few years, we have witnessed new battles over sex education in the schools. Despite the fact that sex is a natural, common human activity, it involves a number of entangled moral and legal issues. Whether teengers should or should not engage in sex is a matter of debate, but the fact that they do experiment with sex is undeniable. Some argue that by teaching teenagers about-safer sex practices we can increase the probability that if they do have sexual intercourse, they will not become infected with the HIV; while others argue that sex education increases promiscuity. Whether such education will increase the likelihood that they will become sexually active is a moralistic response to a reality that defies objectivity. Sex is both a major theme in modern society and a taboo, a behavior not to be discussed or displayed openly. Overcoming the moral indignation associated with drug use and gay behavior, as well as societal beliefs and customs regarding sex, is necessary in order to more fully address the epidemic and to prevent its further spread.

Clearly, there will be continued controversy over interventions directed toward reducing risk of infection and spread of HIV. However, basic to any such efforts will be information about risky behavior in general, sexual behavior, drug use, developmental stages, and so on. More complete understanding of behavioral factors that may alter the effectiveness of interventions or the long- and short-term adoption of preventive recommendations is necessary and must be considered both independently and in the context of the AIDS pandemic.

THE CROSS-CULTURAL PERSPECTIVE AND POLICY IMPLICATIONS

Sociological and anthropological studies have documented how concepts of health and illness often reflect cultural and subcultural contexts (Conrad & Kern, 1985). The Health Belief Model (Becker, 1974) is one potentially useful model of the relationship between people's health beliefs and health behaviors.

This model hypothesizes that preventive health action in the absence of disease symptoms is influenced by a person's belief that (a) he or she is personally vulnerable to disease, (b) the occurrence of disease will have some moderate to severe effect on his or her life, and (c) the perceived effectiveness of advocated health measures are weighted favorably against his or her perception of the physical and psychological "costs" of the recommended action. Further, the model suggests that sociological variables such as social class and peer influence will affect whether recommended behavior changes are actually made. Cultural and subcultural contexts may also determine the method of education likely to be most effective within a given community. For example, brochures will have little impact on persons who do not read or who do not comprehend the language in which the brochure is written. Similarly, if the person highlighted in a television spot focused on AIDS education has attributes the viewer admires or with which the viewer can identify, the message is much more likely to make a positive impact than if the viewer regards the spokesperson as having dissimilar characteristics, experiences, and/or values (Bandura, 1977).

Understanding the response to AIDS, on both the individual and policy levels, would be enhanced by comparative research on AIDS as a social phenomenon (Bennett, 1987; Nelkin & Hilgartner, 1987; Velimirovic, 1987). For the most part, cost-benefit analysis and other rational planning criteria have generally played a relatively small role in forging various national AIDS policies, compared to reactive decision making stimulated by the highly politicized climate surrounding AIDS (Lee & Moss, 1987). Through their effects on the decisions of elected representatives, public attitudes about AIDS play an indirect but significant role in determining differing national and local funding priorities for education and research. The impact of these differing priorities warrants investigation. Comparative studies would also provide insight into how other countries are dealing with AIDS education and prevention, and the effectiveness of various intervention efforts.

CONCLUSIONS

In this chapter, we have considered some of the issues that should be studied as part of the effort to fight AIDS. In doing so, we have tried to make several points. The blurring of distinctions between basic and applied research that has characterized the emergence of health psychology, community psychology, and other "newer" areas of behavioral science is very much the case in HIV-related research. This work typically has aspects of both, as studies reveal information about basic psychosocial and psychophysiological functioning, as well as provide a basis for intervention, care, and prevention. There are also a number of reasons to study AIDS- or HIV-related processes. Newly available funding, for AIDS-related research is too often a dominant, albeit usually unstated, reason. We have tried, however, to highlight areas where research on a number of non-AIDS-related populations may provide useful data for the effort to curb the spread of the epidemic. When the story is told, however, the most compelling rationale for psychosocial study of AIDS-related issues is that they are crucial to the fight against AIDS. Without such research, the role of psychological variables in the etiology, progression, treatment, and prevention of the disease will not be identified, and the overall effort to combat the disease will be hampered.

REFERENCES

Bandura, A. (1977). *Social learning theory*. Englewood Cliffs, N.J.: Prentice-Hall.

Becker, M. H. (Ed.). (1974). *The health belief model and personal health behavior*. Thorofare, NJ: Slack.

Becker, M. H. and Joseph, J. G. (1988). AIDS and behavioral change to reduce risk: A review. *American Journal of Public Health, 78*, 394-410.

Bennett, F. J. (1987). AIDS as a social phenomenon. *Social Science and Medicine, 25*, 529-539.

Brandt, A. M. (1988). AIDS in historical perspective: Four lessons from the history of sexually transmitted diseases. *American Journal of Public Health, 78*, 367-371.

Brown, L. K., & Fritz, G. K. (1988). Children's knowledge and attitudes about AIDS. *Journal of the American Academy of Child and Adolescent Psychiatry, 27*, 504-508.

Cahill, K. M. (Ed.). (1984). *The AIDS epidemic, 1983*. New York: St. Martin's Press.

Coates, D., & Wortman, C. (1980). Depression maintenance and interpersonal control. In A. Baum & J. E. Singer (Eds.), *Advances in environmental psychology* (Vol. 2, pp. 152-173). Hillsdale, NJ: Lawrence Erlbaum Associates.

Coates, T. J., Temoshok, L., & Mandel, J. (1984). Psychological research is essential to understanding and treating AIDS. *American Psychologist, 39*, 1309-1314.

Cohen, S., & Wills, T. A. (1985). Stress, social support, and the buffering hypothesis: A critical review. *Psychological Bulletin, 98*, 310-357.

Conrad, P., & Kern, R. (Eds.). (1985). *The sociology of health and illness: Critical perspectives* (2nd ed.). New York: St. Martin's Press.

Coolfont Report. (1986). A PHS plan for prevention and control of AIDS and AIDS virus. *Public Health Report, 101*, 341-348.

Dawson, D. A., Cynamon, M., & Fitti, J. E. (1987). AIDS knowledge and attitudes: Provisional data from the National Health Interview Survey: United States, August 1987. *Vital and Advance Data (Health Statistics of the National Center for Health Statistics), 146*, 1-10.

DiClemente, R. J., Zorn, J., & Temoshok, L. (1986). Adolescents and AIDS: A survey of knowledge, attitudes, and beliefs about AIDS in San Francisco. *American Journal of Public Health, 76*, 1443-1445.

Fineberg, H. V. (1988) Education to prevent AIDS: Prospects and obstacles. *Science, 239*, 592-596.

Fink, R. (1987). Changes in public reaction to a new epidemic: The case of AIDS. *Bulletin of the New York Academy of Medicine, 63*, 939-949.

Jemmott, J., & Locke, S. (1984). Psychosocial factors, immunologic mediation, and human susceptibility to infectious diseases: How much do we know? *Psychological Bulletin, 95*, 78-108.

Kegeles, S. M., Adler, N. E., Irwin, C. E. (1988). Sexually active adolescents and condoms: Changes over one year in knowledge, attitudes, and use. *American Journal of Public Health, 78*, 460-461.

Kielcolt-Glaser, J. K. & Glaser, R. (1987). Psychosocial moderators of immune functions. *Annals of Behavioral Medicine, 9*, 16-20.

Kiecolt-Glaser, J. K., Stephens, R. E., Lipitz, P. D., Speicher, C. E., & Glaser, R. (1985). Distress and DNA repair in human lymphocytes. *Journal of Behavioral Medicine, 8*, 311-320.

Lee, P. R., & Moss, A. R. (1987). AIDS prevention: Is cost-benefit analysis appropriate? *Health Policy, 8*, 193-196.

Lui, K., Darrow, W. W., & Rutherford, G. (1988) A model-based estimate of the mean incubation period for AIDS in homosexual men. *Science, 240*, 1333-1335.

Melbye, M., Njelesani, E. K., Bayley, A., Mukelabai, K., Manuwele, J. K., Bowa, F. J., Clayden, S. A., Levin, A., Blattner, W. A., Weiss, R. A. (1986). Evidence for heterosexual transmission and clinical manifestations of human immunodeficiency virus infection and related conditions in Lusaka, Zambia. *Lancet, ii*, 1113-1115.

Navia, B. A., Jordan, B. D., Price, R. W. (1986). The AIDS dementia complex: I. clinical features. *Annals of Neurology, 19*, 517-524.

Nelkin, D., & Hilgartner, S. (1987). Disputed dimensions of risk: A public school controversy over AIDS. *Milbank Quarterly, 64* (Supplement), 118-142.

Padian, N. S. (1987). Heterosexual transmission of acquired immunodeficiency syndrome: International perspectives and national projections. *Reviews of Infectious Diseases, 9*, 947-960.

Padian, N., Marquis, L., Francis, D., Anderson, R., Rutherford, G., O'Malley, P., & Winkelstein, W. (1987). Male to female transmission of human immunodeficiency virus. *Journal of the American Medical Association, 258*, 788-790.

Pape, J. W., Liautand, B., Thomas, F., Mathurin, J-R, St. Amand, M-MA, Boncy, M., Pean, V., Pamphile, M., Laroche, A. C., Dehovitz, J., Johnson, W. D. (1985) The acquired immunodeficiency syndrome in Haiti. *Annals of Internal Medicine, 103*, 674-8.

Price, A. H., Desmond, S., & Kukulka, G. (1985). High school students' perceptions and misperceptions of AIDS. *Journal of School Health, 55*, 107-109.

Quinn, T. C., Glasser, D., Cannon, R. O., Matuszak, D. L., Dunning, R. W., Kline, R. L., Campbell, C. H., Israel, E. Fauci, A. S., & Hook, E. W. (1988). Human immunodeficiency virus infection among patients attending clinics for sexually transmitted diseases. *New England Journal of Medicine, 318*, 197-203.

Rahe, R. H. (1975). Life changes and near-future illness reports. In L. Levi (Ed.), *Emotions: Their parameters and measurements* (pp. 511-530). New York: Raven.

Royse, D., Dhooper, S. S., & Hatch, L. R. (1987). Undergraduate and graduate students' attitudes towards AIDS. *Psychology Reports, 60*, 1185-1186.

Sherr, L. (1987). An evaluation of the UK Government Health Education Campaign. *Psychology and Health, 1*, 61-72.

Simkins, L., Eberhage, M. (1984). Attitudes towards AIDS, herpes II, and toxic shock syndrome. *Psychological Reports, 55*, 779-786.

Simkins, L., & Kushner, A. (1986). Attitudes toward AIDS, herpes II, and toxic shock syndrome: Two years later. *Psychology Reports, 59*, 883-891.

Singer, E., & Rogers, T. F. (1986). Public opinion and AIDS. *AIDS and Public Policy Journal, 1*, 8-13.

Singer, E., Rogers, T. F., & Corcoran, M. (1987). The polls—a report. *Public Opinion Quarterly, 51*, 580-595.

Solomon, G. F., Temoshok, L., O'Leary, A., Zich, J. (1987). An intensive psychoimmunologic study of long-surviving persons with AIDS: Pilot work, background studies, hypotheses and methods. *Annals of the N.Y. Academy of Sciences, 496*, 647-655.

Strunin, L., & Hingson, R. (1987). Acquired immunodeficiency syndrome and adolescents: Knowledge, beliefs, attitudes, and behaviors. *Pediatrics, 79*, 825-828.

Temoshok, L., & Baum, A. (1987). Introduction to special issue on AIDS. *Journal of Applied Social Psychology, 17*, 189-192.

Temoshok, L., Canick, J., Moulton, J. M., Sweet, D. M., Zich, J., Straits, K., Pivar, I., Hollander, H. (1988, June). Distress, coping, and neuropsychological status in men with AIDS-related complex. Paper presented at the IV International Conference on AIDS. Stockholm, Sweden.

Temoshok, L., Solomon, G.F., Jenkins, S., Sweet, D.M. (1989, January). Psychoimmunologic studies of men with AIDS and ARC. Paper presented at the Annual Meeting of the American Association for the Advancement of Science. San Francisco, CA.

Temoshok, L., Sweet, D. M., & Zich, J. (1987). A three-city comparison of the public's knowledge and attitudes about AIDS. *Psychology and Health*, *1*, 43-60.

Temoshok, L., Zich, J., & Green, J. (1987). Editorial: Psychosocial aspects of AIDS. *Psychology and Health*, *1*, 39-42.

Temoshok, Zich, J., Solomon, G.F., Stites, D.P. (1987, June). Intensive psychoimmunologic study of long-surviving persons with AIDS. Paper presented at the III International Conference on Aids. Washington, D.C.

Thompson, L. (1988, March 15). What are the dangers for heterosexuals? *Washington Post Health*, pp. 6-7.

Van de Perre, P., Munyambuga, D., Zississ, G., Bulaler, J.P., Nzaramba, D., & Clumeck, N. (1985). Antibody to HTLV-III in blood donors in Central Africa (letter). *Lancet*, *1*(8424), 336-337.

Velimirovic, B. (1987). AIDS as a social phenomenon. *Social Science and Medicine*, *25*, 541-522.

World Health Organization. (1986). Second meeting of the WHO Collaborating Centres on AIDS: Memorandum from a WHO meeting. *Bulletin of the World Health Organization*, *64*, 37-46.

Zich, J., Temoshok, L. (1987). Perceptions of social support in men with AIDS and ARC: Relationships with distress and hardiness. *Journal of Applied Social Psychology*, *17*, 193-215.

Behavioral Science and Public Health Perspectives: Combining Paradigms for the Prevention and Control of AIDS

2

Deborah L. Rugg
*Centers for Disease Control,
Division of Sexually Transmitted Diseases
Atlanta, Georgia*

Melbourne F. Hovell
*Graduate School of Public Health
San Diego State University*

Louis R. Franzini
*Department of Psychology
San Diego State University*

Acquired immunodeficiency syndrome (AIDS) is a global pandemic. As of January 1988, only seven years after the syndrome was first described by the U.S. Centers for Disease Control (CDC), almost 100,000 cases have been reported in 132 countries around the world [Brunet & Ancelle, 1985; Centers for Disease Control (CDC), 1986; CDC, 1986; World Health Organization (Who), 1988]. The World Health Organization (WHO) estimates the actual number of AIDS cases is probably higher due to underreporting (Mahler, 1986). Although most cases have been reported in the United States, AIDS appears to be increasing rapidly in other countries, especially in central Africa, (Kapita, 1986; Mann, Francis, Quinn, et al., 1986; Quinn, Mann, Curran, & Piot, 1986). In addition to cases of AIDS, three to five times as many (300,000 to 500,000) people have symptoms related to infection with the immuno-deficiency virus (HIV). Another five to ten million people around the world are believed to be asymptomatic carriers of HIV (Mahler, 1986). U.S. Surgeon

General Koop has predicted 100 million deaths worldwide by the end of the century, if no cure or vaccine is found.

In addition to the obvious public health consequences, the AIDS pandemic certainly will have pervasive social, economic, political, and legal ramifications. Several characteristics of the AIDS epidemic and the action of the virus create unique risks and heightened fears:

1. Many of the estimated 1.5 million infected people (in the United States) are unaware that they are capable of spreading the virus.
2. The incubation period for the virus may be as long as 10 years.
3. Tests for the antibody to the AIDS virus produce a small percentage of false negatives, thereby missing an ongoing and unsuspected source of infection.
4. Variations of the original HIV have already been reported.
5. The lag time between the time of infection and the production of measurable antibodies in the blood may allow an infected individual to transmit the virus unknowingly.
6. Accurate sexual behavior and IV drug use histories may not be available for certain transient sexual partners, generating additional risks.
7. Behaviors most relevant to preventing the spread of the virus (unprotected intercourse, sharing of needles by drug users, and disdain for using condoms) are extraordinarily difficult to modify.

In recent months, the U.S. Public Health Service (U.S. Public Health Service, 1986), the National Academy of Sciences (Institute of Medicine, National Academy of Sciences, 1986), the World Health Organization (Meyer, 1986), the California Department of Health Services (State of California, Department of Health Services, 1986), and the U.S. Surgeon General (U.S. Surgeon General, 1986) have issued major reports on AIDS. They all emphasize, in the absence of a vaccine, our most powerful tools to prevent and control the spread of AIDS will be information and education prevention campaigns. All prevention efforts will need to be designed with each of these characteristics of the epidemic in mind.

This chapter describes two diverse perspectives, behavioral science and public health, and how their paradigms may be integrated to facilitate the prevention and control of AIDS.

A COMBINING OF PARADIGMS

The Public Health Perspective

The key elements of a public health approach to a health crisis are: 1) it is triggered by a health event; 2) the broad population is the unit of interest, rather than the individual; 3) the investigation of the problem and the choice of solution are empirically derived by empirical epidemiological means (i.e., through systematic observation and description of the phenomenon, eschewing theoretical models of causal mechanisms); 4) intervention is predominantly focused on primary prevention and the prevention of secondary infections (i.e., from the infected to the uninfected); 5) interventions, once identified, are implemented immediately; 6) interventions are often of a direct regulatory nature, focused at the public policy level without involving individual decision-making; and, finally, 7) the public health model is based on the tripartite epidemiological construct of the host-agent-environment (Runyan, DeVellis, DeVellis, & Hochbaum, 1982).

The public health perspective has been extended beyond studying and treating large groups to the concept of "applied significance." Most risk conditions, such as obesity, alcohol and drug consumption, exposure to toxins, etc., affect a large proportion of the population but at relatively low individual levels, whereas only a small proportion of the population has a high level of the risk condition (Rose, 1985). With AIDS, only a minority of the population is currently considered at high risk (e.g., homosexual or bisexual males and IV drug users), whereas a larger proportion of the population is at low risk.

Using available data, we estimate less than one percent of the U.S. population has been exposed to HIV (Figure 2.1). This reveals a serious public health policy question. Should one spend necessarily limited resources on intervention to reduce difficult-to-change, risky sexual and drug abuse behavior in very high risk individuals (Kelly & St. Lawrence, 1986), or should one intervene to reduce the more moderate risk level of the larger population? Should one divide resources to address both needs, but possibly less effectively overall?

Traditionally, the public health approach has been to obtain the greatest effect for the population by directing intervention to the at-risk proportion of the population. However, with some AIDS prevention activities (such as a national AIDS brochure mailout), all segments of society are being targeted. The behavioral science literature suggests such diffuse approaches are often ineffective due to a lack of precision and clarity in their conceptualization. Rather, targeted and well-conceived intervention strategies are required, considering the level of risk of the target population, as well as the cultural differences.

Individuals who are at highest risk of HIV infection have multiple, unprotected anonymous sexual encounters or frequently share IV drug needles; they may require sustained and expensive interventions in order to greatly reduce their risk of contracting or spreading the disease. Educational sessions or mass media campaigns are unlikely to result in a sustained change in these habits. In the past, this would have been the sole domain of mental health and drug treatment research and services. Today it is an area being addressed by public health agencies as well, since the individual behaviors involved carry major public health significance. To find solutions to these problems a clear and

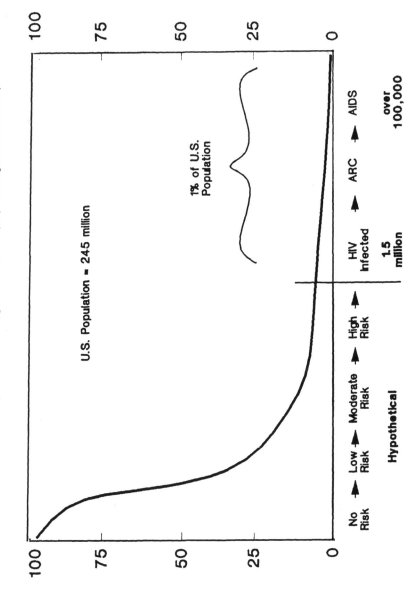

FIG. 2.1. Population-based diagram of AIDS risk (all percentages are estimates).

FIG. 2.2. Relative risk conceptual bar graph. Source: San Francisco AIDS Foundation.

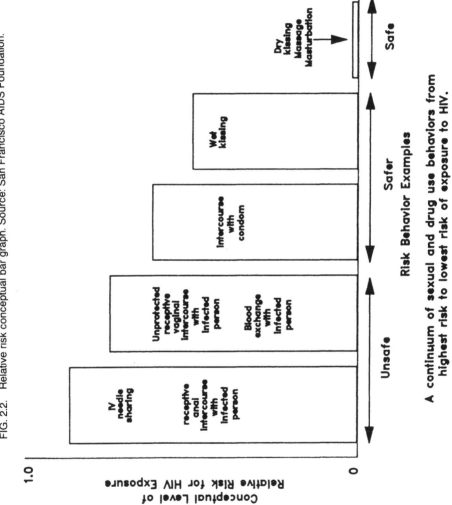

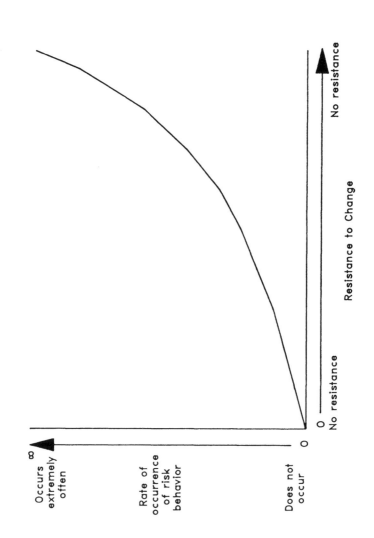

FIG. 2.3. Conceptual graphic representing resistance to change in relation to rate of occurrence of behavior.

22

comprehensive conceptualization of the problem, the target and the solution will be necessary. Additionally, on a national scale, the mental health, public health, and drug treatment fields must combine paradigms and integrate their focus in an unparalleled disease prevention effort. For only a well orchestrated, comprehensive, interdisciplinary approach will end this epidemic.

An Integration of Epidemiological Paradigms With Learning Theory

The concept of a relative risk continuum has been applied to the behaviors involved in the transmission of AIDS. Some behaviors are "safer" than others, and level of risk increases with frequency of occurrence (Figure 2.2). The strength of the behavior and its theoretical resistance to change are also associated with the frequency of the behavior, as is suggested in Figure 2.3. As the frequency of the behavior increases, so does its theoretical resistance to change. This is likely, due to the increased amount of reinforcement being provided. Single session interventions are unlikely to affect such behaviors.

Resources should be used where they can have the greatest impact on controlling the HIV epidemic and protecting the overall population. Based on this concern and learning theory models of behavior, public health interventions for the majority of the population need to facilitate maintenance of existing healthy lifestyles, discourage initiation of risky behaviors, and reduce misinformation, fear, and prejudice. Reducing faulty beliefs and fears will require innovative approaches, since many beliefs are firmly held and are not affected by scientific facts or logic. Traditional health-education strategies (e.g., distribution of pamphlets) are likely to be ineffective in this regard (Rugg, Hovell, & Ito).

Certain risk subgroups, however, e.g., some adolescents, bisexual and homosexual males, and heterosexually active adults, should be targeted for intensive prevention efforts focusing on behavioral and social skills modification. These intensive interventions might include: 1) systematic use of contingent powerful reinforcements (including social reinforcements), 2) behavioral and social skills training, and 3) the persuasive information normally included in health education programs.

Clearly, AIDS prevention efforts must be delivered to a large number of people. The usual methods for reaching a large number of people rely on standardized educational procedures and mass media. Another cost effective approach involves many individuals providing a limited intervention which cumulatively results in benefits for a large number of people. For instance, it has been estimated that over two million smokers would quit if physicians would simply encourage them to do so (Russell, Wilson, Taylor, & Baker, 1979). Such an intervention would be incidental to medical office visits, yet could have a tremendous effect on disease prevention. This approach could also yield major results with AIDS. For example, if every physician, public health official, and school health educator as well as STD and drug treatment counselor, would repeatedly discuss the use of condoms with sexually active clients, the spread of AIDS and other sexually transmitted diseases might be greatly reduced. By expanding this discussion to include a social learning theory perspective, we can begin to identify the factors which not only initiate behavior change, but also maintain behavior change—both in risk behaviors and in health behaviors.

Social Learning Theory and Behavior Modification

Learning theories concentrate on observable and measurable learned behaviors. Change methods are derived from basic principles of theory and repeated experimental research. Operational definitions and careful pre- and post-treatment assessments and follow-ups are hallmark features of this approach.

In behavioral learning theories, it is assumed that learning occurs via any of the following paradigms: operant conditioning, classical conditioning, or modeling. Operant learning involves the systematic contingent application of rewards and punishments to increase or decrease given behaviors, respectively. Classical conditioning produces learning via repeated pairings of the desired response with a previously neutral simulus. Modeling paradigms produce new learning via a symbolic or live demonstration of the desired behavior. Combinations of these paradigms, for example, rewarding novice efforts to duplicate a modeled response, can quickly produce long-lasting performances (Bandura, 1979; Baer, Wolf, & Risley, 1968; Skinner, 1953). Social learning theory is a combination of operant and modeling principles, with some inclusion of self-referent cognitions (i.e. perception of self-efficacy) (Bandura, 1977a; Bandura, 1977b).

The past two decades have seen the advance of a technology of behavior modification based on operant conditioning and social learning theory. This technology has emphasized individual behavior and research methods best suited to the experimental control of individual behavior (Sidman, 1960). Research and program descriptions have been reported extensively in literature where feedback (e.g., Geary, Hovell, & Black, 1985), reinforcement procedures (e.g., Schumaker, Hovell, & Sherman, 1977), modeling/imitation procedures and shaping techniques (e.g., McGarr, & Hovell, 1980) are used to establish new behaviors. These studies have many characteristics in common. One of these is that the environmental variables manipulated to control behavior have been directly related in time (proximal factors) to the target behavior. As behavioral science/behavioral analysis is applied more to health risk behavior change and disease prevention, more distant variables such as learning history, prerequisite skills, and the behavior of others (distal factors) become important and are incorporated into the model (Abrams, Elder, Carleton, & Artz, 1986).

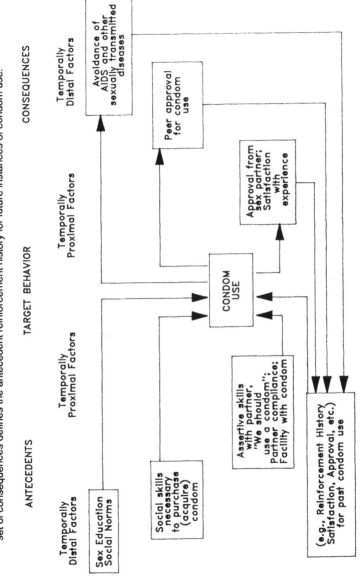

FIG. 2.4. Antecedents and consequences theoretically responsible for condom use behavior. Note: The entire set of consequences defines the antecedent reinforcement history for future instances of condom use.

ANTECEDENTS   TARGET BEHAVIOR   CONSEQUENCES

Temporally Distal Factors   Temporally Proximal Factors   Temporally Proximal Factors   Temporally Distal Factors

Sex Education
Social Norms

Social skills necessary to purchase (acquire) condom

Assertive skills with partner, "We should use a condom"; Partner compliance; Facility with condom

CONDOM USE

Approval from sex partner; Satisfaction with experience

Peer approval for condom use

Avoidance of AIDS and other sexually transmitted diseases

(e.g., Reinforcement History Satisfaction, Approval, etc.) for past condom use

Implications for Condom Use

Unprotected, receptive anal intercourse with an infected partner is one of the behaviors of greatest risk for transmission of HIV (CDC, 1986). Consistent and proper condom use will help to reduce transmission of HIV. Therefore, these two behaviors will be used to illustrate the application of basic learning theory and social learning theory to the prevention of AIDS. Relatively few individuals regularly use condoms (Darrow, 1987; Population Information Program, 1982), probably because most of the population has not attained sufficient reinforcement for condom use. The temporally related antecedents and consequences of condom use are important components of a behavioral model. One might speculate that condom use in many cases has resulted in adverse consequences, such as fear, anxiety, reduced sensation, embarrassment, or ridicule. A flow chart of the important determinants of condom use behavior are diagrammed in Figure 2.4.

Examination of this figure shows that reinforcement history is a powerful component of this model. Both antecedents and consequences may occur immediately prior to or after a given response. The extension of this field now focuses equal attention to the more distal influences on behavior, even though these may be less easily influenced by the behavioral scientist. Attention to more distal factors may be critical for determining variables responsible for maintenance of behavior and prevention of relapse (Marlatt, & Gordon, 1985). Clearly, *maintaining* healthy behavior is a primary goal of behavioral AIDS prevention. Public health officials will need to devise ways to incorporate large scale behavioral reinforcement systems into AIDS prevention and control programs that encourage and enhance long-term behavioral change. These reinforcement systems will need to range from development of social support networks to financial incentives such as explicit rebates, lottery based rewards, or other monetary reinforcements. Such incentive systems could be established to facilitate the prerequisite purchase behavior. Purchasing a condom is a complex task affected by environmental and behavioral factors (Figure 2.5). The policy of providing reinforcement systematically for these prerequisite behaviors as the target behavior is shaped is derived directly from operant learning theory (Skinner, 1953).

Social modeling learning paradigms can then be combined with these contingency management techniques in the following way: 1) explicit social role models (especially peers and "heroes") demonstrate the desired beliefs and behaviors in one-to-one communications, small groups, live theater, or mass media; and then 2) role-play situations are devised where corrective feedback techniques are used to establish and reinforce the complex social and behavioral skills necessary to purchase a condom or perform safer sex. The advertising industry could play a role by providing models not only for purchase of condoms, but also for the *social approval to use condoms* once purchased.

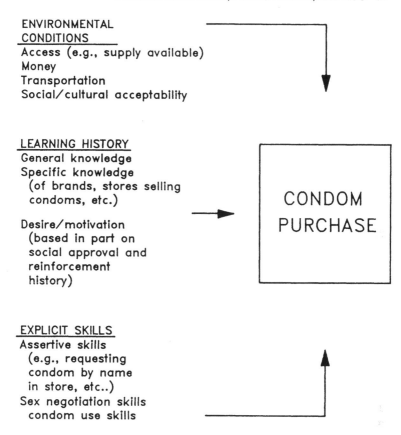

FIG. 2.5.   Prerequisite conditions and skills for condom purchase.

Models of social approval, when widespread and repeated frequently by national media sources, may evoke personal approval on an individual basis, thereby establishing powerful social reinforcement for disease prevention attitudes and behavior. This will ultimately effect the change of actual and perceived social norms, so that eventually it will be socially unacceptable *not* to use condoms and/or engage in safer sex.

Implicatians for Anal Intercourse

A second example of social learning theory applied to AIDS risk reduction examines frequent, anonymous unprotected receptive anal intercourse. Those who choose to continue this behavior, even under aversive conditions (e.g., societal disapproval or the threat of disease), are likely to be quite resistant to change. The public health interventions necessary to successfully modify this sexual behavior pattern must be designed to compete with a powerful reinforcement history. The social and sexual pleasures derived from this behavior are essentially immediate. Punitive control factors, including fear of disease or death, are unlikely to be effective, due to the delay of the punishment gradient. Short-term consequences typically prevail over long-term consequences (Skinner, 1953).

The most influential strategy for behavior change in this situation, which is derived from operant behavior theory, is the differential reinforcement of other (DRO) behavior technique (Skinner, 1953). The DRO technique would encourage reinforcement of safer behaviors which are incompatible with the high risk unprotected anal intercourse behavior (such as intercourse with a condom, oral sex, kissing, massage, masturbation, etc.). Positive assertive communication skills between partners are a prerequisite and contribute initially to facilitating these behavior changes.

Thus, all three paradigms of learning from behavior theory are applicable in this illustration. The acquisition of assertive behaviors (purchasing, using, and insisting on condoms) occurs via observational learning procedures, that is, modeling based on social learning theory. Reinforcement of condom use by partners and society is a major operant technique. Finally, classical conditioning effects emerge when positive emotional experiences are repeatedly paired with the safer sexual behaviors.

Sustaining Change in AIDS Risk Behaviors

Application of behavioral science strategies to AIDS risk behavior change maintenance is complicated by the moral overtone that has traditionally accompanied discussions of sexually transmitted diseases. Health professionals' traditional beliefs of single cause/single cure and the remnants of 18th century rationalism, i.e., that simply providing information will produce behavioral change in patients, also contribute (Brandt, 1985). Brief prescriptions of antibiotics or surgery are expected to stop the disease process permanently, with no need for a long-term or repeated intervention (Ng, Davis, Manderscheid, & Elkers, 1979).

Where this single cause/single cure model has been applied to AIDS risk behavior, the implication has been that one brief and temporary intervention is all that is needed to produce a change in risk behavior and sustain that change. Reliance on HIV antibody counseling/testing to produce sustained behavior change is a case in point, even though it was intended to be only one step in a series of follow-up interventions. Much of health education has also followed this logic. In the traditional health education approach, information and education about the disease process has been emphasized as a rational basis for adopting protective behavior or discontinuing established risk behavior (Prue, Wynder, Scharf, & Resnicow, 1987).

With regard to AIDS, the long-term consequences of high-risk behavior are life threatening. However, the immediate and ongoing reinforcing consequences are powerful. Without eliminating the "natural" reinforcement for risk behaviors or providing reinforcement for the alternatives, the protective and healthy safer sex behaviors are not likely to be developed and sustained. We recommend a complete "behavioral change" analysis of the specific steps involved in risky sexual behaviors and then providing for social reinforcements for the establishment of the prerequisite skills. The social skills involved in choosing a sexual partner, and being assertive regarding the type of sexual activity to be engaged in, involve complex behavioral chains.

Successful AIDS risk reduction will require individuals to learn social and behavioral skills which are a prerequisite to performing safer sex behaviors. These behaviors include obtaining a condom, using a condom properly, requesting your partner to use a condom, saying "no" to any risky sex, and determining your partner's current sexual activity, past sexual history, and serostatus. These assertive skills need to be taught, practiced, and reinforced, especially in the young as they explore their sexuality. It will also require the specific knowledge and component skills necessary to properly and consistently use a condom, since proper condom use is a complex behavior (CDC Condoms for Prevention of Sexually Transmitted Diseases, 1988).

The following Centers for Disease Control (CDC) recommendations for proper use of condoms to reduce the transmission of sexually transmitted diseases (STD) are based on current information:

1. Latex condoms should be used because they offer greater protection against viral STD than do natural membrane condoms.

2. Condoms should be stored in a cool, dry place out of direct sunlight.

3. Condoms in damaged packages or those that show obvious signs of age (e.g., those that are brittle, sticky, or discolored) should not be used. They cannot be relied upon to prevent infection.

4. Condoms should be handled with care to prevent puncture.

5. The condom should be put on before any genital contact to prevent exposure to fluids that may contain infectious agents. Hold the tip of the condom and unroll it onto the erect penis, leaving space at the tip to collect semen, yet assuring that no air is trapped in the tip of the condom.

6. Adequate lubrication should be used. If exogenous lubrication is needed, only water-based lubricants should be used. Petroleum or oil-based lubricants (such as petroleum jelly, cooking oils, shortening, and lotions) should not be used since they weaken the latex.

7. Use of condoms containing spermicides may provide some additional protection against STD. However, vaginal use of spermicides along with condoms is likely to provide even greater protection.

8. If a condom breaks, it should be replaced immediately. If ejaculation occurs after condom breakage, the immediate use of spermicide has been suggested. However, the protective value of postejaculation application of spermicide in reducing the risk of STD transmission is unknown.

9. After ejaculation, care should be taken so that the condom does not slip off the penis before withdrawal; the base of the condom should be held while withdrawing. The penis should be withdrawn while still erect.

10. Condoms should never be reused.

The Behavior of Others and Social Networks

Purchasing a condom may also include the complex social behavior of other people related to a "target" person and his/her behavior. The paradigm then begins to encompass social ecology models of behavior (Wahler, & Graves, 1983; Wahler, House, & Stamberg, 1976). The behavior of teachers, friends, lovers, or family members serves as incidental antecedent and consequent events. Their behavior may be a cue which signals reinforcing or punishing stimuli for an individual's specific behavior. Moreover, considerable variation is likely to occur across individual "audience" members (and across time for a single audience member) in his/her reactions to a given person's behavior. With this complexity added to the model, it is important to understand the learning histories of the predominant audience members whose behavior, in turn, influences the target individual's behavior.

This suggests that social relationships and social networks may also become extremely important in our understanding of the epidemiology of AIDS and critical for the control of the epidemic worldwide. Target or "bridge" individuals who are infected, highly mobile, and practice high-risk behaviors, will need to be the focus of a worldwide strategy for controlling AIDS. Klovdahl, (1985) asserts that modern communities might be more accurately classified and defined by diffuse social networks than by discrete geographic boundaries. A social network may be diffuse and far-reaching, even global, and this necessitates a broadening of perspectives on issues surrounding prevention and control of an infectious agent. Epidemiological and National Center for Health Statistics research do not now lend themselves to this concept of community. However, social network data may be useful in identifying persons who are likely to have been exposed to the virus and may not know it, especially if they become carriers (i.e., they have asymptomatic or subclinical infections). The procedures for testing this hypothesis and the nonrandomness of a disease cluster within a social network have been developed (Klovdahl, 1985). These procedures suggest that the rate of transmission of a disease is, in part, a function of the size of the social network, as well as the level of intimacy of the contacts.

FUTURE DIRECTIONS

The urgent demand for information, education, and prevention campaigns has arisen out of our inability to cure or immunize against AIDS. Three important tasks face behavioral scientists specializing in AIDS prevention. The first task is to direct intensive applied research for high-risk individuals to develop a means of obtaining and maintaining changes in the behaviors that put them at high risk for AIDS. The second is to develop a social learning theory-based AIDS prevention system for moderate risk people which provides for both factual information and reliable social and personal reinforcements for producing and maintaining the desired behavior changes. On a population basis, even limited intervention, if clearly conceptualized, targeted, and directed at a large number of people can serve to reduce the cumulative risk. The third is to design innovative media efforts to educate the low risk population to reduce misinformation, fear, and prejudice. Public health and medical professionals and the media should cooperate with behavioral scientists to implement effective systems for AIDS-prevention education. All must expect the behavioral interventions to be long-term efforts in order to maintain the behavior changes necessary to prevent the transmission of HIV. The behavioral scientists also need to establish realistic expectations in themselves and in other health professionals, educators, and the general public of the potential impact of these infections in reducing the spread of infection.

CONCLUSION

Social and behavioral sciences have long studied risk-taking and health behavior patterns (e.g., Hall, Rugg, Tunstall & Jones, 1984; Hovell, Elder, Blanchard, & Sallis, 1986; Hunt, Barnett, & Branch, 1971; Gentry & Matarazzo, 1981; Matarazzo, 1980; Pomerleau & Brady, 1979; Stone, Adler, & Cohen, 1979). This knowledge may be directly applicable to the prevention and control of AIDS. A growing interest between fields of public health and behavioral science to combine their respective paradigms should enhance the effectiveness of disease prevention strategies. Traditionally, these efforts have found social learning theory programs to be the most successful in the prevention and control of chronic diseases such as coronary heart disease (Elder, Hovell, Lasater, Wells, & Carleton, 1985; Farquhar, Maccoby, Wood, Alexander, et al., 1977). It is most reasonable to expect that expanded social learning theory will be even more critical for the prevention and control of AIDS.

REFERENCES

Abrams, E., Elder, J., Carleton, R., & Artz, L. (1986). A comprehensive framework for conceptualizing and planning organizational health promotion programs. In M.F. Cataldo & T.J. Coates (Eds.), *Health and industry: A behavioral medicine perspective*: New York: Wiley.

Baer, D. M., Wolf, M. M., & Risley, T. R. (1968). Some current dimensions of applied behavior analysis. *Journal of Applied Behavior Analysis, 1*, 91-97.

Bandura, A. (1969). *Principles of behavior modification.* New York: Holt, Rinehart and Winston.

Bandura, A. (1977a). Self-efficacy: Toward a unifying theory of behavior change. *Psychological Review, 84*, 191-215.

Bandura, A. (1977b). *Social learning theory.* New York: Holt, Rinehart and Winston.

Brandt, A. (1985). *No magic bullet: A social history of venereal disease in United States since 1880.* New York: Oxford Press.

Brunet, J. B., & Ancelle, R. A. (1985). International occurrence of the acquired immuno-deficiency syndrome. *Annals of Internal Medicine, 103*, 670-674.

Centers for Disease Control. (1986a). Additional recommendations to reduce sexual and drug abuse-related transmission of HTLV-III/LAV. *Morbidity and Mortality Weekly Reports, 35*(10), 152-155.

Centers for Disease Control. (1986b). Update: Acquired immunodeficiency syndrome—Europe. *Morbidity and Mortality Weekly Reports 35*(3), 35-46.

Centers for Disease Control. (1986c). Update: Acquired immunodeficiency syndrome—United States. *Morbidity and Mortality Weeky Reports, 35*(2), 1, 18-21.

Centers for Disease Control. (1988). Condoms for prevention of sexually transmitted diseases. *Morbidity and Mortality Weekly Reports, 37*(9), 133-137.

Darrow, W. W. (1987, February 20). *Condom use and use-effectiveness in high-risk populations.* Adapted from a presentation to the conference "Condoms in the Prevention of Sexually Transmitted Diseases." Atlanta, GA.

Elder, J. P., Hovell, M. F., Lasater, T. M., Wells, B. L., & Carleton, R. A. (1985). Applications of behavior modification to community health education: The case of heart disease prevention. *Health Education Quarterly, 12*, 151-168.

Farquhar, J. W., Maccoby, N., Wood, P. O., Alexander, J. K., Breitrose, H., Brown, B. W., Jr., Haskell, W. L., Mever, A. J., Nash, J. D., & Stern, M. P. (1977). Community education for cardiovascular health. *Lancet, I*, 1192-1195.

Geary, D. C., Hovell, M. F., & Black, D. R. (1985). Behavioral and medical monitoring for hypertension control: A counselor feedback and consulting mode. *Patient Education and Counseling, 7*, 77-85.

Gentry, W., & Matarazzo, J. (1981). Medical psychology: Three decades of growth and development. In C. K. Prokop & L. A. Bradley (Eds.), *Medical psychology* (pp. 5-15). New York: Academic Press.

Hall, S., Rugg, D., Tunstall, C., & Jones, R. (1984). Preventing relapse to cigarette smoking by behavioral skill training. *Journal of Consulting and Clinical Psychology, 52*, 372-382.

Hovell, M. F., Elder, J. P., Blanchard, J., & Sallis, J. F. (1986). Behavior analysis and public health perspectives: Combining paradigms to effect prevention. *Education & Treatment of Children, 9*, 287-306.

Hunt, W. A., Barnett, L. W., & Branch, L. G. (1971). Relapse rates in addiction programs. *Journal of Consulting and Clinical Psychology, 27*, 455-456.

Institute of Medicine, National Academy of Sciences. (1986). *Confronting AIDS: Directions for public health, health care and research.* Washington, D.C.: National Academy Press.

Kapita, B. M. (1986, June 23-25). *AIDS in Africa.* Paper presented at the International Conference on AIDS, Paris.

Kelly, J. A., & St. Lawrence, J. S. (1986). Behavioral intervention with AIDS. *The Behavior Therapist, 6*, 1231-125.

Klovdahl, A. S. (1985). Social networks and the spread of infectious diseases: The AIDS example. *Social Science & Medicine, 21*, 1203-1216.

Mahler, H. (1988, June 23-25). *Opening address.* Presented at the International Conference on AIDS, Paris.

Mann, J. M., Francis, H., Quinn, T., Asila, P. K., Bosenge, N., Nzilambi, N., Bilaik., Tamfum, M., Ruti, K., Piot, P., McCormick, J., Curran, J. W. (1986). Surveillance for AIDS in a Central African city: Kinshasa, Zaire. *Journal of the American Medical Association, 255*, 3255-3259.

Marlatt, G., & Gordon, J. (1985). *Relapse prevention: Maintenance strategies in the treatment of addictive behaviors.* New York: Guilford Press.

Matarazzo, J. (1980). Behavioral health and behavioral medicine: Frontiers for a new health psychology. *American Psychologist, 35,* 807-817.

McGarr, R., & Hovell, M.R. (1980). In search of the sandman: Shaping an infant to sleep. *Education & Treatment of Children, 3,* 173-182.

Meyer, A. (1986, July 3). *WHO meeting on AIDS education* (information memorandum). Washington, DC: U.S. Agency for International Development.

Ng, L. K. Y., Davis, D. L., Manderscheid, R. W., & Elkers, J. (1979). Toward a conceptual formulation of health and well-being. In P. I. Ahmed & G. V. Coelho (Eds.), *Toward a new definition of health: Psychosocial dimensions* New York: Plenum Press.

Pomerleau, O., & Brady, J. (Eds.). (1979). *Behavioral medicine: Theory and practice.* Baltimore: Williams & Wilkins.

Population Information Program, The Johns Hopkins University. (1982). Update on condoms—products, protection, promotion. *Population Reports,* Series H, Number 6.

Prue, D. M., Wynder, E. L., Scharf, L. S., & Resnicow, K. A. (1987). Health education and behavioral analysis. *Education & Treatment of Children, 10,* 19-32.

Quinn, T. C., Mann, J. M., Curran, J. W., & Piot, P. (1986). AIDS in Africa: An epidemiological paradigm. *Science, 234,* 955-963.

Rose, G. (1985). Sick individuals and sick populations. *International Journal of Epidemiology, 14,* 32-38.

Rugg, D., Hovell, M., & Ito, S. (Unpublished Manuscript). *Innovative approaches to AIDS education: The impact of live theater.*

Runyan, C. W., DeVellis, R. F., DeVellis, B. M., & Hochbaum, G. M. (1982). Health psychology and the public health perspective: In search of the pump handle. *Health Psychology, 1,* 169-180.

Russell, M. A. H., Wilson, C., Taylor, C., & Baker, C. D. (1979). Effects of general practitioners' advice against smoking. *British Medical Journal, 2,* 231-235.

Schumaker, J. B., Hovell, M. F., & Sherman, J. A. (1977). Analysis of daily report card and parent-managed privileges in the improvement of adolescents' classroom performance. *Journal of Applied Behavior Analysis, 10,* 449-464.

Sidman, M. (1960). *Tactics of scientific research: Evaluating experimental data in psychology.* New York: Basic Books.

Skinner, B. F. (1953). *Science and human behavior.* New York: Free Press.

State of California, Department of Health Services, Office of AIDS. (1986, March). *Recommendations for antibody tresting.*

Stone, G., Adler, N., & Cohen, F. (1979). *Health psychology.* San Francisco: Jossey-Bass.

U.S. Public Health Service. (1986, June 4-6). *Plan for the prevention and control of AIDS and the AIDS virus.* Report of the Coolfont Planning Conference. Berkeley Springs, WV.

U.S. Surgeon General. (1986). *Report on acquired immune deficiency syndrome.* Washington, DC: U.S. Government Printing Office.

Wahler, R. G., & Graves, M. G. (1983). Setting events in social networks: Ally or enemy in child behavior therapy. *Behavior Therapy, 14,* 19-36.

Wahler, R. G., House, A. E., & Stamberg, E. E. (1976). *Ecological assessment of child problem behavior.* New York: Pergamon Press.

World Health Organization. (1988). *Cases of AIDS reported as of 1 January 1988.* Geneva, Switzerland: Author.

Target Groups for Preventing AIDS Among Intravenous Drug Users

3

Don C. Des Jarlais
Samuel R. Friedman
New York State Division of Substance Abuse Services
and
Narcotic and Drug Research, Inc.

INTRODUCTION

With the continuing difficulties in developing either effective treatment or a vaccine for AIDS, there has been increasing emphasis on trying to prevent infections through behavior change of persons at risk for human immunodeficiency virus (HIV) infection. The response of IV drug users to the threat of AIDS will be critical to the future spread of HIV in the U.S. Intravenous drug users are the second largest group of persons to have developed AIDS and the primary source of heterosexual and perinatal transmission in the United States. There is a commmon stereotype of the "drug addict" in the United States that hinders AIDS prevention efforts in two ways. Like all stereotypes, it is frequently an inaccurate image of the actual behavior of persons addicted to either heroin or cocaine (and more frequently inaccurate for persons injecting these drugs without being addicted), and it does not present the variety of different subgroups among persons injecting illicit drugs. AIDS prevention strategies will be facilitated through targeting different subgroups of IV drug users and designing specific strategies for those different groups.

In this chapter, we will identify different target groups of IV drug users for AIDS prevention efforts; present available evidence about behavior change in these groups; and then briefly discuss how to prevent transmission of HIV to heterosexual partners who are not themselves IV drug users, and to the children of IV drug users.

35

EPIDEMIOLOGY

HIV is transmitted among IV drug users primarily through the sharing of the equipment ("works") used for injecting drugs (Cohen et al, 1985; Weiss et al, 1985; Friedland et al. 1985. The virus can also be transmitted through heterosexual activity (Redfield et al, 1985; Luzi, Ensoli, Turbessi, Scarpati, & Aivti, 1985). IV drug users are the primary source of heterosexual transmission of AIDS in the United States: 60 percent (163/273) of the heterosexual transmission cases reported to the Centers for Disease Control through April 18, 1986 involved an IV drug user as the likely source of the virus (A. Hardy, personal communication, 1986).

The virus can also be transmitted to children perinatally (Lapoint, Michaud, Pekovik, Chausseau, & Dupuy, 1986). IV drug use in a parent is the major risk for AIDS among children in the United States, accounting for slightly over half (150 of 278) of pediatric AIDS cases (reported through April 18, 1986; A. Hardy, personal communication, 1986).

The New York City metropolitan area has by far the greatest concentration of IV drug users who have developed AIDS. There have been 1,869 cases of AIDS in IV drug users from New York and 490 from New Jersey reported to the U.S. Centers for Disease Control through April 18, 1986. There were an additional 781 cases from a total of 37 different states, and 147 cases from Europe through December 31, 1985 reported to the European Coordinating Center (A. Hardy, personal communication, 1986; IV drug users who also have male homosexuality as a risk factor—1,568 in the U.S. and 35 in Europe—are not included in these totals).

While the actual cases of AIDS among IV drug users have so far been concentrated in the New York area, studies of HIV seroprevalence (indicating infection by the virus) show a great potential for cases throughout the United States and Western Europe. Research in Edinburgh (Robertson et al, 1986) and Italy (Angarano et al, 1985) show seroprevalence rates of greater than 50%, while studies from Zurich (Schupbach et al, 1985) and the Federal Republic of Germany (W. Hoeckmann, personal communication, 1986) show rates between 20% and 40%. Studies in San Francisco and Chicago show approximately 10% seroprevalence in those cities (Spira et al, 1985), while studies from Washington, D.C. and New Orleans show 7% and 2% respectively (H. Ginzburg, personal communication, 1986).

Studies using historically collected blood indicate that the virus can spread relatively rapidly among IV drug users in a community. We examined serum samples from IV drug users collected from 1969 through 1984 for New York City. Testing of these samples showed no presence of HIV antibody in samples from 1969 through 1976. The first seropositive sample was collected in late 1978. There was then a rapid rise, from approximately 20% seropositive in samples collected in late 1978 and 1979, to 40% seropositive in samples collected in 1980, and 50% in samples collected in the following years (Novick, Kreek, Des Jarlais et al., in press).

Similar rapid spread of HIV among IV drug users appears to have occurred in Edinburgh. Seroprevalence rates in the Robertson et al. (1986) study went from essentially zero to 50 percent in less than two years. In contrast, seroprevalence rates in San Francisco appear to have held around 10 percent through 1985 (R. Chaisson, personal communication, 1986). This epidemiologic research shows both an opportunity and a great need for immediate efforts to prevent the virus from saturating IV drug use groups in many different communities.

THE IV DRUG USE SUBCULTURE

Successful prevention efforts will need to be based on an understanding of the social psychology and physiology of IV drug use. The scientific literature on these topics is immense, so we will confine our review to those aspects we believe are most closely related to preventing AIDS.

There is a common misconception that IV drug users have no social organization. A multi-billion-dollar industry, however, does not persevere without some forms of social organization. IV drug use has been traditionally described as a "subculture" within sociological and anthropological research (e.g., Agar, 1973; Combs, Fry, & Lewis, 1976; DuToit, 1977; Johnson, 1980; Weppner, 1977). While the concept of "subculture" does not have an overly precise definition, it is used to denote a distinct group with its own set of values, roles, and status allocation that exists within a larger society (Johnson, 1973, 1980). From the perspective of its members, participating in the subculture is a meaningful activity, rather than a psychopathology, an "escape from reality," or an "illness" (Preble & Casey, 1969).

Although there is considerable regional and ethnic variation, IV drug use clearly constitutes a deviant subculture within the U.S. (Agar, 1973). Possession and sale of drugs are violations of the law, as are many of the activities undertaken to obtain money for purchasing the drugs. In addition to legal differences between IV drug users and members of conventional society, there is an empathy barrier. Most members of conventional society, even those who use illicit drugs, have great difficulty imagining themselves injecting drugs or doing what IV drug users are believed to do to obtain money for drugs. Most members of conventional society find it easier to empathize with victims of drug-related crime than with IV drug users. Thus, IV drug users are not just considered different, but are often objects of fear, mistrust, hostility, scorn, and, to a limited extent, pity. This psychological and social distance between the IV drug use subculture and conventional society contributes to a climate of generalized mistrust between the two groups.

There is a precarious balance between trust and mistrust among IV drug users themselves. They need a degree of interpersonal trust so that they can conduct the business of acquiring drugs, equipment, and locations for injecting, and for social validation of the worth of "getting high." But they also have a widespread mistrust of other IV drug users. Among the many reasons for this mistrust are competition for scarce goods (drugs and the money to buy them), use of informants by law-enforcement agencies, carryover of the "hustling" (use of deception and/or limited violence to obtain money) of "straights" (non-drug users) to the hustling of other drug users, and the use of violence to settle disputes.

Another very important limitation on trust among IV drug users is their varying commitment to the values of the subculture. As with any subculture, new members are not expected to be fully socialized into the group. It is also quite difficult to be a "successful" IV drug user in terms of obtaining money and drugs, avoiding the law, and maintaining some positive relationships with non-users (particularly family and sexual partners) without becoming "strung out" from excessive drug use. Because of these great difficulties, many IV drug users will at least temporarily attempt to stop injecting drugs, either on their own or by entering a treatment program. Persons who enter treatment are usually seen as having failed at being IV drug users, and (at least temporarily) lose the respect and trust of those who continue injecting drugs. Persons who succeed in treatment also come to denigrate current IV drug users so that the mistrust becomes mutual.

IV drug users rely on oral communication. There are few written documents and few print channels of communication. They rely on the spoken word for two main reasons: Since much of what they do is illegal, written documents would be incriminating; and many of them have difficulty with reading and writing. Part of the oral nature of the subculture is a specialized argot. While some terms have been incorporated into the slang of conventional society (e.g., "O.D." for overdose), the argot generally tends to limit communication between members of the subculture and conventional society.

It should be noted that, prior to AIDS, death was already a frequent occurrence within the IV drug use subculture. Estimates of the annual death rate among IV drug users not in treatment range from 3.5% to 8% (Des Jarlais, 1984). Although AIDS clearly poses a threat of a protracted, painful, and often socially isolated death (compared to the rapid, painless death associated with an overdose), there is some tendency to generalize the fatalistic acceptance of death within the subculture to AIDS. AIDS, however, represents a more frequent and qualitatively different way of dying. It serves as much greater motivation for behavior change than any previous health threat associated with IV drug use.

The sharing of works is deeply embedded in the IV drug use subculture. Such sharing serves both social bonding and economic functions. Sharing among "running partners" (persons who cooperate to obtain drugs and the money needed to purchase them) can symbolize their cooperative effort. The legally restricted supply of sterile needles and syringes for injection also encourages multiple users for the same works. (See Des Jarlais, Friedman, & Strug, 1986, for a more complete discussion of the roles of needle sharing within the pre-AIDS IV drug use subculture.) Reducing some types of needle sharing (e.g., the purely pragmatic use of rented works in a "shooting gallery" will be easier than reducing the sharing among running partners or sexual partners, where a close social bond is involved.

The most difficult situation in which to prevent the use of possibly contaminated works occurs when an IV drug user is experiencing withdrawal symptoms (Des Jarlais, et al., 1986). While narcotic withdrawal is not life threatening, it includes anxiety and severe physical discomfort. Injection of a narcotic will provide almost instantaneous relief. Thus, when an IV drug user is undergoing withdrawal and has the drug to inject, he or she will be severely tempted to use whatever works are readily available.

In general, the characteristics of IV drug use as a deviant subculture necessitate specifically designed prevention programs. The differences and hostility between the subculture and conventional society make cooperativeefforts between public-health authorities and IV drug users difficult. Language and literacy problems reduce the potential effectiveness of written communications. The generalized mistrust within the subculture makes collective self-organization to promote the health of the group as a whole difficult (Friedman & Des Jarlais in press; Friedman, et al., in press). The fact that there are many aspects of the IV drug use subculture that make AIDS prevention difficult should not, however, be used as a rationale to justify not making prevention efforts.

CURRENT FINDINGS ON BEHAVIOR CHANGE AMONG IV DRUG USERS

In addition to skepticism based on the social and physiological reasons that make AIDS prevention difficult, there are common stereotypes that IV drug users are concerned only about drugs and/or are basically "self-destructive" and not likely to respond to prevention efforts. These stereotypes create a great inertia against AIDS prevention efforts. The extent to which these beliefs were true prior to AIDS is a matter of considerable disagreement, but they certainly should not be generalized to the AIDS epidemic.

AIDS has created a new and qualitatively different fear of death among IV drug users. This type of death is protracted, usually painful, and often preceded by social isolation. Dying from AIDS has none of the elements of escapism that can be seen in an overdose death.

A number of recent studies indicate that the majority of IV drug users can be expected to change their behavior in order to avoid exposure to the AIDS virus.

In the fall of 1984, we collected data from a sample of New York City IV drug users in treatment, regarding their knowledge of AIDS and responses to the epidemic (Friedman, et al., in press). These subjects had not received any special education/prevention programming at the time of data collection. Essentially all of the subjects knew of AIDS, and over 90 percent knew that it could be transmitted through the sharing of needles for injecting drugs. Fifty-nine percent reported that they had changed their behavior in order to reduce the likelihood of being exposed to the virus. The major changes in behavior were greater use of sterile needles, greater cleaning of previously used needles, and reduction in the sharing of needles.

Selwyn and colleagues (Selwyn, Cox, Feiner, Lipshutz, & Cohen, 1985; P. Selwyn, personal communication, 1986) more recently conducted a study of AIDS knowledge and behavior change among patients in a methadone maintenance program and in a detention center detoxification program. The findings were similar: 97% were aware that sharing needles could transmit AIDS, and over 60% reported that they had changed their drug/needle use in order to reduce the risk of developing AIDS.

Evidence of behavior change among IV drug users in response to AIDS is not confined to self-reports of IV drug users in treatment. Evidence for the increase in use of sterile needles in New York City has also come from interviews with persons selling needles in the "copping areas" (areas where drugs can be purchased) and from the emergence of a market in "counterfeit" sterile needles in which a used needle is washed out and placed in the original package, which is then resealed (Des Jarlais, Friedman, & Hopkins, 1985). "Free" sterile needles, in the forms of 2-for-1 sales and free needles with purchases of $25 and $50 bags of heroin, are now being offered as a marketing tactic in New York City (Des Jarlais & Hopkins, 1985).

Only preliminary data are available from studies of AIDS-related behavior change outside of New York City. These studies also support the idea that IV drug users will change their behavior because of AIDS. In New Jersey, where there have been 538 cases of AIDS among heterosexual IV drug users and 81 cases among homosexual male IV drug users (through May 1, 1986), the threat of the disease has become one of the major reasons for entering treatment. Approximately half of IV drug users entering treatment since the last half of 1985 reported that AIDS was one of their reasons for entering treatment (J. French, personal communication, 1986).

There have been only 18 cases of AIDS among IV drug users in San Francisco (through April 1986, with gay males who inject drugs excluded), and the seroprevalence is estimated to be approximately 10% (R. Chaisson, personal communication, 1986). Yet even here, ethnographic research with IV drug users not in treatment shows that the majority know of the disease and realize that it can be transmitted through sharing works. A "substantial minority" have already reduced their sharing of works in order to avoid exposure to the virus (Biernacki & Feldman, 1986).

The current research on behavior change among IV drug users thus consistently supports the idea that many of them will modify their behavior in order to avoid exposure to the AIDS virus. These changes have occurred prior to formal AIDS prevention programs aimed at IV drug users and suggest that more extensive prevention efforts would produce greater risk reduction.

PREVENTION TARGET GROUPS

While IV drug users can generally be considered to form a single subculture with some geographic and ethnic variations, we want to emphasize the need for targeting different subgroups within the subculture. As noted above, individual IV drug users have varying commitment to the subculture at different points in time, and AIDS prevention efforts will be more effective if they utilize these different levels of commitment.

IV Drug Users in Treatment

IV drug users in treatment programs are among those with the least commitment to the subculture, although they must still be considered at risk for exposure to HIV. Many will drop out of treatment prior to successful completion, and many in ambulatory treatment will continue to inject drugs despite being in treatment. The injection of cocaine is a particular problem for persons in ambulatory treatment, since at present there is no effective chemotherapy that blocks the effects of cocaine. IV drug users in treatment are also more easily reached with information about AIDS than those not in treatment.

A critical part of AIDS prevention among IV drug users in treatment is prior education efforts for the staff of the treatment programs. All staff in contact with persons at increased risk need to be able to provide accurate basic information about AIDS. This includes the viral causation of AIDS, the long latency period, early symptoms, the fact that clinical AIDS is only the most severe manifestation of HIV infection, and the specifics of the modes of transmission of the virus. They should know that causal contact does not transmit the virus and that the traditional means of cleaning needles and syringes (rinsing with nonsterile water) do not kill the virus. Finally, they should know the "safe sex" guidelines relevant to prevention of homosexual and heterosexual transmission.

Staff should never be sources of misinformation. They need to maintain credibility with persons at increased risk and may permanently lose credibility if they appear to be spreading misinformation. In the rapidly changing AIDS field, with the frequent news stories that do not provide full explanations of various "new findings," this can be difficult. Staff need to have a sense of what they do *not* know about AIDS, as well as what they do know. The treatment program as a whole will need a resource/referral source through which difficult questions can be answered.

Staff need more than just knowledge; they should be able to communicate the information accurately, without embarrassment and without either sensationalizating or denying the seriousness of AIDS. This means having "worked through" their own emotional reactions to the epidemic, including fears that they themselves might contract the illness through casual contact or from their own previous IV drug use, and the emotional reactions that AIDS evokes even in persons not at risk for viral exposure.

Admitting that clients or patients in treatment are at risk for IV drug use is difficult for many treatment program staff, since it may seem to undermine the basic treatment message that drug abuse problems can be overcome. This does not, however, justify the absence of AIDS education/prevention activities. Many drug-abuse treatment clients either drop out of treatment or inject drugs at some level while in treatment. One cannot ignore the opportunity of providing needed information while they are in treatment. For residential programs, the most opportune time for such prevention/education efforts may be at intake, where the knowledge can serve to enforce the motivation not to inject drugs. For ambulatory treatment programs, where clients and patients must be considered at risk for injecting drugs while in treatment, prevention/education at intake and periodically throughout treatment would be appropriate.

To be most effective, prevention efforts for persons at increased risk will involve more than sharing information. The modes of transmission of the virus involve private behaviors, and the disease is quite capable of arousing strong emotions. In this situation, education about AIDS may easily merge with counseling about transmission-related behavior. Even drug-abuse treatment staff who are competent to provide counseling on drug injection may not be competent to provide counseling about sexual and in utero transmission of HIV. They should, however, be able to recognize when a client or patient needs counseling in these areas and be able to make an appropriate referral.

While it is necessary to provide AIDS education/prevention to persons in drug-abuse treatment, controlling the epidemic will require prevention efforts aimed at those who are not in treatment. Relatively few illicit drug injectors are in treatment at any point in time, and once the virus becomes established in a geographic area, many IV drug users will be exposed before they come to treatment. Thus, it will be necessary to mount effective IV drug use-AIDS prevention efforts outside of treatment settings.

Persons at Risk for Initiation into IV Drug Use

The ideal point for prevention of AIDS among IV drug users would be to prevent initiation into IV drug use. This would not only prevent needle-sharing transmission of HIV, it would also prevent the many other health and social problems associated with IV drug use. Educational programs about the dangers of AIDS and IV drug use have been developed in New York City for use in junior and senior high schools. While we support the development of these programs, we also feel that they are not likely to be greatly effective. First, drug-prevention programs based on fear arousal have not been successful in the past (Schaps, DiBartolo, Palley, & Churgin, 1978), particularly if the fear is associated with a low probability event. Second, many persons who eventually become IV drug users drop out of school well before they make decisions about injecting drugs.

Prevention programs targeted at reducing initiation into IV drug use may have to operate outside of school settings. They include discussions of experiences with non-injected drugs as part of the behavioral processes that lead to drug injection. Such programs may need to focus on teaching skills needed to resist social pressures to begin injecting drugs (similar to the cigarette-smoking prevention programs that focus on teaching social skills to resist initiation into cigarette smoking; e.g., Botvin & Eng, 1980; Botvin, Eng, & Williams, 1980). Such programs undoubtedly would be more expensive than the in-school programs. They would also pose some difficult policy/strategic questions: Should they focus only on drug injection (the AIDS danger), or should they be broader and include any use of such drugs as cocaine and heroin, or broader still and focus on any illicit drug use? Preventing non-injected drug abuse is a valid public health goal in itself, but may dilute efforts to reduce the AIDS-specific problem of initiation into drug injection.

Current IV Drug Users Who Would Enter Treatment

Fear of AIDS, among other reasons will undoubtedly lead significant numbers of IV drug users to seek treatment for their drug use. For the U.S. as a whole, however, the availability of treatment was significantly less than the demand prior to the AIDS epidemic. Expanding the treatment system could significantly reduce transmission of HIV among IV drug users. Users who had not been exposed would greatly reduce their chances of being exposed, and users who had already been exposed would greatly reduce their chances of exposing others. The economics of treating AIDS (currently estimated to be between $100,000 and $150,000 per case; Hardy, 1986) versus providing drug-abuse treatment (approximately $3,000 per patient year) also argues for expansion of the treatment network.

Unfortunately, there are real factors other than finances that currently limit the availability of drug-abuse treatment. Drug-abuse treatment has general approval within American society, but is particularly subject to the "NIMBY" (not in my backyard) phenomenon. In addition, methadone maintenance treatment, which tends to be the most acceptable treatment modality to large numbers of IV drug users, also tends to have the least degree of in-my-neighborhood acceptance. Any public association of IV drug use with AIDS is likely to increase the difficulties in finding acceptable locations for new drug-abuse treatment programs. Finally, if there is to be a significant reduction of HIV transmission through increased treatment, the program expansion will have to be on a large scale. Based on our New York experience, we would estimate that there are approximately four IV drug users not in treatment for every one currently in treatment. Thus, to control HIV transmission among IV drug users through additional treatment would require a massive expansion of the treatment system.

IV Drug Users Who Do Not Wish to Enter Treatment

Many current IV drug users wish to reduce their chances of exposure to HIV but will not enter treatment or refrain from all drug injection. (As noted above, there are also IV drug users in treatment but who also will continue some level of drug injection. Much of this section also applies to them.) Even though many IV drug users will not eliminate their drug injection, they will nevertheless reduce sharing of works and/or increase their use of sterile works as a way of reducing their risk of developing AIDS.

Whether legal restrictions on the sale of sterile hypodermic needles should be reduced in order to reduce transmission of HIV among IV drug users has been the subject of much public discussion in New York, New Jersey, and other states. There are only 11 states in the country that require prescriptions for the purchase of hypodermics (National Association of Boards of Pharmacy, 1983). Increasing the legal availability of hypodermic needles has received some support among public-health officials, but it has generally been opposed by law-enforcement officials, who predict that it would lead to greater IV drug use.

The actual effects of increasing the legal availability of sterile needles are unknown. Almost no data have been collected on the relationship between the legal availability of sterile needles and levels of IV drug use prior to the AIDS epidemic; and we have serious doubts that such earlier data can be generalized to the epidemic situation. The actual effects of an increased legal availability on reducing HIV transmission and levels of IV drug use may depend greatly on the specific methods of changing the legal availability and the simultaneous presence of other AIDS prevention efforts.

A second method of attempting to reduce HIV transmission among IV drug users who are not ready to enter treatment would be education on not sharing needles and on how to properly "clean" needles in order to kill HIV. Printed materials containing this information (after emphasizing that stopping drug injection is the only certain method of avoiding HIV exposure) are being used in several states. Some of these materials have been criticized as "encouraging IV drug use." Again, only empirical study will show the extent to which such educational materials and training reduce HIV transmission or affect levels of IV drug use.

Heterosexual Partners and Children of IV Drug Users

Space limitations do not permit a full discussion of the complex questions related to preventing AIDS among the heterosexual partners and children of IV drug users, but we will outline some of the relevant issues. As discussed in the earlier section on epidemiology, IV drug users are the primary source of HIV transmission to heterosexual partners and children in the United States.

Both the heterosexual partners and children are relatively large groups. A study of sexual relationships of male IV drug users in New York City found that almost 80 percent of them had their primary sexual relationship with women who did not inject drugs themselves. The size of the female heterosexual partner population was estimated to be at least half the size of the IV drug use population (Des Jarlais et al, 1984). IV drug users also have considerable numbers of children. A recently completed New York Study of the children of methadone maintenance patients found an average of almost two children per patient, and a quarter of the patients indicated that they expected to have additional children (Deren, 1985). The incidence of surveillance-definition AIDS in both heterosexual partners and children has been low, compared to the numbers of partners and children at risk—which suggests that these modes of transmission may be less likely to lead to AIDS than drug injection—but the incidence follows the same exponential increase as the cases in IV drug users (Des Jarlais, Chamberland, Yancovitz, Weinberg, R. Friedman in press).

Preventing AIDS among the sexual partners and children of IV drug users will clearly be a necessary part of overall public-health control of the epidemic.

The behavior changes needed to prevent heterosexual and in utero transmission are at least as complex and difficult as those associated with drug-injection transmission. Disruption of ongoing sexual relationships and forgoing having children would involve considerable psychological costs and would require more intensive prevention resources than are needed for dissemination of information. Until more is known about the probabilities of heterosexual and in utero transmission, it is difficult to provide any guidelines for the trade-offs of risk reduction and psychological costs. The same "safer sex" guidelines used for homosexual transmission (e.g., avoidance of bodily fluid transfer and anal intercourse, use of condoms), and, for women who are HIV antibody positive, postponing voluntary pregnancies until more is known about transmission to children, would seem to be minimal recommendations for prevention in the heterosexual partners and children groups.

The prevention of in utero transmission is one clear case where HIV antibody testing may be of specific use. Women who are contemplating pregnancy should be provided with the opportunity for voluntary testing, with strict protection of the confidentiality of the results.

ETHNIC AND RACIAL DIFFERENCES

At several places in this chapter, we have noted that ethnic differences among IV drug users will have to be considered in prevention efforts. These ethnic differences are intellectually separate from, but confounded with, social class factors. In general, the delivery of prevention services to minority groups has been inadequate in the United States, and the problems are likely to be at least as great for AIDS, if not greater. The subject of ethnicity and AIDS is sufficiently complex to justify a separate article, so we will make only a few comments here.

Compared to their percentage of the total population, Blacks and Hispanics are overrepresented among AIDS cases in the U.S. as a whole. This is particularly true for the IV drug-related cases, of which 80 percent have occurred among Blacks and Hispanics (A. Hardy, personal communication, 1986).

There is a great lack of information on how best to incorporate ethnicity and racial considerations into AIDS prevention efforts for IV drug users and their sexual partners. Printed materials about AIDS and IV drug use have been translated into Spanish, and Black and Hispanic ex-addicts have worked as health educators for IV drug users. Information is needed on what else should be done. Much of the needed knowledge may be specific to local geographic areas. Questions for "needs assessment" research include (1) the extent to which AIDS is perceived to be a disease of gay white males and/or of IV drug users and/or of heterosexuals; (2) attitudes toward the various "safer sex" practices; (3) the social integration of IV drug users within the ethnic group and the larger community, including how attitudes toward IV drug users combine sympathy, fear, and denial of a problem; and (4) the integration of the ethnic minority into the larger community, which may involve increased discrimination against the group as a potential outcome of a perceived association between the group and AIDS.

SEX DIFFERENCES

Sex differences in planning AIDS-IV drug use prevention programs are also sufficiently complex to deserve a full analysis, so we will make only limited comments here. To some extent, gender considerations interact with ethnic considerations, since sex roles vary across ethnic groups. There are some factors that are similar across ethnic groups. In many ethnic groups, a woman who injects drugs is more highly stigmatized than a man who injects drugs, including the assumption that a woman who injects drugs is also a prostitute. Conflict between drug use and child-rearing responsibilities may be more intense for women in many ethnic groups. Many women who inject drugs are dependent on a male sexual partner as a source of drugs and share drug-injection equipment primarily with that man. Since the woman is likely to have less power in the relationship, taking precautions against HIV transmission—both via shared drug equipment and heterosexual activity—may be particularly difficult if the man objects.

How best to incorporate ethnic/racial and sex differences in AIDS prevention programs is an area where additional research is urgently needed. Given the rapidity with which HIV can spread among IV drug users, using seroconversion rates as the outcome measures in evaluating prevention efforts that incorporate ethnic and sex differences may be too costly in time and money. It will often be more appropriate to use focus groups and self-reported behavior changes to evaluate potential effectiveness.

DISCUSSION

Research has not yet demonstrated what are the most effective means of preventing AIDS among IV drug users, but there are several tentative generalizations that seem to hold. First, the mass media seem to be able to convey the basic information that AIDS is deadly and that it can be spread through the sharing of equipment for injecting drugs. (Pamphlets and posters can supplement the mass media for this message.) This basic information will produce a significant amount of behavior change among IV drug users, but probably not enough to do more than slow the spread of the virus within the group and prevent exposure in a small minority of IV drug users.

Secondly, prevention and education campaigns need to include very specific information. Some of the behavior changes that IV drug users report undertaking to avoid AIDS may not be effective. For example, methods of cleaning needles such as rinsing with water or using a wire to remove clotted blood are not sufficient to kill HIV. If IV drug users are to sterilize their equipment, they will have to be taught the specific information needed to do so.

A third generalization about prevention/education programs for IV drug users is that they should incorporate face-to face communication. The use of ex-addicts as health educators is currently under way in New Jersey, New York, Maryland, and the Netherlands. The use of current or ex-addicts should make it easier to communicate the specific details noted above, permit the recipient of the information to ask clarifying questions, and avoid the literacy and argot problems found among many IV drug users. Face-to-face communication would also permit the health educator to modulate the emotional tone of the message in accord with the response of the recipient. The seriousness of AIDS needs to be stressed, but not to the point where so much anxiety is aroused that denial becomes the dominant response.

A final aspect of preventing AIDS among IV drug users concerns the perceived conflict between preventing AIDS and "encouraging drug use." Some form of this conflict will probably occur among almost all groups active in preventing AIDS among IV drug users, from public-health officials to drug-abuse treatment staff to ex-addict health educators.

SUMMARY

In the absence of any effective treatment or vaccine, control of the AIDS epidemic must be through prevention efforts. Since IV drug users constitute the second largest risk group in the United States and are the primary source of transmission to heterosexual partners and children, overall control of the epidemic will require control within the IV drug use group.

Because of the social organization of IV drug users in the U.S., there are greater constraints on prevention efforts with this group than with others. Present research, however, shows that IV drug users in New York City and elsewhere do modify their behavior in response to the threat of AIDS. Even so, efforts at prevention that have begun with the IV drug use subculture need to be reinforced by programs undertaken by public-health and drug-abuse treatment and prevention personnel.

Persons at risk for HIV exposure through IV drug use do not constitute a homogeneous group. Different prevention activities need to be targeted to these different groups. Special prevention efforts also need to be devised for persons who have not yet started IV drug use, heterosexual partners (who do not themselves inject drugs), and potential parents who may have been exposed to HIV.

Public-health efforts aimed at preventing AIDS among IV drug users may be limited by perceptions that some AIDS prevention efforts may actually "encourage" illicit drug use. Such perceptions may be held both among the general public and among some members of the drug-abuse treatment/ prevention community. At present, relevant data on the accuracy of these perceptions are almost nonexistent. AIDS has created a qualitatively different risk of death associated with IV drug use, and previous beliefs about what does and does not encourage IV drug use cannot safely be generalized to the AIDS situation. The dilemma about preventing adverse health consequences of drug use versus "encouraging" drug use can be applied to any treatment of adverse health consequences of drug use (e.g., using naloxone to treat acute overdoses). AIDS, however, magnifies the scale of the dilemma on several dimensions—it is specific to IV drug use rather than all forms of drug use; some successful prevention can probably be achieved without any overall reduction in drug injection (e.g., reducing the use of contaminated needles); the adverse consequences may occur after successful elimination of IV drug use, thus undermining the hope needed in drug-abuse treatment programs; and the fatal consequences are not limited to the drug user, but may also include sexual partners and children.

Specific approaches to these prevention policy questions will vary according to the different target groups for preventing AIDS among IV drug users, the extent to which HIV has spread among the local IV drug users, the feelings of individual prevention workers, the philosophy of the sponsoring organization, and the local political climate. The problem is certainly large enough to permit a wide variety of approaches, and there are not yet sufficient data to identify the single "best" prevention approach. Individuals working to prevent AIDS among IV drug users, their sexual partners, and their children need to believe in the validity of what they are personally doing, but will also need to be able to keep an open mind to forthcoming data showing the relative effectiveness of the different approaches. In the meantime, the AIDS problem is of sufficient urgency that we should be trying and assessing a wide variety of prevention programs.

ACKNOWLEDGMENTS

Support for the preparation of this chapter was provided by grant DA 03574 from the National Institute on Drug Abuse. The chapter is based on an article in the *Journal of Applied Social Psychology*.

REFERENCES

Angarano, G., Pastore, G., Monno, L., Santantonio, F., Luchera, N., & Schiraldi, O. (1985). Rapid spread of HTLV-III infection among drug addicts in Italy. Lancet, *8467*(II), 1302.

Cohen, H. W., Marmor, M., Des Jarlais, D. C., Spira, T., Friedman, S. R., & Yancovitz, S. et al. (1985, April). *Behavioral risk factors for HTLV-III/LAV seropositivity among intravenous drug abusers.* Paper presented at the International Conference on Acquired Immunodeficiency Syndrome (AIDS), Atlanta, Georgia.

Des Jarlais, D. C., Chamberland, M. E., Yancovitz, S. R., Weinberg, P., & Friedman, S. R. (1984). Heterosexual partners: A large risk group for AIDS [letter]. *Lancet, 8415,* 1346-1347.

Des Jarlais, D. C., Friedman, S. R., Spira, T. J., Zolla-Pazner, S., Marmor, M., Holzman, R., Mildvan, D., Yancovitz, S., Mathur-Wagh, U., Garber, J., El-Sadr, W., Cohen, H., Smith, D., & Kalyanaraman, V. S. (1986). A stage model of HTLV-III LAV infection in intravenous drug users. In L. S. Harris (Ed.), *NIDA research monograph 67. Problems of drug dependence. 1985. Proceedings of the 47th Annual Scientific Meeting. The Committee on Problems of Drug Dependence, Inc.* (pp. 328-334).

Friedland, G. H., Harris, C., Small, C. B., Shine, D., Moll, B., Darrow, W., & Klein, R. S. (1986). Intravenous drug abusers and the Acquired Immune Deficiency Syndrome (AIDS) demographic, drug use and needle sharing patterns. *Archives Internal Medicine, 145,* 837-840.

Friedman, S. R., Des Jarlais, D. C., Sotheran, J. L. Garber, J., Cohen, H., & Smith, D. (1987). AIDS and self-organization among intravenous drug users. *International Journal of the Addictions, 22,* 201-220.

Hardy, A. M., Rauch, K., Echenberg, D., Morgan, W. M., & Curran, J. W. (1986). The economic impact of the first 10,000 cases of acquired immunodeficiency syndrome in the United States. *Journal of the American Medical Association, 255*(2), 209-211.

Lapoint, N., Michaud, J., Pekovic, D., Chausseau, J. P., & Dupuy, J. M. (1986). Transplacental transmission of HTLV-III virus [letter]. *New England Journal of Medicine, 312*(20), 1325-1326.

Luzi, G., Ensoli, B., Turbessi, G., Scarpati, B., & Aiuti, F. (1985, November 2). Transmission of HTLV-III infection by heterosexual contact. *Lancet, II,* 1018.

Marmor, M., Des Jarlais, D. C., Friedman, S. R. Lyden, M., & El-Sadr, W. (1985). The epidemic of Acquired Immunodeficiency Syndrome (AIDS) and suggestions for its control in drug abusers. *Journal of Substance Abuse Treatment, 1,* 237-247.

Novick, D. M., Kreek, M. J., Des Jarlais, D. C., Spira, T. J., Khuri, E. T., Ragunath, J., Kalyanaraman, V. S., Gelb, A. M., & Miescher, A. (1986). Antibody to LAV, the putative agent of AIDS, in parenteral drug abusers and Methadone-maintained patients: Therapeutic, historical and ethical aspects. In L. J. Harris (Ed.), *Problems of drug dependence 1985.* (Research Monograph 67, pp. 318-320). Rockville, MD: National Institute on Drug Abuse.

Redfield, R. R., Markham, P. D., Salahuddin, S. Z., Wright, D. C., Sarngadharan, M. G., & Gallo, R. C. (1985). Heterosexually acquired HTLV-III/LAV disease. *Journal American Medical Association, 254,* 2094-2096.

Robertson, J. R., Bucknall, A. B. V., Welsby, P. D., Roberts, J. J. K., Inglis, M. M., Peutherer, J. F., & Brettle, R. P. (1986). Epidemic of AIDS related virus (HTLV-III/LAV) infection among intravenous drug users. *British Medical Journal, 292,* 527-529.

Schupbach, J., Haller, O., Vogt, M., Luthy, R., Joller, H., Oelz, O., Popovic, M., Sarngadharan, M. G., & Gallo, R. C. (1985). Antibodies to HTLV-III in Swiss patients with AIDS and pre-AIDS and in groups at risk for AIDS. *New England Journal of Medicine, 312*(5), 265-270.

Spira, T. J., Des Jarlais, D. C., Bokos, D., Onichi, R., Kiprov, R., & Kalyanaraman, V. S. (1985, April). *HTLV-III/LAV antibodies in intravenous drug users: Comparisons of high and low risk areas for AIDS.* Presented at the International Conference on the Acquired Immune Deficiency Syndrome (AIDS), Atlanta, GA.

Weiss, S. H., Ginzburg, H. M., Goedert, J. J., Biggar, R. J., Mohica, B. A., Blattner, W. A. et al. (1985). *Risk for HTLV-III exposure and AIDS among parenteral drug abusers in New Jersey.* Presented at the International Conference on the Acquired Immunodeficiency Syndrome (AIDS). Atlanta, GA (April 14-17, 1985).

Adolescents and AIDS: Current Research, Prevention Strategies, and Policy Implications

4

Ralph J. DiClemente
School of Medicine
Department of Epidemiology and International Health
University of California

INTRODUCTION

Since its recognition in 1981 (Gottlieb, Schroff, Schanker, Weisman, Fan, Wolf, & Saxon, 1981; Masur, Michelis, Greene, Onorato, Vande Stouwe, Holzman, Wormser, Brettman, Lange, Murray, & Cunningham-Rundles, 1981; Siegal, Lopez, Hammer, Brown, Kornfeld, Gold, Hassett, Hirschman, Cunningham-Rundles, Adelsberg, Parham, Siegal, Cunningham-Rundles, & Armstrong, 1981), acquired immunodeficiency syndrome (AIDS) has rapidly become a serious problem which has spread to all continents of the world (DiClemente, Boyer, Mills, & Helquist, 1988). Recent advances in anti-retroviral therapies have produced promising, new therapeutic agents (Yarchoan & Broder, 1987), although, at present, there is no cure for AIDS.

Attributable, in large part, to the lack of an effective therapy for the disease, primary prevention has become increasingly more important in combating the AIDS epidemic (Stone, Grimes, & Magder, 1986). In the United States, as well

ADOLESCENTS AT—RISK: THE SCOPE OF THE PROBLEM

Adolescents between the ages of 13 and 19 comprise almost 10% of the United States population, accounting for approximately 25 million persons (Bureau of the Census, 1986). Estimates vary widely on the proportion of adolescents who are sexually active. Depending on the survey, anywhere from 50% to 70% of adolescents report being sexually active by 19 years of age (Alan Guttmacher Institute, 1981; Harris, 1986; Hofferth, Kahn, & Baldwin, 1987; Zelnik & Kanter, 1980). Of sexually active adolescents, only 47% and 25% of females and males, respectively, report using condoms as a primary contraceptive method (Harris, 1986). More alarming, one-third to one-quarter of sexually active adolescents never use any form of contraception (Alan Guttmacher Institute, 1981).

Longitudinal data collected at three timepoints (1971, 1976, and 1979) suggest that the proportion of adolescents who are sexually active is increasing for all ages from 15 to 19, with the greatest increase observed for 16-year-old White females. In 1971, for example, approximately 15% of 16-year-old-White females were sexually active. By 1979, the proportion of 16-year-old females who reported being sexually active had more than doubled, increasing to 32% (Zelnik & Kanter, 1980). Evidence suggests that this trend toward earlier initiation of sexual intercourse is continuing with greater numbers of adolescents projected to engage in sexual activity at increasingly younger ages. Two emerging trends have been identified which increases the likelihood of risk for HIV infection in this population. First, data indicate that adolescents below the age of 14 show the greatest increase in rate of initiation of sexual activity relative to other ages (Kovar, 1979), and, second, data indicate a growing trend toward increased numbers of sexual partners among adolescents (Hass, 1979; Zelnik & Kanter, 1977).

Adolescents and AIDS

AIDS is uncommon among adolescents. At present, adolescents between the ages of 13 and 19 account for less than one percent of all diagnosed cases of AIDS in the United States (Centers for Disease Control, 1989). Relying on the prevalence of diagnosed cases of AIDS among adolescents as a guide to formulating and developing risk-reduction educational programs may, however, severely underestimate the threat and, perhaps, the prevalence of infection within this population. The number of adolescent AIDS cases is a poor surrogate marker for estimating the prevalence of HIV infection. With an incubation period reported to be as long as 7 years (Curran, Morgan, Hardy, Jaffe, Darrow, & Dowdle, 1985), adolescents who are infected may not manifest symptoms until their twenties. This actuarial procedure may obscure the fact that a number of cases acquired their infections as teenagers. A more accurate marker for projecting the future rate of HIV infection in the adolescent population may be the rates of sexually transmitted diseases.

Prevalence of Sexually Transmitted Diseases Among Adolescents

Epidemiologic data on the prevalence of sexually transmitted diseases (STDs) among this population suggest that adolescents are at increased risk of HIV infection (Cates & Rauh, 1985; Fichtner, Aral, Blount, Zaidi, Reynolds, & Darrow, 1983; Hein, 1987; O'Reilly & Aral, 1985; Shafer et al., 1984). National data on the prevalence of gonorrhea among sexually active females show that those between the ages of 10 to 14 and 15 to 19 had the highest rates of infection compared to older age groups. Strikingly, the rates for females in the younger age group, 10 to 14, and those females 15 to 19 years of age are very similar—approximately 3,500 cases per 100,000 sexually active females. Similar data regarding syphilis and chlamydia reveal that the highest rates occur among adolescents, despite the impression that STDs are a problem particularly endemic to the adult population (Bell & Hein, 1984; Hein, 1987). Further, findings indicate that the rate of STDs declines exponentially past the age of 19 (Bell & Holmes, 1984). The evidence suggests that a substantial proportion of adolescents engage in high-risk behaviors associated with the acquisition and transmission of STDs; for example, engaging in unprotected sexual intercourse, which is directly related to the risk of HIV infection. In an overarching assessment of the scope of this problem, the National Institute of Allergies and Infectious Disease Study Group (1980) found that STDs are the most pervasive, destructive, and costly communicable disease problem confronting adolescents (Kroger & Wiesner, 1981).

Need for School-Based AIDS Prevention Programs

In the absence of an effective vaccine or curative therapy, a coordinated and systematic school-based HIV prevention program providing knowledge about risk factors associated with the transmission of HIV infection could be a significant factor in preventing the spread of infection among this population (National Academy of Sciences, 1986; U.S. Department of Health and Human Services, 1986). Despite the growing concern and awareness of the need to develop and implement HIV prevention programs with the nation's public school system, few school systems presently provide AIDS education as part of the formal curriculum, and, of those school systems that provide some form of AIDS education, few have conducted careful evaluations, if any, to identify program effectiveness (McCormick, 1987).

Adolescents' Knowledge About AIDS

There are little data assessing adolescents' knowledge of AIDS and risk of HIV infection. The limited evidence we have suggests that adolescents, even within an AIDS epicenter (DiClemente, Zorn, & Temoshok, 1987a), are not sufficiently informed about the cause, transmission, and, especially, the prevention of HIV infection. An early large-scale survey conducted with 1,326 high-school-age adolescents in San Francisco reported that 92% of the adolescents surveyed could accurately identify the primary route of HIV transmission as sexual intercourse, however, only 60% were aware that using condoms during sexual intercourse could reduce the risk of infection (DiClemente, Zorn, & Temoshok, 1986; DiClemente, Zorn, & Temoshok, 1987b). This suggests that a large proportion of adolescents are not taking the appropriate preventive measures to reduce risk of HIV infection, even though they are well aware that sexual intercourse is a primary route of disease transmission. Recent evidence suggests that minority adolescents, in comparison to their White peers, are less knowledgeable about AIDS, overall, and particularly uninformed about the effectiveness of condoms as a protective barrier to prevent infection (DiClemente, Boyer, & Morales, 1988). Unfortunately, adolescents have not changed sexual practices nor methods of contraception as a result of the AIDS epidemic (Kegeles, Adler, & Irwin, 1988; Strunin & Hingson, 1987). Thus, although evidence indicates that condoms are an effective method for prohibiting the transmission of HIV (Van de Perre, Jacobs, & Sprecher-Goldberger, 1987; Conant, Hardy, Sernatinger, Spicer, & Levy, 1986), the usefulness of this method for controlling the spread of HIV infection is limited by adolescents' awareness of the effectiveness of condoms and their use during sexual intercourse.

Objectives of School-based HIV Prevention Programs

To make a reasonably well-informed decision about risk behaviors associated with HIV acquisition, adolescents need timely, accurate, and unbiased information. Good decisions are less probable when formulated in an informational vacuum, or when made with inadequate or incorrect information. The objective of HIV prevention programs should be to encourage health-promoting behaviors and eliminate or reduce high-risk sexual and drug-related behaviors. Adolescents cannot be coerced into changing behavior patterns; but, by providing clear and developmentally appropriate information, and the social skills necessary to resist referent-group pressures, we can provide an impetus which, as a direct consequence, may result in the postponement, reduction, or elimination of high-risk behaviors.

Development of School-based HIV Prevention Programs

School-based HIV prevention programs, culturally sensitive and age appropriate, provided the most practical approach for controlling the spread of infection among adolescents (Hafner, 1988; DiClemente, Boyer, & Mills,

1987). To be comprehensive in scope, school-based HIV prevention programs should include three primary components. First, there is a pressing need for standardized curricula for high schools (grades 9–12) and middle schools (grades 6–8). The curricula should be designed to increase students' knowledge of AIDS, prevent the initiation of and/or reduce high-risk sexual and drug practices associated with disease transmission, and dispel misconceptions about causal transmission which result in unnecessary anxiety and fear about personal susceptibility. A second component, previously neglected, is the need for teacher training to instruct teachers in the most effective methods for communicating curricula information to adolescents. Third, programs should be evaluated, short and long term, to determine effectiveness.

Development of School-based HIV Prevention Curricula

To achieve maximal effectiveness, HIV prevention curricula must incorporate the most recent medical information about AIDS and HIV infection. The curricula should include information about the cause, acquisition, treatment, and prevention of AIDS. Identification and discussion of known risk factors is also a high priority. In addition, curricula should clearly and unequivocally dispel myths and misconceptions about HIV acquisition; especially the often-cited myths related to casual contagion of AIDS. Adolescents who harbor these misconceptions have reported unnecessarily high and, at times, debilitating levels of fear and anxiety regarding their personal susceptibility to HIV infection. Dispelling such misconceptions may, therefore, reduce unnecessary fear and anxiety that divert adolescents' attention from actual modes of HIV transmission as well as decreasing the potential for stigmatization of segments of the population most adversely affected by the AIDS epidemic. Finally, HIV prevention curricula must go beyond conveying information and dispelling AIDS myths. They must foster decision-making skills (especially as they relate to the potential for engaging in unsafe sexual or drug practices), resistance training, and self-esteem enhancement to combat peer pressure to engage in risk-taking behaviors. They must also promote coping strategies that permit adolescents to exercise a "range of options" for risk management in avoiding high-risk activities, while not isolating themselves from their peers or alienating their peers.

Sexual behavior patterns, more than any other behavior, are difficult to modify. Historically, single-point interventions (administered at one time point), have not been effective in changing behavior. What is needed is a well-planned HIV prevention program which will be administered over time to achieve maximal effect over the course of an adolescent's school career. Repeated exposure offers a greater probability for effecting behavior modification as well as reinforcing previous HIV risk-reduction behavioral changes.

Teacher Training

As teachers deliver AIDS information, they, too, must be trained and educated about AIDS and other STDs and trained to communicate this information. Unfortunately, teachers who feel uncomfortable discussing sexuality and specific sexual behaviors, which they may personally consider offensive, are not likely to be effective communicators or facilitators of frank, open discussions. In-service training should be conducted within each school on a regular basis. Training should include basic AIDS education and a personal assessment of values and attitudes toward sexuality in general and homosexuality in particular. Overcoming these personal biases and inhibitions is crucial to fostering an atmosphere where adolescents are encouraged to candidly discuss such a sensitive personal topic as their sexual behavior.

Evaluation of HIV Prevention Programs

Programs should be adequately evaluated to assess effectiveness in increasing adolescents' knowledge about AIDS and HIV infection and reducing high-risk behaviors. Evaluation should be conducted both short and long term to assess decrement in knowledge as a means of identifying informational gaps or changes in the frequency or type of high-risk behaviors that may increase risk of HIV infection. Monitoring changes in adolescents' knowledge and attitudes permits timely and rapid modification or augmentation of the program by incorporating new information, thereby maintaining maximal program effectiveness.

Efficacy of School Health-Education Programs

When health-education programs are designed to be developmentally appropriate and pertinent to adolescents' lifestyles, they have been effective in increasing knowledge of health-promoting behaviors (Kirby, 1980; Thomas, Long, Whitten, Hamilton, Fraser, & Askin, 1985), and, more importantly, in reducing some of these behaviors (Zelnik & Kim, 1982). Evidence from the School Health Education Evaluation, the most comprehensive health-education evaluation conducted in the United States, demonstrates that adolescents' participation in health-education curricula results in significant changes in knowledge, attitudes, and frequency of self-reported risk behaviors (Connell, Turner, & Mason, 1985). Furthermore, health-promoting changes increase in direct proportion to the amount of instruction provided in the curriculum (Connell & Turner, 1985).

Directly relevant, recent findings from the San Francisco Comprehensive AIDS Program Evaluation (CAPE), a study of middle- and high-school AIDS curricula using a pretest–postest design, showed that students who received AIDS instruction were significantly more knowledgeable about AIDS relative to a comparable control group. Of particular importance, there was a substantial increase in knowledge about the efficacy of using condoms during sexual intercourse as a means of preventing HIV infection for students in the AIDS instruction group. At baseline, approximately 70% of the adolescents correctly reported that condoms could reduce their risk of HIV infection. At posttest, after 3 consecutive days of AIDS education, almost 92% of the instruction group were aware of the value of condoms. Further, students in the instruction group reported significantly fewer misconceptions regarding casual contact as a mode of HIV acquisition. The control group did not show any significant gain in knowledge or decrease in the number of misconceptions about casual contact (DiClemente, Pies, Stoller, Straits, Haskin, Oliva, & Rutherford, in press). Similar findings have been reported from Rhode Island (Brown, Fritz, & Barone, in press) and Seattle (Miller & Downer, 1988). In the pilot study of Brown and his colleagues (in press), students reported more hesitancy towards high-risk behaviors, although the changes were modest. Further studies must incorporate behavioral measures such as sexual and drug-related behaviors within the evaluation design to assess whether changes in AIDS knowledge and self-protective attitudes translate into concomitant changes in health-promoting behaviors (Becker & Joseph, 1988).

At present, two studies have reported on adolescents' changes in sexual behavior in response to the AIDS epidemic. In a population-based survey, approximately 15% of adolescents responding to a telephone interview reported changing their sexual behavior as a consequence of the threat of AIDS (Strunin & Hingson, 1987). Another clinic-based study assessing condom use at two time points, found that adolescents were not likely to increase condom use over a 1-year time period (Kegeles, Adler, & Irwin, 1988). Other studies suggest that among high-risk groups most severely affected by the epidemic, health-education programs stressing sexual risk reduction have been successful in reducing those behaviors most associated with HIV infection (Carne, Johnson, Pearce, Smith, Tedder, Weller, Loveday, Hawkins, Williams, & Adler, 1987; Martin, 1987; McKusick, Wiley, Coates, Stall, Saika, Morin, Charles, Horstman, & Conant, 1985; Winkelstein, Samuel, Padian, Wiley, Lang, Anderson, & Levy, 1987). Preliminary findings have also been reported documenting health-promoting behavior changes as a consequence of HIV prevention campaigns in heterosexual populations (Winkelstein, Samuel, Padian, & Wiley, 1987).

DEVELOPMENT, IMPLEMENTATION, AND EFFECTIVENESS OF HIV PREVENTION PROGRAMS: PUBLIC POLICY PERSPECTIVES

Currently, there is no general consensus regarding the need or desire for the implementation of school-based HIV prevention programs. Assuming that school-based HIV prevention programs should be implemented as the most feasible intervention strategy for controlling the dissemination of HIV infection among the adolescent population, public policymakers will need to satisfactorily confront and resolve two primary issues: will HIV prevention programs be mandated and will there be centrally developed curricula? Both issues will create a maelstrom of controversy, simply because they "go against the grain" of current educational policies in the United States. Presently, educational policy in the U.S. is established on a local level, with each individual school district and local school board responsible for defining breadth of study requirements and establishing guidelines and policy specifying subject matter acceptable for instruction. This is less true for senior high schools, although there is considerable regional variation in the control local school boards exhibit with respect to formulating educational curricula. In the U.S., therefore, local control of educational policy is an inveterate tradition. Surmounting this well-established tradition will not be a simple task, however.

Mandatory HIV Prevention Programs

Perhaps the most controversial policy decision confronting school officials, health educators, and local public-health officials is whether school-based HIV prevention programs should be mandated (DiClemente, 1988). Given the epidemiologic data on the prevalence of sexually transmitted diseases and unintended teen pregnancies among this population, any program in which adolescents have an opportunity to avoid HIV prevention education jeopardizes their health and the welfare of society in general. School systems, therefore, must not only provide HIV prevention programs, but must also make these programs compulsory. Without compulsory programs, we are creating a window of vulnerability through which many adolescents will leave school inappropriately informed about the risks of unsafe sex and drug practices. Any policy that permits adolescents to avoid exposure to HIV prevention programs is, in my estimation, irresponsible and is a disservice to those we profess to protect.

On the surface, such a policy seems Draconian in nature. On closer examination, however, there is ample precedent for implementing mandated HIV prevention programs. To draw a loose analogy, most states require adolescents wishing to drive motor vehicles to satisfactorily complete a competency examination, including a demonstration of both knowledge and manual skills. If, as a society, we mandate that adolescents not be permitted to drive without demonstrating a predetermined level of competency, plus additional follow-up assessments to assess stability of competency over time, then should any program that requires demonstrating a similar degree of "AIDS competency" be considered unusual or coercive in nature? There are, of course, mitigating instances when such programs may be considered offensive to some parents and adolescents as well as infringing upon parental control. The data, quite to the contrary, suggest that adolescents feel it is important to include HIV prevention programs as part of the formal school curriculum. Based on the study conducted in San Francisco (DiClemente, Zorn, & Temoshok, 1986) an overwhelming proportion of the adolescents surveyed (approximately 88%) consider prevention education to be an important informational component that should be included in the school curriculum. Parents also approve of school-based AIDS instruction. A national poll found that 91% of parents surveyed approve of the inclusion of AIDS prevention education in the classroom (Meade, 1987; National Broadcasting Company, 1987).

Obviously, guaranteeing that students can express a certain level of AIDS knowledge does not, ipso facto, guarantee that they will avoid high-risk behaviors associated with HIV acquisition. Knowledge alone has not been demonstrated to be a powerful mediator of behavior change, however, it is a prerequisite for change (Zimbardo & Ebbesen, 1970; Hecker & Ajzen, 1983). Knowledge, from this perspective, is necessary but not sufficient to promote behavior change among adolescents without incorporating other health education strategies. Ideally, a comprehensive AIDS education program will include peer-directed discussion and support groups to encourage and promote an atmosphere for initiation and maintenance of behavior change. Likewise, resistance training and role playing of potentially high-risk situations in the classroom can assist adolescents in developing a repertoire of responses for rejecting overtures to engage in risk-taking behaviors. Thus, increasing adolescents' knowledge about AIDS will serve as a cornerstone upon which other more creative and proactive prevention strategies can be overlaid enhancing decision-making skills directed towards facilitating health-promoting behavior changes.

With respect to the issue of infringement on parental control of the child's education, mandatory HIV prevention programs do not, necessarily, require instruction within the framework of the classroom. For instance, parents who object to their child receiving HIV education in the context of the classroom may withdraw the child from such a program; thus, effectively invoking parental control. Because the adolescent will be required to demonstrate competency on an examination, however, parents may have to assume more responsibility for providing the appropriate HIV instruction comparable to that which would be received through the school curriculum. Obviously, this is not an optimal solution for either the adolescent or the parents.

At the moment, there is much discussion and little consensus on the issue of providing school-based HIV education, irrespective of whether or not such education will be mandated. However, mandatory HIV prevention education is necessary, and the form these programs assume will be the focus of much heated debate. A key component within an HIV prevention program is curricula as they form the substance of what will be communicated to adolescents.

Mandated HIV Prevention Curricula

Separate, though related issue is the the argument for mandated HIV prevention curricula. This issue extends beyond whether or not local communities
will be mandated to provide school-based programs. The issue, most suc-
cinctly phrased, is whether school-based HIV prevention programs will primarily be developed within the local community by indigenous public-health
authorities, educators, civic leaders, clergy, etc., or whether a more uniform
program is perhaps more appropriate to guarantee equality of AIDS instruction across diverse geographic areas.

Acknowledging differences in the incidence rate, level of knowledge, and
fear of AIDS between geographic areas (DiClemente, Zorn, & Temoshok,
1987a), if we are to ensure uniformity of information across communities, this
suggests that centrally developed school-based HIV prevention curricula
would be most appropriate and advantageous. As noted in an earlier section,
whether adolescents reside in San Francisco or Toledo, they are at risk for HIV
infection by virtue of engaging in behaviors associated with disease transmission. Irrespective of their residence, adolescents in low-incidence areas should
be exposed to a standardized school-based HIV prevention program which
ensures that if they migrate to other areas of the U.S. they will be as well
informed as their peers in high-incidence areas.

Although the situation described above is the most patently obvious, there
are, of course, many instances in which adolescents residing within the same
community but attending different schools may receive totally different HIV
prevention programs. In fact, there are instances where one adolescent may
receive some form of HIV prevention instruction and another adolescent residing nearby, but attending a different school, may not receive any instruction
at all. Thus, differences in the type and depth of HIV prevention education
may exist within a community as well as across diverse communities. Development of a standardized school-based HIV prevention program does not
imply that community differences are unimportant and that such differences
do not warrant considerable attention. One tenet for effective program development is that school-based AIDS prevention programs design curricula that
are age appropriate, flexible to suit language abilities, and culturally sensitive
(DiClemente, Boyer, & Mills, 1987). To accommodate these recommendations, standardized school-based HIV prevention programs and core curricula
may be developed, and the curricula modified according to local input. This
point may require clarification. Clearly, it suggests that local input into curricula development may enhance the substance and effective communication
of HIV information for adolescents residing in a particular community. In this
manner, public-health interest is satisfactorily served, and individual communities can extend their curricula as they deem appropriate to their needs, while
maintaining a basic level of HIV instruction. Thus, every adolescent will be

guaranteed to receive fundamental information about AIDS, and those communities that prefer to augment the school-based HIV prevention program or core curricula are, of course, free to do so.

CONCLUSION

We can prevent the spread of HIV infection among the adolescent population. To do so, however, we must vigorously educate adolescents about high-risk sexual and IV drug practices and dispel misconceptions, such as the myth that AIDS can be spread by casual contact. Teachers play a vital role in this mission. Properly trained, they can become powerful change agents in influencing adolescents to avoid high-risk practices. Well-designed and executed evaluations will permit constant monitoring of program effectiveness, as well as identification of new gaps in knowledge. And, perhaps most important, public policy must mandate HIV prevention programs so they reach all adolescents, whether they reside in high-density AIDS epicenters like San Francisco and New York City or in communities which are, at present, considered low-risk areas.

If we are to successfully confront the challenge of AIDS, HIV risk-reduction programs targeted at adolescents will play a major role. Adolescents' health and the welfare of society in general depend on the prompt development and implementation of these programs. Only by mounting a systematic and concerted school-based HIV prevention education campaign will we be able to combat the growing threat of increased morbidity and mortality among the adolescent population.

REFERENCES

Alan Guttmacher Institute. (1981). *Teenage pregnancy: The problem that hasn't gone away*. New York: The Alan Guttmacher Institute.

Becker, M. H., & Joseph, J. G. (1988). AIDS and behavioral change to reduce risk: A review. *American Journal of Public Health, 78*, 394–410.

Bell, T., & Hein, K. (1984). The adolescent and sexually transmitted disease. In K. K. Holmes, P. Mardh, P. F. Sparling, & P. Wiesner (Eds.), *Sexually transmitted diseases*. New York: McGraw-Hill.

Bell, T. A., & Holmes K. K. (1984). Age-specific risks of syphilis, gonorrhea, and hospitalized pelvic inflammatory disease in sexually experienced U.S. women. *Sexually Transmitted Diseases, 11*, 291–295.

Brown, L. K., Fritz, G. K., & Barone, V. J. (in press). The impact of AIDS education on junior and senior high school students: A pilot study. *Journal of Adolescent Health Care*.

Bureau of the Census (1986). Projections of the population of the United States. *Current Population Reports. Series 25*, No. 952.

Carne, C. A., Johnson, A. M., Pearce, F., Smith, A., Tedder, R. S., Weller, I. V. D., Loveday, C., Hawkins, A., Williams, P., & Adler, M. W. (1987). Prevalence of antibodies to Human

Immunodeficiency Virus, gonorrhea rates, and changed sexual behavior in homosexual men in London. *Lancet*, 1, 656-658.

Cates, W., & Rauh, J. L. (1985). Adolescents and sexually transmitted disease: An expanding problem. *Journal of Adolescent Health Care*, 6, 257-261.

Centers for Disease Control. (1987). AIDS weekly surveillance report, September 20, 1987. Atlanta: Centers for Disease Control.

Conant, M., Hardy, D., Sernatinger, J., Spicer, D., & Levy, J.A. (1986). Condoms prevent transmission of AIDS-associated retrovirus. *Journal of the American Medical Association*, 255, 1706.

Connell, D. B., & Turner, R. R. (1985). The impact of instructional experience and the effects of cumulative instruction. *Journal of School Health*, 55, 324-331.

Connell, D. B., Turner, R. R., & Mason, E. F. (1985). Summary of the findings of the School Health Evaluation: Health promotion effectiveness, implementation, and costs. *Journal of School Health*, 55, 316-321.

Curran, J. W., Morgan, W. M., Hardy, A. M., Jaffe, H. W., Darrow, W. W., & Dowdle, W. R. (1985). The epidemiology of AIDS: Current status and future prospects. *Science*, 229, 1352-1357.

DiClemente, R. J. (1988). Policy perspectives on the implementation and development of school-based AIDS prevention education programs in the United States. *AIDS & Public Policy Journal*, 3, 14-16.

DiClemente, R. J., Boyer, C. B., & Mills, S. (1987). Prevention of AIDS among adolescents: Strategies for the development of comprehensive risk-reduction health education programs. *Health Education Research*, 2, 287-291.

DiClemente, R. J., Boyer, C. B., Mills, S., & Helquist, M. (1988). Prevention of Acquired Immune Deficiency Syndrome: International perspectives. *Health Education Research*, 3, 3-5.

DiClemente, R. J., Boyer C. B., & Morales, E. (1988). Minorities and AIDS: Knowledge, attitudes and misconceptions among Black and Latino adolescents. *American Journal of Public Health*, 1, 55-57.

DiClemente, R. J., Pies, C., Stoller, E., Straits, C., Haskin, J., Oliva, G., & Rutherford, G. (in press). Evaluation of school-based AIDS curricula in San Francisco. *Journal of Sex Research*.

DiClemente, R. J., Zorn, J., & Temoshok, L. (1986). Adolescents' and AIDS: A survey of knowledge, beliefs and attitudes about AIDS in San Francisco. *American Journal of Public Health*, 76, 1443-1445.

DiClemente, R. J., Zorn, J., & Temoshok, L. (1987a). Adolescents' knowledge of AIDS near an AIDS epicenter. *American Journal of Public Health*, 77, 876-877.

DiClemente, R. J., Zorn, J., & Temoshok, L. (1987b). The association of gender, ethnicity, and length of residence in the Bay Area to adolescents' knowledge and attitudes about the Acquired Immune Deficiency Syndrome. *Journal of Applied Social Psychology*, 17, 216-230.

Fichtner, R. R., Aral, S. O., Blount, J. H., Zaidi, A. A., Reynolds, G. H., & Darrow, W. W. (1983). Syphilis in the United States: 1967-1979. *Sexually Transmitted Diseases*, 10, 77-80.

Gottlieb, M. S., Schroff, R., Schanker, H. M., Weisman, J. D., Fan, P. T., Wolf, R. A., & Saxon, A. (1981). Pneumocytis carinii pneumonia and muscosal candidiasis in previously healthy homosexual men: Evidence of a new acquired cellular immunodeficiency. *New England Journal of Medicine*, 305, 1425-1431.

Hafner, D. W. (1988). AIDS and adolescents: School health education must begin now. *Journal of School Health*, 58, 154-155.

Harris, L. (1986). *American teens speak: Sex, myths, TV and birth control*. The Planned Parenthood Poll. New York, NY: Planned Parenthood Federation of America, Inc.

Hass, A. (1979). *Teenage sexuality: A survey of teenage sexual behavior*. New York: Macmillian.

Hecker, B. I., & Ajzen, I. (1983). Improving the prediction of health behavior: An approach based on the theory of reasoned action. *Academy of Psychology Bulletin*, 5, 11-19.

Hein, K. (1987). AIDS in adolescents: A rationale for concern. *New York State Journal of Medicine, 87,* 290–295.

Hofferth, S. L., Kahn, J. R., & Baldwin, W. (1987). Premarital sexual activity among U.S. teenage women over the past three decades. *Family Planning Perspectives, 19,* 46–49.

Kegeles, S. M., Adler, N. E., & Irwin, C. E. (1988). Sexually active adolescents and condoms: Changes over one year in knowledge, attitudes and use. *American Journal of Public Health, 78,* 460–461.

Kirby, D. (1980). The effects of school sex education: A review of the literature. *Journal of School Health, 50,* 559–563.

Kovar, M. (1979). Some indicators of health-related behavior among adolescents in the United States. *Public Health Reports, 94,* 109–118.

Kroger, F., & Wiesner, P. J. (1981). STD Education: Challenge for the 80's. *Journal of School Health, 51,* 242–246.

Martin, J. L. (1987). The impact of AIDS on gay male sexual behavior patterns in New York City. *American Journal of Public Health, 77,* 578–581.

Masur, H., Michelis, M. A., Greene, J. B., Onorato, I., Vande Stouwe, R. A., Holzman, R. S., Wormser, G., Brettman, L., Lange, M., Murray, H. W., & Cunningham-Rundles, S. (1981). An outbreak of community-acquired *Pneumocystis carinii* pneumonia: initial manifestation of cellular immune dysfunction. *New England Journal of Medicine, 305,* 1431–1438.

McCormick, K. (1987). AIDS instruction becomes a troubling test of courage for local school boards. *American School Board Journal, March,* 25–30.

McKusick, L., Wiley, J. A., Coates, T. J., Stall, R., Saika, G., Morin, S., Charles, K., Horstman, W., & Conant, M. A. (1985). Reported changes in the sexual behavior of men at risk for AIDS, San Francisco, 1982–84—the AIDS Behavioral Research Project. *Public Health Reports, 100,* 622–629.

Meade, J. (1987). What parents should know when AIDS comes to school. *Children, April,* 59–65.

Miller, L., & Downer, A. (1988). AIDS: What you and your friends need to know: A lesson plan for adolescents. *Journal of School Health, 58,* 137–141.

National Academy of Sciences. (1986). *Confronting AIDS.* Washington, DC: National Academy Press.

National Broadcasting Company. (1987, January 16). NBC news poll results. New York: Author.

National Institute of Allergies and Infectious Disease Study Group. (1980). Sexually transmitted diseases: Summary and recommendations. Washington, DC: U.S. Department HEW, National Institutes of Health.

O'Reilly K. R., & Aral S. O. (1985). Adolescence and sexual behavior: Trends and implications for STD. *Journal of Adolescent Health Care, 6,* 262–272.

Shafer, M., Beck, A., Blain, B., Dole, P., Irwin, C., Sweet, R., & Schacter, J. (1984). Chlamydia trachomatis: Important relationships to race, contraception, lower genital tract infection, and Papanicolaou smear. *Journal of Pediatrics, 104,* 141–146.

Siegal, F. P., Lopez, C., Hammer, G. S., Brown, A. E., Kornfeld, S. J., Gold, J., Hassett, J., Hirschman, S. Z., Cunningham-Rundles, C., Adelsberg, B. R., Parham, D. M., Siegal, M., Cunningham-Rundles, S., & Armstrong, D. (1981). Severe acquired immunodeficiency in male homosexuals, manifested by chronic perianal ulcerative herpes simplex lesions. *New England Journal of Medicine, 305,* 1439–1444.

Stone, K. M., Grimes, D. A., & Magder, L. S. (1986). Primary prevention of sexually transmitted diseases. *Journal of the American Medical Association, 255,* 1763–1766.

Strunin, L., & Hingson, R. (1987). Acquired immunodeficiency syndrome and adolescents: Knowledge, beliefs, attitudes and behaviors. *Pediatrics, 79,* 825–828.

Thomas, L. L., Long, S. E., Whitten, K., Hamilton, B., Fraser, J., & Askin, R. V. (1985). High school students' longterm retention of sex education information. *Journal of School Health, 53,* 274–278.

United States Department of Health and Human Services. (1986). *Surgeon General's Report on AIDS*. Washington, DC: Author.

Van de Perre, P., Jacobs, D., & Sprecher-Goldberger, S. (1987). The latex condom, an efficient barrier against sexual transmission of AIDS-related viruses. *AIDS, 1*, 49-52.

Winkelstein, W., Samuel, M., Padian, N. S., & Wiley, J. A. (1987). Selected sexual practices of San Francisco heterosexual men and risk of infection by the human immunodeficiency virus. *Journal of the American Medical Association, 257*, 1470-1471.

Winkelstein, W., Samuel, M., Padian, N. S., Wiley, J. A., Lang, W., Anderson, R. E., & Levy, J. A. (1987). The San Francisco Men's Health Study: III. Reduction in human immunodeficiency virus transmission among homosexual/bisexual men, 1982-1986. *American Journal of Public Health, 76*, 685-689.

Yarchoan, R., & Broder, S. (1987). Development of antiretroviral therapy for the acquired immunodeficiency syndrome and related disorders. *New England Journal of Medicine, 316*, 557-564.

Zelnik, M., & Kanter, J. F. (1977). Sexual and contraceptive experience of young unmarried women in the United States, 1976 and 1971. *Family Planning Perspectives, 9*, 55-62.

Zelnik, M., & Kanter, J. F. (1980). Sexual activity, contraceptive use and pregnancy among metropolitan-area teenagers. *Family Planning Perspectives, 12*, 230-231.

Zelnik, M., & Kim, Y. J. (1982). Sex education and its association with teenage sexual activity, pregnancy and contraceptive use. *Family Planning Perspectives, 14*, 112-120.

Zimbardo, P., & Ebbesen, E. B. (1970). *Influencing attitudes and changing behavior*. Reading, MA: Addison-Wesley.

Assessing the Costs and Benefits of an Increased Sense of Vulnerability to AIDS in a Cohort of Gay Men

5

Jill G. Joseph
Department of Epidemiology
University of Michigan

Susanne B. Montgomery
Department of Health Behavior and Health Education
University of Michigan

David G. Ostrow
Department of Psychiatry & Institute for Social Research
University of Michigan

John P. Kirscht
Department of Health Behavior and Health Education
University of Michigan

Ronald C. Kessler
Institute for Social Research & Department of Sociology
University of Michigan

John Phair
Northwestern Medical School

Joan Chmiel
Northwestern Medical School

The first cases of acquired immunodeficiency syndrome (AIDS) were reported in 1981 (Centers for Disease Control, 1981), and by early 1984 several research groups had reported isolation of the putative agent, now known as human immunodeficiency virus (HIV; Barre-Sinoussi et al., 1983; Levy, Hoffman, Kramer, Landis, Shimabukaro, & Oshiro, 1984; Popovic, Sardgadharan, Read, & Gallo, 1984). The licensure of tests to detect antibodies to HIV was announced on March 1, 1985, and these procedures are now uniformly used for the screening of donated blood in the United States (Centers for Disease Control, 1985). HIV antibody testing is also being applied in clinical and at-risk populations. For a variety of reasons, it has been suggested, and even urged, that at-risk individuals learn their HIV antibody status (Centers for Disease Control, 1987; Goedert, 1987). While some proponents of such policies have an explicitly political agenda, most hope to motivate and facilitate behavioral changes in vulnerable populations. It is generally argued that those who obtain their HIV antibody results will have a better understanding of their potentially increased risk for AIDS and, therefore, will be more likely to undertake behavioral risk reduction. Nonetheless, concerns continue to be expressed about several issues related to testing. These include the accuracy and/or predictive value of HIV antibody testing, the duration of the latency between infection and seroconversion, and the potentially adverse psychological consequences of positive test results. More fundamentally, little published information is available which directly assesses, specifically, the effects of HIV antibody testing or, more generally, the effects of an increased sense of vulnerability to AIDS.

There is available, however, an extensive literature on threatening health communications and on the role of risk perception in relation to behavior. While this research may be applicable to the area of HIV testing, it has, in most instances, dealt with much less distressing situations. Threatening messages have been studied in relation to cigarette smoking, screening for heart disease, TB tests, driving, compliance with medication regimens, dieting to reduce obesity, etc. (Sutton, 1982). Typically more threatening messages, linked with higher levels of fear, have been associated with greater likelihood of following recommendations. However, a number of investigators believe that if the level of threat is too great, especially coupled with a lack of efficacious action, the reaction may well be to ignore, distort, or avoid the threat (Rogers & Mewborn, 1976). After a thorough review of the work on fear-arousing communications, Beck & Frankel (1981) concluded that beliefs concerning the controllability of a threat, both in terms of the availability of an effective response and the personal ability to take this action, are the key consideration. Thus, the relationship of threat to subsequent behavior must take account of several other factors.

It is reasonably well established that perceptions of risk of disease or trauma vary considerably among people and that they may show little correspondence to epidemiological findings (Harris & Guten, 1979; Kirscht, Haefner, Kegeles, & Rosenstock, 1966); for example, many smokers accept the association between use of cigarettes and disease, but do not believe themselves to be personally vulnerable (Pechacek & Danaher, 1979). Weinstein (1984) has documented an "optimistic bias" in people's judgments concerning their own susceptibility to health threats. It must be remembered that beliefs concerning

risk reflect subjective interpretations, arrived at through information processing that is limited and potentially biasing (Kahneman, Slovic, & Tversky,
1982); these beliefs are linked to the psychological processes through which
the individual seeks to control both emotions and dangers (Leventhal, Meyer,
& Nerenz, 1980). Thus, beliefs about risks may show little correspondence to
"objective" information, and acting to change risk is a complex process that is
affected by a number of other factors. Furthermore, an increased sense of
health risk has been demonstrated in other situations to be associated with
potentially negative consequences, including a decreased sense of personal
control (Taylor, 1983) and apparently adverse behavioral or psychological
changes (MacDonald, Sackett, Haynes, & Taylor, 1984).

As suggested earlier, much less is specifically known concerning the effects
of a sense of risk for AIDS and/or positive HIV serologic tests. Previous work
by our group demonstrated that risk perceptions in a cohort of homosexual men
are biased "optimistically" and are unrelated to behavioral risk reduction after
multivariate adjustment for sociodemographic variables and components of a
health belief model (Joseph et al., 1987). In spite of the lack of any relationship
to behavioral changes, an increased perception of personal risk of AIDS was
nonetheless associated with subsequent psychological distress. These results
were observed during the six-month interval between the first and second
biannual assessments (1984–1985). Somewhat contradictory findings are
reported from a similar cohort in San Francisco; those men with a visual image
of AIDS deterioration were more likely to have reduced numbers of sexual
partners in both cross-sectional and longitudinal analyses (it is assumed here
that such an image increases one's sense of personal risk; McKusick, Horstman,
& Coates, 1985a; McKusick et al., 1985b). Similarly, belief in vulnerability and
perception of oneself as a member of a high-risk group were associated with
risk reduction in multivariate analyses of cross-sectional data from a sample of
64 gay male physicians living in Southern California (Klein, Sullivan, Wolcott,
Landsverk, Namir, & Fawsy, 1987). On the other hand, the same factors were
not associated with changes in sexual behavior among a sample of gay male
college students studied in a similar fashion. Valdeserri and others reported
results from a group intervention for homosexual men seeking HIV antibody
testing results which indicated that 67% of the participants perceived themselves to be vulnerable to AIDS prior to the intervention, and 72% following the
intervention (Valdeserri et al., 1987). They report concomitant increases in
positive attitudes regarding specific safer-sex recommendations, although no
causal link between the increased sense of vulnerability and these changes can
be established. The few reports assessing the effects of HIV antibody testing
and notification are equally disparate in both methodology and conclusions
(Farthing et al., 1987; Fox et al., 1988; Coates et al., 1988).

In this chapter, we assess the relationship of perceived risk to both behavioral risk reduction (potential benefits) and psychological distress (potential

costs). In order to more comprehensively address this question, the results of two complementary investigations undertaken in the same cohort of gay men will be presented. In the first, an index describing perceived risk of AIDS is analyzed for its relationship to behavior and distress. These analyses were conducted in the 524 men seen at all four semiannual assessments during a two-year period. In the second, the behavioral and psychological effects of learning HIV serologic status will be described. These analyses were conducted among approximately 560 men in the cohort who completed the third and fifth assessments. The specific methods for the two investigations and the results of this work will be described separately.

GENERAL METHODS

Participants

Participants in this study were recruited from a group of approximately 1,000 homosexual men enrolled in the Multicenter AIDS Cohort Study (MACS). This longitudinal epidemiologic study has been designed to investigate the natural history of HIV infection and AIDS in several cohorts of homosexual men (Chmiel et al., 1987; Kaslow & Ostrow, 1985). Biannual study visits are used to obtain a medical history, provide a physical examination focused on symptoms of infection, and collect specimens for laboratory and serologic examinations. Participants in the Chicago MACS were invited to enroll in the psychosocial investigations (termed the Coping and Change Study or CCS) between June 1984 and August 1985. Approximately 95% of MACS participants agreed to take part in the supplemental psychosocial study, with 90% returning the initial questionnaire. Results reported here are confined to those men not diagnosed with AIDS. As described elsewhere (Emmons, Joseph, Kessler, Wortman, Montgomery, & Ostrow, 1986), this cohort is largely white (92%), in their mid-30s, well-educated (average educational attainment = 16.3 years), and with a mean income of approximately $24,500 in 1984–1985. At the time of the initial survey, 51.9% of the men reported that they were involved in a "primary relationship" with another man, and over 95% reported that they were primarily or exclusively homosexual. Although it cannot be assumed that participants in this study are representative of all homosexual males living in Chicago, participants do resemble members of their risk group who have been diagnosed with AIDS and cohorts being studied at other sites (Martin, 1987; McKusick et al., 1985b). As discussed in greater detail below, participants were not aware of their HIV antibody status until the second year of the study.

Research Procedures

As described in our earlier work, a psychosocial questionnaire was developed for use in this population (Joseph et al., 1984). This self-administered questionnaire provides a range of behavioral and psychosocial data, as well as routine sociodemographic information. Participants were given this question-naire when they visited the study center for each semiannual MACS visit, but took it home for completion approximately two weeks later. This delay was incorporated into the study design in order to avoid overestimating the impact of AIDS and the extent of the stress in the cohort. Pretesting suggested that such overestimation might occur because MACS examinations were asso-ciated with increased attention to the issue of AIDS and consequent increases in psychological distress. Participants were also asked to complete the ques-tionnaire in private at home, a setting more typical of their daily functioning. As implied above, both biomedical and psychosocial data were obtained every six months. These sequential assessments will be referred to as Survey 1 (S1), Survey 2 (S2), etc.

Behavioral Assessment

Participants in the CCS are asked to report the frequency and types of recep-tive homosexual activity as practiced with a variety of male partners, ranging from one's primary sexual partner to anonymous sexual partners. This struc-tured, self-administered questionnaire inquires about behavior during the preceding month, a period of time which pretesting suggested is sufficiently short to permit accurate recall, but long enough to reduce the intraindividual variability in sexual behavior. In order to meaningfully include the variety of sexual behaviors which could lead to HIV exposure, a summary Behavioral Risk Index (BRI) was constructed, as shown in Table 5.1. Four categories of sexual behavior were described, ranging from celibacy to the practice of recep-tive anal intercourse unprotected by condom usage with multiple sexual partners. If there were ambiguities in a participant's questionnaire responses

TABLE 5.1
Behavioral Risk Index

No Risk:	Celibate
Low Risk:	If monogamous, no receptive anal intercourse or receptive anal intercourse with condom use
	OR
	If non-monogamous, no receptive anal intercourse
Modified High Risk:	If monogamous, receptive anal intercourse without condom use
	OR
	If non-monogamous, receptive anal intercourse with condom use
High Risk:	Non-monogamous receptive anal intercourse without condom use

(for example, if participants declined to provide information regarding condom usage during receptive anal activities), it was always assumed that they fell into the highest risk category applicable. It was necessary to make such assumptions in less than 3% of the cases.

Incident seroconversion data between S_1 and S_4 were compared to this risk index and shown to range from 0 per 100 person-years in the celibate group to 14 per 100 person-years in the highest risk group, with intermediate rates for the low-risk (1.75 per 100 person-years) and modified high-risk (10.9 per 100 person-years) groups. This suggests that the self-reported behavioral data provide a valid summary measure of receptive sexual practices which are more or less safe.

Assessment of Psychological Distress

The psychosocial questionnaire also assessed social and emotional functioning in a variety of ways. Items from a frequently used and well-validated inventory, the Hopkins Symptom Check List (HSCL), were included to generate screening scores for somatization, obsessive-compulsive behavior, interpersonal sensitivity, depression, and anxiety (Derogatis, Lipman, Rickels, Uhlenhuth, & Covi, 1974). Separate scores for each of these subscales were analyzed, as well as a total HSCL score which described global distress. Reliability coefficients for these indices at S_1 ranged from 0.75 to 0.90.

Statistical Methods

Standard univariate and multivariate statistical techniques were used to estimate the relationship between perceived risk or HIV antibody testing and each of the outcome measures. Analyses not reported here examined the impact of including health status as a predictor variable and of removing outliers from the behavioral analyses. Neither the structure nor the magnitude of the association between independent and dependent measures was influenced by these alterations in the analyses. They are, therefore, not reported.

PERCEIVED AIDS RISK
IN RELATION TO BEHAVIOR AND DISTRESS

Psychosocial Assessment

The psychosocial questionnaire obtained data in two different ways regarding perceived risk of AIDS. The first question ("Considering all the different factors that may contribute to AIDS, including your own past and present behavior, what would you say are your chances of getting AIDS?") asked the respondent to report his absolute risk of AIDS; the second ("When you compare yourself to the average gay man, what would you say are your chances of getting AIDS?") focused on comparative risk assessment. A combined-risk index summed the scores for each participant on the absolute and comparative risk measures and ranged from one (minimum) to nine (maximum). Indices were also developed describing core components of a model predicting health behavior. Alpha-reliability coefficients were calculated for these indices and, as reported elsewhere, were satisfactory (Emmons et al., 1986). A detailed description of coding procedures is available to interested readers upon request. In addition, age, income, education, race, and participation in a primary relationship were used to assess sociodemographic status.

Results

The two questions which constitute the perceived-risk measure are shown in Table 5.2 with response frequencies noted. In evaluating these results, it is important to consider that slightly over 40% of the cohort were HIV seropositive at entry into the study, reflecting recruitment procedures designed to provide sufficient cases of AIDS during the study period. Indeed, this cohort has contributed approximately 10% of all AIDS cases in Chicago, providing further evidence of sexual histories which placed them at considerable risk for HIV infection. Nonetheless, the cohort appeared to optimistically underestimate their risk of AIDS with less than 15% ever believing that they had at least a "large chance" of being diagnosed with the syndrome. This effect is particularly apparent in response to the comparative risk question. Over 50% of the cohort responded at each semiannual survey that their chances of getting AIDS were lower than that of other gay men. Furthermore, despite the evolution of the AIDS epidemic during the two years described here, there was remarkably little change in risk appraisals during this period of time.

A summary measure of perceived risk was constructed by adding together each participant's response to the questions described in Table 5.2. This yielded

TABLE 5.2
Prevalence of Perceived Risk: Absolute and Comparative Measures S1–S4 ($N = 524$)

What are your chances of getting AIDS?	S1	S2	S3	S4
Almost certain will not get AIDS or small chance	43.4%	41.0%	31.8%	32.4%
Some chance	49.2%	47.5%	54.9%	55.6%
Almost certain will get AIDS or large chance	7.4%	11.5%	13.3%	12.0%

Compared to other gay men, what are your chances of getting AIDS?	S1	S2	S3	S4
Much lower or a little lower	54.8%	57.1%	51.8%	55.3%
About the same	33.6%	31.2%	35.9%	33.3%
Much higher or a little higher	11.6%	11.7%	12.3%	11.4%

TABLE 5.3
Prevalence of Perceived Risk: Summary Score
S1–S4 (N = 524)

	S1	S2	S3	S4
x̄	4.78	4.68	4.70	4.66
S.D.	0.87	0.82	0.74	0.76
Range	1–8	2–7	3–7	3–7

scores with a theoretical range from one to nine although, as shown in Table 5.3, the observed ranges were considerably more constrained. Thus, in addition to a probable optimistic bias, there appears to be a tendency to moderate risk perception away from either extreme appraisal. It is also apparent that when considered in this fashion, the mean level of perceived risk is quite stable across the two-year observational period. Additional analyses examined the relationship of age (<35/>35), race (white/non-white), and education (no college/some college) to perceived risk at S1 through S4. There were no significant differences between any of these groups at any of the assessments.

The relationship between perceived risk and the more objective behavioral risk index was then examined, as shown in Table 5.4. Analysis of variance techniques were used to perform all possible pairwise comparisons of mean values at each survey; significant differences are noted. While those at high risk consistently have the highest scores, the mean scores are remarkably similar, given the dramatic differences in behavior across the four groups.

TABLE 5.4
Mean Level of Perceived Risk (± S.D.) in Each Group Defined by the
Behavioral Risk Index: S1–S4

Behavior Risk Index Group	S1	S2	S3	S4
Celibate	4.5 ± 1.1	4.6 ± 0.9	4.6 ± 0.7	4.5 ± 0.7
(N)	(28)	(46)	(60)	(65)
Low Risk	4.7 ± 0.8	4.7 ± 0.8	4.7 ± 0.8	4.7 ± 0.8
(N)	(198)	(216)	(265)	(259)
Modified High Risk	4.7 ± 0.8	4.5 ± 0.7	4.6 ± 0.7	4.7 ± 0.7
(N)	(68)	(88)	(94)	(120)
High Risk	4.9 ± 0.8	4.8 ± 0.8	4.8 ± 0.8	4.8 ± 0.8
(N)	(190)	(142)	(74)	(44)

Notes: Significant Difference in Perceived Risk Scores.

High >	High >	High >
Celibate (p = .01)	Mod. High (p < .01)	Celibate (p = .04)
Low Risk (p < .01)		
Mod. High (p = .01)		

These serial cross-sectional data cannot, of course, distinguish between components of perceived risk which arise from more remote events or behaviors. If those in the lowest-risk categories had sexual histories which included high-risk behaviors, this might explain the similarity of the four groups (although it would leave unexplained the general tendency to underestimate risk). Nor can these data distinguish the potentially mutual effects of behavior and perceptions on each other. For example, it is unclear whether those at lower risk might have been motivated by their risk perceptions to practice safer sexual activities.

In order to examine this question, a regression model was constructed which compared: (1) those consistently celibate or at low behavioral risk as assessed on the BRI for each of the four surveys (29.9% of the cohort); and (2) all others in the cohort. This group of "all others" was heterogeneous, but each individual reported modified high- or high-risk behavior at one or more surveys. Predictor variables were perceived risk, other components of a health belief model, sociodemographic characteristics, and appropriate dummy variables to describe behavior at S1. The inclusion of such dummy variables is necessary as behavior at S1 is associated both with concurrent perceptions or attitudes (predictor variables) and with future behavior (outcome variable). These associations would lead to confounding and overestimation of the relationship between predictor and outcome variables. In order to control for this potential effect, the dummy variables describing behavior at S1 were included in the regression model. Earlier reports describe the rationale for construction of health belief variables and their coding (Emmons et al., 1986; Joseph et al., 1986). The examined regression model, therefore, estimates the relationship between perceived risk and long-term behavior after taking account of other potentially relevant psychosocial variables, sociodemographic status, and initial behavior. The outcome variable was coded so that "0" represented the adverse outcome (higher-risk sexual behavior) and "1" the desirable outcome (long-term, lower-risk behavior). Thus, the interpretation of the regression coefficients is straightforward: positive coefficients indicate that the predictor variable is associated with desirable behavioral risk reduction, and negative coefficients indicate the opposite.

Table 5.5 displays the results of the multivariate regression with the entire model after excluding all variables which did not satisfy an arbitrary criterion value of $p < .10$ for inclusion. In both cases, the relationship between perceived risk and behavioral risk reduction is a *negative* one. That is, those who perceive themselves to be at higher risk for AIDS are *less* likely to have long-term, lower-risk behavior. Only in the limited model, however, does this relationship achieve statistical significance. There is, then, no evidence in this cohort that an increased sense of risk is advantageous. It is, on the other hand, the availability of social norms supportive of behavioral change and two measures of perceived stress which predict continuously lower-risk behavior.

TABLE 5.5
Relationship of Perceived Risk and Other Components of a
Health Belief Model to Long-term Receptive Sexual Behaviors
(Consistently Lower Risk versus All Others)

	Full Model		Reduced Model	
	B		B	
Perceived risk	-.027	$(p < .1)$	-.030	$(p < .05)$
AIDS knowledge	.009		—	
Perceived virulence	$-.184 \times 10^{-3}$		—	
Perceived behavioral efficacy	-.009		—	
Belief in alternative health practice	.056		—	
Difficulties with sexual impulse control	-.015		—	
Reliance on biomedical technology	-.043		—	
Supportive social norms	.069	$(p < .01)$	.078	$(p < .001)$
Stress of AIDS	.002	$(p < .001)$	.001	$(p < .05)$
Stress of behavioral change	.030	$(p < .1)$	.033	$(p < .05)$
Age	.007	$(p < .01)$	.007	$(p < .01)$
Income	$.159 \times 10^{-6}$		—	
Education	.028	$(p < .01)$	.034	$(p < .001)$
Race	.267	$(p < .05)$	.262	$(p < .01)$
Primary relationship	.035		—	

In addition, those who are older, who have more education, or who are white
were also more likely to be in the lower-risk group during the two years of
observation.

Earlier work by our group had demonstrated that increased perceptions of
risk may be associated with adverse psychological effects (Joseph et al., 1987).
This possibility was examined in cross-sectional and longitudinal analyses
which used five HSCL subscales as measures of distress. Both analysis of
variance and multiple regression techniques were employed, the latter including baseline assessment of the subscale as a covariate. Not reported further,
these results revealed no relationship between received risk and distress.

EFFECTS OF LEARNING SEROLOGIC TEST RESULTS

Failure to adequately assess perceived risk of AIDS might explain the failure
to detect a positive association with behavioral risk reduction. Perhaps the
index described above imperfectly represents men's appraisal of risk, in which
case a more direct assessment would provide increased validity and, therefore,
improve analytic sensitivity. In the investigation which follows, actual HIV
antibody test results are used to assess, in another fashion, the benefits and
costs of a heightened perception of personal risk for AIDS.

HIV antibody testing using both standard ELISA and Western Blot methods was conducted in the cohort using blood samples collected at the semiannual MACS medical examinations. However, participants in the MACS were recruited prior to federal policies mandating notification regarding HIV serologic test results. Participants could, therefore, choose whether or not they wished to learn their test results. All participants were initially offered the opportunity to do so in late 1985, following S3. A careful protocol was followed which included pre- and post-counseling, necessary referral, and use of a sealed envelope to "blind" the research physician assisting in notification of the test results unless informed by the participant himself. By June 1987, approximately 150 men of the 474 who were seen at each of the first five surveys had elected to receive their test results. Thus, those who did not receive test results can be compared among both the seropositive and seronegative participants.

Results

Analyses not reported here examined differences between those who chose to receive their test results and those who did not. There were no significant sociodemographic or behavioral differences between the two groups at baseline, although a higher percentage of those obtaining results was seropositive (34% versus 29%).

As shown in Table 5.6, behavior at S3 was compared with behavior at S5 in order to describe change during the intervening year in four groups: antibody-positive men who *did* versus antibody-positive men who *did not* receive their test results; antibody-negative men who *did* versus antibody-negative men who *did not* receive their test results. Overall, positive change is virtually uniform; however, receiving test results did not significantly influence any measure of behavioral risk reduction. This is true for both the specific comparisons shown in Table 5.6 and in multivariate regressions which included

TABLE 5.6
Results of Receiving HIV Antibody Results:
Change in Behavior Between S3 and S5

	Antibody Positive		Antibody Negative	
	Results Received	Results Not Received	Results Received	Results Not Received
Behavior	67	156	88	242
Celibacy	+3%	+1%	+1%	+3%
Anonymous partners	-6%	-2.5%	-5%	-5%
Any receptive anal intercourse	-1%	0	-4%	-5%
Condom use during receptive anal intercourse	+41%	+25%	+25%	+7%

the baseline level of behavior as a covariate. However, at least for condom usage, notification appears to have had an appreciable impact and statistical power may be insufficient to detect this effect.

The potential "costs" of receiving test results were assessed by constructing the same comparisons, using the five HSCL subscales as measures of outcome (somatization, obsessive-compulsive, interpersonal sensitivity, depression, and anxiety). There were increases in all of these measures of distress among those receiving positive test results when compared to seropositive men not receiving results; the increase in depression achieved statistical significance. On the other hand, those who found out that they were seronegative generally demonstrated improvements in levels of distress, and this effect was significant for somatization. These univariate findings were confirmed by the use of multivariate regression which took account of baseline mental health, effectively removing the potential confounding discussed earlier. It is especially compelling that mean interval from notification to S5 was six months, so that these are longer-term, rather than immediate, effects.

DISCUSSION

Results reported here have explored the potential benefits and costs of a sense of being at risk for AIDS. In this cohort of gay men, personal risk appraisal appears to be optimistic and largely unrelated to concurrent self-reports of sexual behavior. Whether a global risk index or specific notification regarding HIV antibody status is examined, there is no evidence of a beneficial effect on behavioral risk reduction. On the contrary, those who feel themselves to be at increased risk are less likely to consistently engage in lower-risk behavior across a two-year observational period. There is no evidence that this generalized perception of risk is associated with increased psychological distress. Receiving HIV positive serologic test results does, however, lead to subsequent increases in depression not observed in seropositive men who remain unaware of their status.

These results need to be tempered by an appreciation of the unique characteristics of the cohort. It is advantaged, both with respect to socioeconomic status and exposure to AIDS risk-reduction materials. Cohort members are certainly likely to be highly motivated and concerned with the AIDS crisis in order to participate so consistently in the long-term biomedical and psychosocial studies. For those less aware of their potentially increased AIDS risk or less familiar with risk-reduction guidelines, a heightened sense of personal risk (with or without HIV antibody testing) may be useful. This issue requires further careful evaluation.

We also recognize that this is an observational study, rather than an experimentally manipulated intervention trial. In the latter setting, it would be possible to more fully evaluate the mechanisms which might link alteration in risk perceptions to subsequent behavioral or psychological effects. Certainly there is an urgent need for both observational and intervention studies in other populations. Special emphasis should be given to research with younger, minority, and less-educated participants which these findings identify as less likely to establish and maintain long-term, low-risk behaviors.

In spite of such cautions, these results suggest that an uncritical enthusiasm for testing or other techniques designed to create a sense of vulnerability to AIDS might be inappropriate. Those formulating policy to routinize or mandate testing need to consider carefully the full array of available information. There is no evidence in this cohort of beneficial effects from a sense of risk, while some deleterious effects on both mental health and behavior were observed. We suggest that global perceptions of increased risk might easily be transformed into a sense of hopelessness and helplessness in dealing with the AIDS epidemic or personal behavior. At a minimum, it seems evident that behavioral risk reduction is complex, related to multiple social and psychological phenomena, and unlikely to be the straightforward result of a single event or attitude.

ACKNOWLEDGMENTS

This work was supported by funding from the National Institute of Mental Health (2 RO1 MH39346-02A1) and the University of Michigan for the Coping and Change Study, and by the National Institute of Allergy and Infectious Diseases for the Chicago Multicenter AIDS Cohort Study N01-AI-32535, with partial funding by the National Cancer Institute.

Special appreciation is expressed to participants in these concurrent studies whose continuing assistance makes this research possible. Please refer questions and comments to Jill G. Joseph, Ph.D., Department of Epidemiology, School of Public Health, University of Michigan, 109 Observatory Street, Ann Arbor, MI 48109.

REFERENCES

Barre-Sinoussi, F., Chermann, J., Rey, F., Nugeyre, M., Chameret, S., Gruest, J., Dauguet, C., Axler-Blin, C., Vezinet-Brun, F., Rouzioux, C., Rosenbaum, W., & Montagnier, R. (1983). Isolation of a T-lymphotropic retrovirus from a patient at risk of acquired immunodeficiency syndrome (AIDS). *Science, 220,* 861-871.

Beck, K., & Frankel, A. (1981). A conceptualization of threat communication and protective health behavior. *Social Psychology Quarterly, 44,* 204-217.

Centers for Disease Control. (1981). Kaposi's sarcoma and *Pneumocystis* pneumonia among homosexual men—New York City and California. *Morbidity and Mortality Weekly Reports,* 30(250), 305.

Centers for Disease Control. (1985). Screening donated blood and plasma for antibody to the virus causing acquired immunodeficiency syndrome. *Morbidity and Mortality Weekly Reports, 34*, 1-4.

Centers for Disease Control. (1987). Recommendations for prevention of the transmission of HIV. *Morbidity and Mortality Weekly Reports*, Supplement.

Chmiel, J., Detels, R., Kaslow, R., Van Raden, M., Kingsley, L. A., & the MACS Group (1987). Factors associated with prevalent human immunodeficiency virus (HIV) infection in the Multicenter AIDS Cohort Study. *American Journal of Epidemiology, 126*, 568-577.

Coates, T. J., Morin, S., & McKusick, L. (1988). Consequences of AIDS antibody testing. *CME Syllabus and Proceedings, American Psychiatric Association Annual Meeting, 141* (Abstract, p. 240).

Derogatis, L., Lipman, R., Rickels, K., Uhlenhuth, E., & Covi, L. (1974). The Hopkins Symptom Checklist (HSCL): A self report symptom inventory. *Behavioral Science, 19*, 1-15.

Emmons, C., Joseph, J., Kessler, R., Wortman, C., Montgomery, S., & Ostrow, D. (1986). Psychological predictors of reported behavior change in homosexual men at risk for AIDS. *Health Education Quarterly, 13*, 331-345.

Farthing, C. F., Jesson, W., Taylor, H. L., Lawrence, A. G., & Gazzard, B. G. (1987). The HIV antibody test: Influence on sexual behavior of homosexual men. *Proceedings III International Conference on AIDS*, (Abstract, p. 2).

Fox, R., Odaka, N. J., Brookmeyer, R., & Polk, B. F. (1987). Effect of HIV antibody disclosure on subsequent sexual activity in homosexual men. *AIDS, 1*, 241-246.

Harris, D., & Guten, S. (1979). Health protective behavior: An exploratory study. *Journal of Health and Social Behavior, 20*, 17-29.

Joseph, J., Emmons, C., Kessler, R., Wortman, C., O'Brien, K., Hocker, W., & Schaefer, C. (1984). Coping with the threat of AIDS: An approach to psychosocial assessment. *American Psychologist, 39*(1), 1297-1302.

Joseph, J., Montgomery, S., Emmons, C., Kessler, R., Ostrow, D., Wortman, C., O'Brien, K., Eller, M., & Eshleman, S. (1986). Magnitude and determinants of behavioral risk reduction: Longitudinal analysis of a cohort at risk for AIDS. *Psychology and Health, 1*, 73-96.

Joseph, J., Montgomery, S., Emmons, C. A., Kirscht, J., Kessler, R., Ostrow, D., Wortman, C., O'Brien, K., Eller, M., & Eshlemen, S. (1987). Perceived risk of AIDS: Assessing the behavioral and psychosocial consequences in a cohort of gay men. *Journal of Applied Social Psychology, 17*, 216-230.

Kahneman, D., Slovic, P., & Tversky, A. (1982). *Judgment under uncertainty: Heuristics and biases*. Cambridge: Cambridge University Press.

Kaslow, D., Ostrow, D., and the Multicenter AIDS Cohort Study. (1987). The Multicenter AIDS Cohort Study (MACS): Rationale, organization, and selected characteristics of the participants. *American Journal of Epidemiology, 126*, 310-318.

Kessler, R., & Greenberg, D. (1981). *Linear panel analysis: Quantitative models of change*. New York: Academic Press.

Kirscht, J., Haefner, D., Kegeles, S., & Rosenstock, I. (1966). A national study of health beliefs. *Journal of Health and Human Behavior, 7*, 248-254.

Klein, D., Sullivan, G., Wolcott, D., Landsverk, J., Namir, S., & Fawsy, F. (1987). Changes in AIDS risk behaviors among homosexual male physicians and university students. *American Journal of Psychiatry, 144*, 742-747.

Leventhal, H., Meyer, D., & Nerenz, D. (1980). The common-sense representation of illness danger. In S. Rachman (Ed.), *Medical psychology* (Vol. 2, pp. 218-253). New York: Pergamon Press.

Levy, J., Hoffman, A., Kramer, S., Landis, J., Shimabukaro, J., & Oshiro, L. (1984). Isolation of lymphocytopathic retroviruses from San Francisco patients with AIDS. *Science, 225*, 840-842.

MacDonald, L., Sackett, D., Haynes, R., & Taylor, D. (1984). Labelling in hypertension: A review of the behavioral and psychological consequences. *Journal of Chronic Diseases, 37*(12), 933-942.

Martin, M. (1987). The impact of AIDS on gay male sexual behavior patterns in New York City. *American Journal of Public Health, 77,* 578-581.

McKusick, L., Wiley, J., Coates, T., Stall, R., Saika, G., Morin, S., Charles, K., Horstman, W., & Conant, M. (1985). Reported changes in the sexual behavior of men at risk for AIDS. San Francisco, 1982-1984—the AIDS Behavioral Research Project. *Public Health Reports, 100,* 622-629.

McKusick, L., Horstman, W., & Coates, T. J. (1985). AIDS and sexual behavior reported by gay men in San Francisco. *American Journal of Public Health, 7,* 493-496.

Pechacek, T., & Danaher, B. (1979). How and why people quit smoking: A cognitive-behavioral analysis. In P. Kendall & S. Hollon (Eds.), *Cognitive behavioral intervention: Theory, research, and procedures* (pp. 389-423). New York: Academic Press.

Popovic, M., Sardgadharan, M., Read, E., & Gallo, R. (1984). Detection, isolation and continuous production of cytopathic retroviruses (HTLV-III) from patients with AIDS and pre-AIDS. *Science, 224,* 497-500.

Rogers, R., & Mewborn, C. (1976). Fear appeals and attitude change: Effects of a threat's noxiousness/probability of occurrence and the efficacy of coping responses. *Journal of Personality and Social Psychology, 34,* 54-61.

Sutton, S. (1982). Fear-arousing communications: A critical examination of theory and research. In J. Eiser (Ed.), *Social psychology and behavioral medicine* (pp. 303-338). New York: John Wiley and Sons.

Taylor, S. (1983). Adjustment to threatening events: A theory of cognitive adoption. *American Psychologist, 38*(11), 1161-1173.

Valdesseri, R. O., Lyter, D. W., Kingsley, L. A., Leviton, L. C., Schofield, J. W., Huggins, J., Ho, M., & Rinaldo, C. R. (1987). *New York State Medical Journal, 87,* 272-287.

Weinstein, N. (1984). Why it won't happen to me: Perceptions of risk factors and susceptibility. *Health Psychology, 3,* 431-457.

Misperception Among Gay Men of the Risk for AIDS Associated With Their Sexual Behavior*

6

Laurie J. Bauman
Karolynn Siegel
Department of Social Work
Memorial-Sloan Kettering Cancer Center

INTRODUCTION

From the time it was determined that AIDS was communicable through intimate sexual contact, the principal public health strategy for limiting the spread of the disease has been education—to disseminate information concerning the sexual practices implicated in transmitting the AIDS virus (HIV). Campaigns to reach people at highest risk for AIDS—homosexual men, IV drug users, and sexual partners of high-risk individuals—have included brochures, one-to-one counseling, mass-media advertising campaigns, and public lectures. Many of the strategies designed to persuade those at high risk to adopt safer-sex practices were based on conceptual models of the factors associated with the adoption of preventive health practices, such as the Health Belief Model (HBM; Leventhal, Meyer, & Nerenz, 1980; Leventhal, Safer, & Panagis, 1983), the Fear-Drive Model (Leventhal et al., 1983), and the Dual-Process Model (Leventhal et al., 1983).

The Health Belief Model is the conceptual framework most widely used to explain health-related preventive behaviors (Kirscht, 1983). According to this model, the dimensions that influence the adoption of a health action are: (1) perceived susceptibility or vulnerability to developing a health problem; (2) perceived severity of the illness; (3) perceived benefits of the change; (4) perceived barriers or possible negative effects of the change; and (5) cues or a stimulus to change, such as a symptom or a health communication (Janz & Becker, 1984). The Fear-Drive Model posits that "the fear produces subjective discomfort or tension which motivates action" (Leventhal et al., 1983).

*This chapter was originally published in *Journal of Applied Social Psychology,* 1987, Vol. 17, No. 3, pp. 329-350. Copyright 1987 by V. H. Winston & Sons, Inc. Reprinted with permission.

The Dual-Process Model views fear as an effective motivating factor when it is associated with the health threat itself, but, under some circumstances (e.g., when high fear engenders feelings of hopelessness), behavior may be directed in unexpected ways (e.g., the individual may be less likely to take action). All health communications have the potential to arouse fear and must be crafted to evolve a level of threat that harnesses the motivational force for change without causing despair.

Like the HBM, most models of preventive health behavior include the recognition of one's own vulnerability or at-risk status as a condition of adopting behavior designed to prevent illness. They also consistently highlight the role of anxiety or fear as a motivator of action (Cummings, Becker, & Maile, 1980). In this chapter, we report data from a study of gay men in New York City which was designed to investigate the factors associated with adopting safer-sex practices. In particular, we focus on men's subjective perceptions of the riskiness of their current sexual practices and examine the relative accuracy of these perceptions in light of available epidemiological data on the relative efficacy of different sexual practices as modes of transmission of the AIDS-associated (HIV) virus. We then assess the extent to which men underestimate the degree of risk associated with their sexual behaviors and examine several possible explanations for such inaccurate appraisals of risk.

LITERATURE REVIEW

The factors associated with individuals' appraisals of their risks for experiencing negative events is a growing area of inquiry. Some of the research conducted in this field has studied threats that are not specific to illness and disease, such as natural disasters (Kunreuther, 1979), divorce (Perloff & Farbisz, 1985), or being a victim of a crime (Hindelang, Gottfredson, & Garofalo, 1978; Perloff, 1982; Skogan & Maxfield, 1981; Weinstein, 1980). However, most investigations in this area assess individuals' perceptions of their risks of contracting or dying from a variety of diseases, including diabetes, cancer, heart attack, stroke, pneumonia, leukemia, alcoholism, and venereal disease (Harris & Guten, 1979; Kirscht, Haefner, Kegeles, & Rosenstock, 1966; Knopf, 1976; Lang, 1980; Perloff, 1982; Slovic, Fischhoff, & Lichtenstein, 1976; Weinstein, 1980).

The data from these studies indicate two important patterns. First, perception of vulnerability to an illness is associated with adopting preventive health practices (Becker et al. 1977; Cummings, Jette, Brock & Haefner, 1979; Kasl, 1975). Second, people tend to systematically underestimate the degree to which they are at risk (Harris & Guten, 1979; Kirscht et al., 1966; Larwood, 1978; Robertson, 1977; Weinstein, 1980, 1983, 1984). Weinstein (1980), Harris & Guten (1979), Kirscht et al. (1966), and Perloff (1982) have all found that many more people assess their risk of experiencing a negative event as below-average than assess their risk as above-average.

Several social psychological processes have been suggested to account for this frequently observed phenomenon, which Perloff (in press) refers to as "the illusion of unique invulnerability." These are: (1) unrealistic optimism (Weinstein, 1980, 1982, 1984); (2) health belief schema (Morgan & Spanish, 1985); and (3) defensive coping mechanisms (e.g., denial) to manage anxiety (Weinstein, 1977).

Unrealistic Optimism

Weinstein (1980) argues that, in general, people tend to think that they are "invulnerable," that they will not be victims of undesirable life events. It is usually extremely difficult to evaluate objectively the accuracy of a given individual's assessment of his/her risk for experiencing a specific event (since so many complex factors go into such an assessment). However, it is possible to detect unrealistic optimism on a group level by asking individuals to assess their risk relative to other individuals like themselves. If more people rate their risk below average than above average, this is evidence of unrealistic optimism.

Weinstein (1980) used this strategy in researching the mechanisms associated with unrealistic optimism. He found that people tend to believe that a negative event is less likely to happen to them than to others. This is, in part, a reflection of defense mechanisms, or "wishful thinking," in which people distort reality in a positive direction in order to avoid the anxiety that would result from a more realistic view (Kirscht et al., 1966; Perloff & Farbisz, 1985; Weinstein, 1977). However, Weinstein found that cognitive distortions, such as selective recall or flawed information processing, also contributed to unrealistic optimism. For example, negative events that are perceived to be within the subject's control are particularly subject to unrealistic optimism. This is so because in evaluating their risk, people recall the behaviors they have engaged in to avoid the occurrence of such an event. However, they are much more likely to remember their own efforts than they are to remember and take into account that many other people have also undertaken such efforts. He also found that people judge their risk by using stereotypes, consistent with the "representativeness" heuristic (Kahneman & Tversky, 1972). That is, people tend to imagine a stereotype of the kind of person to whom a specific negative event might occur, such as AIDS, and compare themselves to that stereotype. Because they tend to view themselves as deviating greatly from the stereotype, they manifest unrealistic optimism in assessing their own risk.

Attempts to reduce unrealistic optimism by increasing subjects' awareness of their risk factors did not succeed; in fact, it substantially increased optimistic bias (Weinstein, 1983). After reviewing a long list of risk factors (of which they had relatively few), most subjects tended to believe that they were at even less risk than others. This seems to be due to their assumption that others have more risk factors and have initiated fewer preventive health behaviors. However, when the number of risk factors and types of health practices of "typical" peers were described to subjects prior to their relating their own risk relative to others, unrealistic optimism was not observed.

Weinstein's work demonstrates that cognitive processes, as well as defense mechanisms, are associated with an unrealistically optimistic assessment of one's risk. Although Weinstein found that unrealistic optimism was particularly likely when events were undesirable (evidence of "wishful thinking"), unrealistic optimism was also demonstrated to be a function of flawed information processing. More specifically, it may be attributed to the fact that people focus on their own circumstances only, and ignore the perspective of others, thereby concluding incorrectly that their chances of experiencing an unwanted event were lower than others' chances.

Health Belief Schema

Laypersons' conceptions about the causes of health and illness have received increasing attention in recent years, but little is known about how people arrive at a "health belief schema," that is, how individuals store, retrieve, and apply information about their health. Morgan and Spanish (1985) conducted research on how people evaluate the importance of different risk factors for heart attacks. They found that people are generally able to describe the widely known risk factors and appear to be moderately well informed. However, they weight these factors differently in applying them to their own behavior and to explaining the occurrence of heart attacks in others.

Health beliefs develop into a schema following a progression of levels of organization of information, from episodes to categories to abstractions (Morgan & Spanish, 1985). Applying this conceptual framework to schema about AIDS, we believe that men begin by collecting episodes or stories about the illness and examples of men who have or have not developed AIDS. They use these bits of information and examples to develop categories, or risk factors, that are associated with contracting the illness. These risk factors are weighted in different ways by different men and are not necessarily congruent with prevailing medical opinion.

Most gay men have been given a great deal of information about the sexual behaviors that put them at risk for AIDS. Previous research (McKusick, Horstman, & Coates, 1985; Research and Decisions Corporation, 1984) and our own work indicates that most gay men are well informed about how the HIV is transmitted during sexual activity. However, according to the literature on health schema, risk factors are weighted differently by individuals when they apply them to their own behavior and when they use them to explain illness in others. Thus, we might expect that gay men would disagree among themselves about which factors put them at most risk and that their assessments might be different from those of medical experts.

Management of Anxiety

Under conditions of high stress or threat, denial is often used to protect against unmanageable anxiety. In recent years, there has been increasing recognition that denial can have positive functions when regulation of emotional distress is critical. It can maintain homeostasis and permit the individual time to marshal coping resources (Chodoff, Friedman, & Hamburg, 1964; Davis, 1963; Hamburg & Adams, 1967; Lazarus, 1981; Lifton, 1964; Mastrovito, 1974; Moos, 1982). As Taylor (1983) points out, the individual's ability to adapt successfully to a threatening event depends, in part, on his/her ability to maintain a set of "illusions" that require that certain facts be interpreted in a positive, optimistic way.

However, denial is not always functional. While it successfully reduces emotional distress, it tends to interfere with taking direct action, which may be necessary in certain situations to optimize other goals, such as safety and survival (Bauman, 1984). Women who discover a breast lump, for example, may find denial to be an effective strategy to reduce their emotional distress, but it may also be a significant factor in delaying medical treatment (Katz, Weiner, Gallagher, & Hellman, 1970).

In the case of AIDS, gay men are faced with apparently contradictory tasks. For their self-preservation, they must adopt fundamental changes in their sexual practices; changes that can have profound implications, not only for their sexual life, but also for their lifestyle patterns and their personal identities as gay men. In order to be sufficiently motivated to initiate and maintain such major changes, they must experience a high degree of threat and, hence, a high degree of anxiety. However, they must also find strategies for managing this enormous anxiety without resorting to denial, for if they did, it would interfere with the maintenance of safer-sex practices. Thus, it may be that gay men must choose between two difficult alternatives. They can choose to adopt safer-sex practices in order to protect their health; but first they must abandon denial of their high-risk status as a coping strategy, which, in turn, leaves them vulnerable to high levels of anxiety. If they manage their anxiety through denial, they undermine their ability to maintain the kinds of changes in their lifestyles that are necessary to avoid infection with the AIDS virus.

Below we present data from a New York City sample of asymptomatic gay men. We compared their subjective assessment of the riskiness of their sexual behaviors to an objective assessment of the actual riskiness of their behaviors. We identify those men who underestimate their risk and examine whether the three factors discussed above—unrealistic optimism, health belief schema, and anxiety—are associated with this misperception.

METHODS

The sample consisted of 160 gay men currently asymptomatic with respect to AIDS. Participants were recruited as part of a longitudinal study of sexual practices among gay men. Respondents were interviewed at two points in time, six months apart. Data presented here were gathered during the second interview, which took place for most men during 1985.

It is not possible to draw a random probability sample of gay men residing in the New York City area, since all members of the population cannot be enumerated and, therefore, a complete sampling frame cannot be con- structed. In an attempt to achieve a sample that provided some repre- sentation from varied segments of the gay community, we recruited subjects through diverse sources: advertisements in gay and non-gay tabloids; notices in the newsletters of gay organizations; fliers distributed in the vicinity of gay bars, discos, and bookstores; announcements at gay social functions; and referrals by community physicians.

The mean age of the respondents was 37 years (23% were in their 20s, 45% in their 30s, and 32% were 40 or older). Approximately 45% earned less than $25,000 per year, and about one third earned $35,000 or more. The sample was generally well educated: Three quarters had completed four or more years of college, with 45% reporting some graduate schooling. Only 6% of the respondents were non-white; 40% were Catholic, 32% were Pro- testant, and 22% were Jewish.

It is difficult to assess the nature of any sampling bias introduced by our recruitment strategy. Martin (1985) has compared the characteristics of five groups of gay men recruited in different ways for a study of the impact of AIDS on the New York City gay community. The groups were: a random sample of the memberships of 48 gay organizations; unsolicited volunteers who learned about the study through articles in gay and non-gay newspapers; personal referrals from members of a pilot sample; men recruited at a street fair held the day of the Gay Pride Parade; and men recruited through a public health clinic. Differences among men drawn from the first four sources were generally small, and the clinic sample differed the most dramatically from all other sources. The sample of (unsolicited) volunteers, which most closely resembles our own, tended to slightly overrepresent whites and residents of Manhattan, but was remarkably similar to all samples (except the clinic sample) in age, income, education, and years of residence in New York City.

In addition to any sampling bias introduced by the recruitment strategy, it is possible that individuals who self-select into studies of this nature differ on important characteristics from the overall gay population. For example, given the present social climate in which even asymptomatic gay men fear discrimination based on their at-risk status, there is an understandable reluctance on the part of some men to identify themselves as gay. Sampling bias from any source can be a problem when the objective is to estimate a population parameter that might be related to those characteristics which are under- or overrepresented. However, for the more limited purposes of the present study, that of examining patterns of relationships among a restricted set of variables, true representativeness is not essential.

Measures

Data were gathered from each respondent through a self-administered questionnaire, and a face-to-face interview with a gay male interviewer. The principal variables used in the analysis and their operationalization are described below.

Objective Appraisal of Risk

As part of the interview, respondents reported how many times and with how many different partners they engaged in a wide range of sexual practices during the most recent typical month. These practices were grouped into three categories, based on the probable risk they presented to the respondent in terms of chance of becoming infected.

Because there is some ambiguity concerning whether specific sexual acts are efficient modes of transmission of the AIDS (HIV) virus, it is difficult to evaluate precisely the epidemiologic risks associated with different behaviors. We have relied on existing epidemiologic studies linking various sexual practices with seropositivity, helper T-cell ratios, and frank AIDS; these studies are not all consistent in their findings, and, due to limitations in research design, some must be regarded as provisional.

The most consistent finding has been the identification of receptive anal intercourse as a behavioral risk factor (Detels et al., 1983; Goedert et al., 1984, 1985; Kingsley et al., 1986; McCusker, Stoddard, Mayer, Cowan, & Groopman, 1986; Marmor et al., 1984; Martin, 1986). However, even here, a few studies have failed to identify a relationship between this practice and HIV-associated conditions (Darrow, Jaffee & Curran, 1983; Jaffee et al., 1983). Some available data suggest that insertive and receptive fisting (Darrow et al., 1983; Goedert et al., 1984; Jaffee et al., 1983; Marmor et al., 1984) and insertive rimming (oral-anal contact; Jaffee et al., 1983) are possible risk factors as well.

Given the inconsistency of available findings and the limitations of the research designs of several studies, it was not possible to rely exclusively on extant epidemiologic data as a basis for classifying the riskiness of our respondents' sexual practices. Therefore, for virtually all practices other than receptive anal intercourse—where the preponderance of evidence strongly supports the classification of this behavior as a high-risk behavior—we categorized behavior as risky, low risk, or safe based on its usual designation in available risk-reduction guidelines. This decision was made for several reasons. First, these guidelines in fact represent the best attempts by knowledgeable professional groups and organizations to interpret the implications of available epidemiologic and clinical evidence. Second, these guidelines are a principal source of information for most gay men regarding the risks associated with different practices. Third, Siegel, Grodsky, and Herman (1986) reviewed a sampling of available safer-sex brochures and found a high degree of agreement across materials in the classification of practices. Finally, risk-reduction guidelines tend to be formulated using the principle that practices which permit the exchange of body fluids in which the virus has been isolated are potentially high-risk behaviors. However, they do tend to reflect available evidence about the relative efficiency of different modes of transmission. For example, most risk-reduction guidelines recognize the available evidence that wet kissing is an inefficient route of transmission. We believe that it is reasonable to rely on the generally agreed-upon classification of different sexual behaviors contained in safer-sex brochures as the basis for objectively classifying the relative riskiness of our respondents' behavior.

Using this criterion, we grouped sexual practices into three categories based on the degree of risk they presented to the respondent's chances of becoming infected by a partner:

(1) *"Risky"* practices, which permit the efficient exchange of blood and semen (partner inserted penis into respondent's anus without using a condom; respondent inserted his penis into partner's anus without using a condom; respondent used his tongue to touch or lick partner's anus; respondent put his partner's feces into mouth; partner inserted his whole hand or fist into respondent's anus; respondent inserted his whole hand or fist into partner's anus; respondent drank partner's urine; respondent's partner ejaculated into his mouth).

(2) *"Low risk"* practices, which probably do not permit the efficient exchange of body fluids (partner used his tongue to touch or lick respondent's anus; respondent inserted his penis into partner's anus while using a condom; partner inserted his penis into respondent's anus while using a condom; partner inserted one or more fingers into respondent's

anus[1]; respondent inserted one or more fingers into partner's anus[1]; respondent ejaculated into partner's mouth; partner put his penis into respondent's mouth without ejaculating; partner engaged in water sports or urinated on respondent; partner inserted a dildo or some other object in respondent's anus).

(3) *"Safe"* practices, which provide virtually no opportunity for the exchange of body fluids (hugging, kissing, mutual masterbation, rubbing penises together manually).

Respondents' present pattern of sexual behavior was characterized as risky, low risk, or safe, based on their reported pattern of sexual practices during a recent typical month. Individuals who engaged in one or more risky practices at least once were classified as risky. Those who engaged in no risky behaviors, but one or more low-risk behaviors at least once were classified as low risk. The remaining respondents who engaged in no risky practices and no low-risk behaviors were classified as safe.

The terms safe, low risk, and risky are used in a relative, not an absolute sense. Those classified in the middle category are engaging in practices that are probably safe, but carry some inestimable risk because of uncertainties that remain concerning the relative efficacy of certain modes of transmission (e.g., saliva) and because certain practices may create the opportunity for infection under certain circumstances (e.g., oral sex in which withdrawal is attempted before ejaculation but some leakage of semen occurs). The term "safe sex" is used in a relative sense to refer to practices which are currently believed to present no risk of infection in the vast majority of instances.

For the present analyses, we did not differentiate between men who engaged in a risky practice or low-risk practice more than once or with more than one partner from those who engaged in that practice only once or with only one individual. This decision was made based on two considerations. First, even if a respondent reported having engaged in such practices only once, or with only one partner, because the time frame asked about was a typical month, it was likely that over the course of an entire year he would have engaged in this practice several times or with several partners. The only

---

[1]There is particular ambiguity about anodigital contact and its potential for transmitting the virus. Most safer-sex brochures do not address this practice specifically, and those which do tend to classify it with fisting as a risky practice. Because less is known about this practice than fisting, we chose to classify it as a low-risk practice, which is the most conservative classification from the point of view of our hypotheses. That is, considering this a low-risk practice makes it less likely that men engaging in this practice would be categorized as underestimating the riskiness of their sexual practices. However, we also repeated the analyses which follow, classifying anodigital contact as risky, and all of the relationships remained the same.

exception would be gay men who had only one partner during the past year. This group, however, accounts for only about 18.5% ($n = 29$) of our sample. Of these, 55% ($n = 16$) were in the risky group. Furthermore, given the long incubation period of AIDS, unless the monogamous relationship was of several years' duration, the partners are probably still best advised to practice safer sex.

Additionally, it has been estimated that in some cities with a large homosexual population, as many as 68% of that population may be infected with the AIDS virus (Curran et al. 1985). Under such circumstances, unsafe sexual contact with even one or a very small number of men carries a substantial risk of infection. For example, using Curran et al.'s (1985) estimate of the prevalence of HIV infections in cities like New York with a large gay population, the chances of being exposed to the virus by engaging in risky sex with one partner during the past year is 68%; with two partners, 90%; and with three partners, 98%. Using a more conservative estimate of 36% (Martin, 1985), the chances of being exposed to the virus with one, two, or three partners are 36%, 59%, and 74%, respectively.

Subjective Appraisal of Risk.

Respondents were asked to rate how risky they thought their current pattern of sexual behavior was in terms of its contributing to their chances of getting AIDS. Ratings were made on a ten-point scale (10 = most risky).

Anxiety.

Anxiety was measured using the anxiety symptom dimension of the Brief Symptom Inventory (BSI). The BSI (Derogatis & Spencer, 1982), a shortened form of the SCL-90-R, is a standardized, widely used scale of 53 items which provides three summary scores, as well as scores on nine primary symptom domains, including anxiety. The items included in the anxiety symptom dimension tap nervousness and tension, panic attacks and feelings of terror, as well as cognitive components involving apprehensive feelings and some somatic symptoms of anxiety.

Likelihood of Developing AIDS.

As a measure of perceived vulnerability to AIDS, respondents were asked to rate their chances, compared to other gay men, of developing AIDS someday. The response categories were below average, average, and above average.

Pattern of Relationships.

Respondents were asked to characterize their pattern of sexual relationships over the past six months. Responses were grouped to create four categories:

celibate, one partner, several regular partners, or multiple primarily anonymous partners.

Sex-Related Behaviors.

Respondents were asked if, during the most recent typical month, they engaged in a number of sex-related practices during the time of their sexual encounters. Although these practices are sometimes encouraged in available risk-reduction guidelines, they provide no protection against infection with the AIDS virus. The behaviors were: washing or showering before a sexual contact; washing or showering after a sexual contact; and inspecting one's partner for sores, lesions, or rashes. Respondents were assigned scores on this variable based on the total number of practices they undertook at least half of the time.

RESULTS

Actual Riskiness and Perceived Riskiness of Sexual Practices

Based on the criteria described above for objectively assessing the riskiness of sexual practices, we found that 42% of the sample engaged in high-risk sexual activities during the most recent typical month, 33% participated in sexual activities that are "probably" safe (low risk), and 25% engaged in only safe-sex practices. Of the 66 men who engaged in risky practices, 31 (47%) engaged in one risky practice, 19 (29%) engaged in two, and 16 (24%) engaged in three or more. These data reflect the distribution of practices in this sample of men only, and should not be assumed to be necessarily representative of the sexual practices of the population of gay men in New York City.

The distribution of men's subjective assessments of the riskiness of their sexual practices (rated on a scale of 1 to 10) was very different. Over three quarters rated the riskiness of their practices at the bottom third of the scale (31% said "1"; 30% said "2"; 18% said "3"; and 12% said "4"). A very small percentage (9%) rated themselves "5" or above on the scale.

Accuracy of Perception of Riskiness of Sexual Practices

In Table 6.1, we present a cross-tabulation of the riskiness ratings respondents assigned to their current sexual practices (subjective assessment) with our assessment of the actual riskiness of their current sexual practices (objective assessment). Those who were engaged in safe sex practices only were quite accurate in their assessment of the riskiness of their practices: 56% rate their risk as 1 on the 10-point scale, and 31% place their risk as 2 or 3. Those practicing probably safe (low-risk) behaviors appropriately tend to rate their

TABLE 6.1
Subjective Risk Assessment by Objective Risk Assessment

		Objective risk assessment			Total	
		Safe % (n)	Low risk % (n)	High risk % (n)	%	(n)
Subjective assessment	1	56 (22)	19 (9)	19 (13)	29	(44)
	2–3	31 (12)	67 (32)	47 (31)	49	(75)
	4–5	8 (3)	10 (5)	17 (11)	12	(19)
	6+	5 (2)	4 (2)	17 (11)	10	(15)
		100 (39)	100 (48)	100 (66)	100	(153)

Kendall's Tau $c = .28$, $p = .0000$.

behavior as slightly more risky: Only 19% assessed their risk as 1, but 67% rated it as 2 or 3. However, those practicing risky sex tend not to rate the riskiness of their practices higher than the low-risk group, and only 17% (11 of 66) place themselves on the upper half of the scale measuring their appraisal of the riskiness of their sexual behavior.

Of most interest to the present investigation are those individuals who are engaged in high-risk activities but who underestimate their risk, for it is this group that does not acknowledge the level of danger inherent in their behavior and is, therefore, likely to be poorly motivated to adopt modifications. We defined all cases falling into the raised cells of Table 6.1 as underestimating their risk.[2] These individuals were participating in risky sex, but believed it to

---

[2]Among the group of men engaging in low-risk sexual practices (n = 48), nine men classified the riskiness of their practices as "1", which may also be construed as an instance of underestimation of risk. However, we chose to limit the group we call "underestimators" to those engaging in clearly risky sexual practices, since these men are of greatest concern for targeting public health interventions and are clearly at the highest risk. In addition, since it is possible that some of the low-risk sexual practices may indeed be safe, we chose to define as underestimating only those men who were clearly in violation of safer-sex guidelines.

be low risk or safe. While the cases falling in these cells ($n = 55$) constitute only 34% of the entire sample, they account for 83% of those engaging in risky sexual behavior.

Factors Associated with Underestimating the Riskiness of Sexual Practices

We examined the relationship of several factors to the accuracy of respondents' assessments of the riskiness of their sexual behaviors. The factors examined were ones suggested by the social psychological literature to be associated with individuals' appraisals of their risk of experiencing threatening events.

Unrealistic Optimism.

First, we examined whether gay men were misperceiving their risks due to unrealistic optimism (Weinstein, 1980). We asked gay men to evaluate their risks of getting AIDS, relative to other gay men. Following Weinstein's (1980) logic, we assessed optimism or pessimism by calculating the mean of this comparative risk variable (below average = -1, average = 0, and above average = +1). If the men's assessments of their risk for getting AIDS are unbiased, then the mean should be zero (i.e., an equal proportion should evaluate their risk as above and below average). If the mean is negative, and significantly different from zero, this is evidence of unrealistic optimism. Since unrealistic optimism has been found in a series of studies and under many conditions, we expected to find it operating in this sample as well. Of the 160 men in our sample, 81 (51%) rated their risk as below average. The mean is -.35%, which differs significantly from zero (Student's t, $p < .05$). Thus, as a group, the gay men in our sample, faced with the threat of AIDS, do tend to exhibit unrealistic optimism in their estimate of their risk of contracting AIDS.

Health Schema.

The second factor we expected to be associated with the accuracy of gay men's assessments of the riskiness of their current sexual practices was their varying beliefs about the factors that influence one's chances of getting AIDS. Many men evidently develop their own personal weighting scheme about which past and present behaviors put them at risk or protect them from developing the disease. We had assessed the level of knowledge concerning risky and safer-sex practices of all the men who participated in the survey at the time of the first interview. Virtually all men were able to recite accurately the recommended guidelines for avoiding infection (although the specificity of their responses varied). After the first interview was completed, we also gave each respondent a copy of risk-reduction guidelines, asked them to review them in our presence, and encouraged them to ask any questions they had regarding the recommendations outlined. Thus, by the second interview, from which the data reported here are taken, we could be relatively sure that all men had been counseled about risk reduction at least once.

We examined two factors likely to be related to beliefs about sexual practices and how those practices might protect them against AIDS. First, we assessed whether those who limited their number of sexual partners to one or a few regular partners were more likely to assess their risky sex practices as safe. Clearly, any gay man who engages in sexual activities that involve the exchange of semen or blood is placing himself at risk. This is true even if he has limited his partners to one or a few men, since, as noted above, a very high proportion of gay men in New York City are estimated to be seropositive.

The data suggest that gay men may believe that limiting themselves to a single partner or restricting contact to a few regular partners can minimize the dangers of risky sexual practices (Table 6.2). A majority of the men who engaged in sex with anonymous partners accurately appraised their practices, whereas men with only one partner or several regular partners were more likely to underestimate their risk. Although safer-sex guidelines almost universally recommend reducing one's number of sexual partners, and "knowing" one's partners, these behaviors by themselves do not eliminate risk when sexual practices which include exchange of semen or blood occur.

Next, we examined whether those who inaccurately appraised the riskiness of their practices were taking precautions which they may have believed would mitigate their risk, but, in fact, probably conferred no protection. We assessed three essentially ineffectual health activities: inspecting one's partner for lesions, showering before sex, and showering after sex. We counted up the

TABLE 6.2
Accuracy of Risk Assessment by Kinds of Sexual Partners[1]

		Patterns of partners			
		One partner	Regular partners	Anonymous partners	Total
Accuracy of risk assessment	Accurate assessment	48%	57%	69%	61%
	Underestimation	52%	43%	31%	39%
		100% $n = 29$	100% $n = 44$	100% $n = 68$	100% $n = 141$

Kendall's Tau $c = -.18, p = .02.$
[1]Celibate men were eliminated from this table.

TABLE 6.3
Accuracy of Risk Assessment by Sex-Related Behaviors

| | | Number of sex-related behaviors | | | | |
		0	1	2	3	Total
Accuracy of risk assessment	Accurate	85%	58%	55%	54%	65%
	Underestimation	15%	42%	45%	46%	35%
		100%	100%	100%	100%	100%
		n = 47	n = 40	n = 47	n = 22	n = 156

Kendall's Tau $c = .26$, $p = .001$.

number of these behaviors engaged in at least half the time they had sex and examined the relationship of the resulting score to accuracy of perception of risk (Table 6.3). Those who had adopted any of these practices were more likely to be inaccurate than those who had not.

Anxiety.

Finally, we examined how anxiety influenced accuracy of men's perceived riskiness of their sexual practices. As we observed above, most of the men engaging in risky sexual behaviors underestimated the extent to which they were putting themselves at risk. If underestimating the riskiness of risky sexual behavior is an attempt to manage anxiety through denial, we would expect to see an empirical relationship between underestimating the riskiness of one's practices and low anxiety. We examine this relationship in Table 6.4, in which anxiety scores have been grouped into three categories; the "high" scores were defined using a t-score cutoff that corresponds to a clinical level of symptomatology.

TABLE 6.4
Accuracy of Risk Assessment by Anxiety

| | | Anxiety | | | |
		Low	Medium	High	Total
Accuracy of risk assessment	Accurate assessment	51%	69%	71%	65%
	Underestimation	49%	31%	29%	35%
		100%	100%	100%	100%
		n = 47	n = 45	n = 63	n = 155

Kendall's Tau $c = -.18$, $p = .02$.

We see that as anxiety decreases, the tendency to underestimate one's risk increases which is consistent with our hypothesis that underestimation of the riskiness of one's sexual practices is, in part, an attempt to manage anxiety.

DISCUSSION

In this chapter, we have reported data suggesting that gay men tend to underestimate the riskiness of their sexual practices. Of the gay men in this sample who engaged in at least one high-risk behavior in a typical month, 83% appraised their behavior to be relatively safe. Since misinformation could be ruled out as a possible reason for their misperception, we explored several other possible explanations.

First, we found that gay men as a group tend to experience unrealistic optimism; that is, to underestimate their own personal vulnerability to AIDS, relative to other gay men. This pattern, which has been identified in other populations and with other kinds of risks, seems to be due to both defensive posturing and cognitive distortion.

We believe that gay men must realistically appraise the riskiness of their behavior in order to experience a sense of vulnerability. Such a realistic assessment is likely to increase their anxiety about their health, which, in turn, will motivate them to initiate and maintain safer-sex practices. Based on Weinstein's work, however, simply listing all possible risk factors, as many safer-sex guidelines do, may have the opposite effect than intended: It may actually increase the likelihood of perceiving onself as at lower risk than others. Therefore, we suggest that risk-reduction guidelines be designed so that, in addition to making men aware of all the risk factors for AIDS, they can derive a score which reflects the probable riskiness of their sexual behaviors. In addition, the scores should be interpretable in terms of epidemiologically established risks for HIV-associated conditions.

Second, we have shown that another mechanism through which men may underestimate the riskiness of their own sexual practices is the nature of the health beliefs they have developed about AIDS. Although all of the gay men we interviewed were able to describe which sexual practices were safe and which were risky, some had weighted the degree of risk associated with their own behavior based on misperceptions, such as the belief that engaging in high-risk sexual practices with one or a few regular partners was a safe compromise. This misperception may possibly be traced to the ambiguous language of most risk-reduction guidelines, which suggests "reducing" the number of partners and "knowing" your partners (Siegel et al., 1986). It may be desirable to review and rewrite safer-sex guidelines to be very specific about the kinds of sexual practices that are always risky (e.g., unprotected anal intercourse) and to emphasize that such practices are dangerous, regardless of the fact that one has limited the number of partners with whom he engages in such practices. Another detected misperception was that undertaking certain behaviors would reduce one's risk (e.g., showering, inspecting one's partner for lesions), when, in fact, they confer no protection. Belief in the efficacy of such precautions is dangerous because it leads to a false sense of security. Gay men who engaged in ineffectual precautions were more likely to believe that their risky sexual practices were safe. This kind of misperception is possibly due, in part, to statements in many risk-reduction guidelines which often do encourage washing and good basic hygiene. It is also likely to be due to the kinds of health-belief schemas men have constructed to explain risks for AIDS. Such models can have a powerful influence on the kinds of behaviors adopted with the expectation of reducing risk. In this case, it may be necessary for safer-sex guidelines to emphasize that behaviors such as showering before and/or after sex, getting adequate sleep, eating well, and exercising regularly do not reduce the risks of infection if one engages in risky behaviors.

More research needs to be initiated on the health-belief schema gay men hold about AIDS in order to understand how misperceptions and risk-factor weightings contribute to the persistence of risky sexual practices. From our experience, in addition to exploring beliefs about the protective value of limiting partners and knowing one's partners, particularly fruitful areas of inquiry might include identifying the other sex-related behaviors men perceive to be protective, but which are not (e.g., the belief that being the active (insertive) partner in anal intercourse is safe).

Additionally, the data suggest an important relationship between anxiety and perception of the riskiness of one's sexual behavior. The data in Table 4 indicate an association between low levels of anxiety and a tendency to underestimate the riskiness of one's sexual practices. The relationship is consistent with models of preventive health behavior. For example, the Health Belief Model posits that an individual must first recognize and acknowledge that he is at risk for AIDS before he will experience heightened anxiety, which, in turn, motivates the adoption of safer-sex practices. Gay men who deny or misperceive that they are at risk for AIDS (i.e., who exhibit unrealistic optimism) experience lower anxiety, which then generates little motivation for practicing safer sex. Therefore, such men continue to engage in high-risk sexual practices. Their denial of the extent to which they are at risk for AIDS also extends to denying that their current sexual behavior puts them at increased risk of infection.

A possible explanation for the relationship between misperception of the riskiness of one's sexual practices and anxiety is also suggested by cognitive dissonance models. When the AIDS epidemic occurred, certain sexual practices of gay men were suddenly defined as dangerous (i.e., potentially life threatening). To acknowledge and confront the fact that their past and present behavior put them at risk for AIDS may have been too threatening for many men. Some, therefore, tended to misperceive or distort the available public health information in ways that permitted them to appraise their behavior as less risky than it actually was. This has the dual effect of minimizing the anxiety that would result if they confronted their increased risk for AIDS due to their past behavior and permitting continuation of risky sexual practices that increase their risk of infection.

In our view, anxiety can be an important motivating force for practicing safer sex and protecting one's health. For this reason, we believe that, consistent with the tenets of the Fear-Drive Model and Dual-Process Model, moderate-fear health-education messages are probably necessary to motivate men to limit their practices to those considered safe. However, the cost of this strategy to gay men in terms of their psychological distress is high. We need to explore ways of helping gay men to successfully accomplish the difficult dual tasks of maintaining a level of anxiety sufficient to motivate safer-sex, while at the same time managing anxiety and maintaining psychological equilibrium.

Further, we need to explore the options for motivating behavioral change in men who use denial to manage anxiety at the expense of their health. Health messages regarding sexual practices may need to be more confrontational in order to reach men who are still practicing risky sex and to help them acknowledge that their practices are risky for AIDS. Our suggestion to score men's risk factors relative to other gay men and in terms of their absolute risks for AIDS may succeed in breaking through some men's denial. However, we expect that, in some cases, more intensive interventions would probably be necessary, in addition to written materials.

Models of preventive health behavior consistently emphasize that individuals must acknowledge that they are at risk before they will initiate and maintain preventive health practices. In this chapter, we have drawn attention to some of the mechanisms through which gay men may misperceive the risk. Although health education has apparently succeeded in communicating the facts about AIDS and how it is transmitted, additional strategies must be developed to help those at high risk to intergrate and apply these facts in ways that will successfully protect them from acquiring and/or transmitting AIDS.

ACKNOWLEDGMENTS

This work was supported by grants from the National Institute of Mental Health (MH39441) and the New York State AIDS Institute (C000577).

REFERENCES

Bauman, L. J. (1984). *Coping, social support and breast cancer: An empirical and theoretical study of the stress process.* Doctoral dissertation, Columbia University. University Microfilms International No. 8427348.

Becker, M. H., Haefner, D. P., Kasl, S. V., Kirscht, J. P., Maiman, L. A., & Rosenstock, I. M. (1977). Selected psychosocial models and correlates of individual health-related behaviors. *Medical Care, 15* (Supplement), 27-46.

Chodoff, P., Friedman, S., & Hamburg, D. A. (1964). Stress, defenses and coping behavior: Observations in parents of children with malignant disease. *American Journal of Psychiatry, 120*, 743-749.

Cummings, K. M., Becker, M. H., & Maile, M. C. (1980). Bringing the models together: An empirical approach to combining variables used to explain health actions. *Journal of Behavioral Medicine, 3*, 123-145.

Cummings, K. M., Jette, A. M., Brock, B. M., &Haefner, D. P. (1979). Psychosocial determinants of immunization behavior in a swine influenza campaign. *Medical Care, 17*, 639-649.

Curran, J. W., Morgan, M. W., Hardy, A. M., Jaffee, H. W., Darrow, W. W., & Dowdle, W. R. (1985). The epidemiology of AIDS: Current status and future prospects. *Science, 229*, 1352-1357.

Darrow, W. W., Jaffee, H. W., & Curran, J. W. (1983). Passive anal intercourse as a risk factor for AIDS in homosexual men. *Lancet, 2*, 160.

Davis, F. (1963). *Passage through crisis: Polio victims and their families.* Indianapolis, IN: Bobbs-Merrill.

Derogatis, L. R., & Spencer, P. M. (1982). *The Brief Symptom Inventory (BSI): Administration, scoring and procedures manual.* Baltimore: Clinical Psychometrics Research.

Detels, R., Schwartz, K., Visscher, B. R., Fahey, J. L., Greene, R. S., & Gottlieb, M. S. (1983). Relation between sexual practices and T-cell subsets in homosexually active men. *Lancet, 1*, 610-612.

Goedert, J. J., Biggar, R. J., Winn, D. M., Greene, M. H., Mann, D. L., Gallo, R. C., Sarngadharan, M. G., Weiss, S. H., Grossman, R. J., Boder, A. J., Strong, D. M., & Blattner, W. A. (1984). Determinants of retrovirus (HTLV-III) antibody and immunodeficiency conditions in homosexual men. *Lancet, 2*, 711-716.

Goedert, J. J., Biggar, R. J., Winn, D. M., Mann, D. L., Byar, D. P., Strong, D. M., DiGioia, R. A., Grossman, R. J., Sanchez, W. C., Kase, R. G., Greene, M. H., Hoover, R. N., & Blattner, W. A. (1985). Decreased helper T lymphocytes in homosexual men: II, sexual practices. *American Journal of Epidemiology, 121*, 637-644.

Hamburg, D. A., & Adams, J. E. (1967). A perspective on coping behavior: Seeking and utilizing information in major transitions. *Archives of General Psychiatry, 17*, 277-284.

Harris, D. M., & Guten, S. (1979). Health-protective behavior: An exploratory study. *Journal of Health and Social Behavior, 20*, 17-29.

Hindelang, M. J., Gottfredson, M. R., & Garofalo, J. (1978). *Victims of personal crime.* Cambridge, MA: Ballinger.

Jaffee, H. W., Keewham, C., Thomas, P. A., Haverkos, H. W., Auerbach, D. M., Guinan, M. E., Rogers, M. F., Spira, T. J., Darrow, W. W., Kramer, M. A., Friedman, S. M., Monroe, J. M., Friedman-Kien, A. E., Laubenstein, L. J., Marmor, M., Safai, B., Dritz, S. K., Crispi, S., Fannin, S. L., Orkwis, J. P., Kelter, A., Rushing, W. R., Thacker, S. B., & Curran, J. W. (1983). National case control study of Kaposi's sarcoma and *Pneumocystis carinii* pneumonia in homosexual men: Part I, epidemiologic results. *Annals of Internal Medicine, 99*, 145-151.

Janz, N. K., & Becker, M. H. (1984). The health belief model: A decade later. *Health Education Quarterly, 11*, 1-47.

Kasl, S. V. (1975). Social psychological characteristics associated with behaviors that reduce cardiovascular risk. In A. J. Enelow & J. Henderson (Eds.), *Applying behavioral science to cardiovascular risk* (pp. 173-180). Dallas: American Heart Association.

Katz, J. L., Wiener, H., Gallagher, T. F., & Hellman, L. (1970). Stress, distress, and ego defenses: Psychoendocrine response to impending breast tumor biopsy. *Archives of General Psychiatry, 23*, 131-142.

Kingsley, L., Rinaldo, C., Ostrow, D., Odaka, N., Visscher, B., & Solomon, R. (1986, June). *Risk factors for seroconversion to LAV/HTLV-III among homosexual men.* Paper presented at the International Conference on AIDS. Paris.

Kirscht, J. P. (1983). Preventive health behavior: A review of research and issues. *Health Psychology, 2,* 279-301.

Kirscht, J. P., Haefner, D. P., Kegeles, S. S., & Rosenstock, I. M. (1966). A national study of health beliefs. *Journal of Health and Human Behavior, 7,* 248-254.

Knopf, A. (1976). Changes in women's opinions about cancer. *Social Science and Medicine, 10,* 191-195.

Kunreuther, H. (1979). The changing societal consequences of risks from natural hazards. *The Annals of the American Academy of Political and Social Science, 443,* 104-116.

Lang, L. (1980). *Sickness as sin: Observers' perceptions of the physically ill.* Unpublished manuscript, University of Massachusetts, Amherst.

Larwood, L. (1978). Swine flu: A field study of self-serving biases. *Journal of Applied Social Psychology, 8,* 283-289.

Lazarus, R. S. (1981). The costs and benefits of denial. In B. S. Dohrenwend & B. P. Dohrenwend (Eds.) *Stressful life events and their contexts* (p. 131-156). New York: Prodist.

Leventhal, H., Meyer, D., & Nerenz, D. (1980). The common sense representation of illness danger. In S. Rachman (Ed.), *Contributions to medical psychology* (Vol. 2, pp. 7-30). New York: Pergamon Press.

Leventhal, H., Safer, M. A., & Panagis, D. M. (1983). The impact of communications on self-regulation of health beliefs, decisions, and behavior. *Health Education Quarterly, 10,* 3-31.

Lifton, R. J. (1964). On death and death symbolism: The Hiroshima disaster. *Psychiatry, 7,* 191-210.

Marmor, M., Friedman-Klein, A. E., Zolla-Pazner, S., Stahl, R. E., Rubenstein, P., Laubenstein, L., William, D. C. Klein, R. J. & Spigland, I. (1984). Kaposi's sarcoma in homosexual men: A seroepidemiological study. *Annals of Internal Medicine, 100,* 809-815.

Martin, J. L. (1985, Nov). *The impact of AIDS on New York City gay men: Development of a community sample.* Paper presented at the 113th annual meeting of the American Public Health Association. Washington, D. C.

Martin, J. L. (1986, June). Demographic factors, sexual behavior patterns, and HIV antibody status among New York City gay men. Paper presented at the annual meeting of the American Psychological Association. Washington, D. C.

Mastrovito, R. C. (1974). Cancer: Awareness and denial. *Clinical Bullentin, 4,* 142-146.

McCusker, J. Stoddard, A., Mayer, K., Cowan, D., & Groopman, J. (1986, June). *Logistic regression modeling of previous and current sexual behavior and HTLV-III/LAV antibody status among asymptomatic homosexual men.* Paper presented at the International Conference on AIDS. Paris.

McKusick, L. Horstman, W., & Coates, T. (1985). AIDS and sexual behavior reported by gay men in San Francisco. *American Journal of Public Health, 75,* 493-496.

Moos, R. H. (1982). Coping with acute health crisis. In T. Millon, C. Green, & R. Meagher (Eds.), *Handbook of clinical health psychology* (pp. 129-151). New York: Plenum Press.

Morgan, D. L., & Spanish, M. T. (1985). Social interaction and the cognitive organization of health-relevant knowledge. *Sociology of Health and Illness, 7,* 401-422.

Perloff, L. S. (1982). *Nonvictims' judgments of unique and universal vulnerability to future misfortune.* Unpublished doctoral dissertation, Northwestern University, Evanston, IL.

Perloff, L. S. (in press). Social comparison and illusions of invulnerability to negative life events. In C. R. Snyder & C. Ford (Eds.), *Clinical social psychological perspectives on negative life events.* New York: Plenum.

Perloff, L. S., & Farbisz, R. (1985, May). *Perceptions of uniqueness and illusions of invulnerability to divorce.* Paper presented at the Midwestern Psychological Association meeting. Chicago.

Research and Decisions Corporation. (1984). *Designing an effective AIDS prevention campaign strategy for San Francisco: Results from the first probability sample of an urban gay male community.* San Francisco: Author.

Robertson, L. S. (1977). Car crashes: Perceived vulnerability and willingness to pay for crash protection. *Journal of Community Health, 3,* 136-141.

Siegel, K., Grodsky, P. B., & Herman, A. (1986). AIDS risk reduction guidelines: A review and analysis. *Journal of Community Health, 11,* 233-243.

Skogan, W. G., & Maxfield, M G. (1981). *Coping with crime.* Beverly Hills, CA: Sage.

Slovic, P., Fischhoff, B., & Lichtenstein, S. (1976). Cognitive processes and societal risk taking. In J. S. Carroll & J. W. Payne (Eds.), *Cognition and social behavior* (pp. 165-184). Hillsdale, NJ: Lawrence Erlbaum Associates.

Taylor, S. E. (1983). Adjustment to threatening events: A theory of cognitive adaption. *American Psychologist,* November, 161-173.

Weinstein, N D. (1977, August). *Coping with environmental hazards: Reactions to the threat of crime.* Paper presented at the American Psychological Association Convention. San Francisco.

Weinstein, N. D. (1980). Unrealistic optimism about future life events. *Journal of Personality and Social Psychology, 39,* 806-820.

Weinstein, N. D. (1982). Unrealistic optimism about susceptibility to health problems. *Journal of Behavioral Medicine, 5,* 441-460.

Weinstein, N. D. (1983). Reducing unrealistic optimism about illness susceptibility. *Health Psychology, 2,* 11-20.

Weinstein, N. D. (1984). Why it won't happen to me: Perceptions of risk factors and susceptibility. *Health Psychology, 3,* 431-457.

Changes in Sexual Behavior Among Gay and Bisexual Men Since the Beginning of the AIDS Epidemic

7

Thomas J. Coates
Division of General Internal Medicine
Center for AIDS Prevention Studies
University of California, San Francisco

Ron D. Stall
Colleen C. Hoff
Center for AIDS Prevention Studies
University of California, San Francisco

EXECUTIVE SUMMARY

The most important public health agenda in AIDS is to prevent more individuals from becoming infected with HIV. Research is an essential component of program development. The research to date has highlighted that important behavior changes have occurred. However, many urban centers have shown less than optimal changes among gay and bisexual men, and data are not available for many other centers. There are few data available on the efficacy of various strategies for behavior change. Research is essential to pinpoint behavior and to implement and evaluate the efficacy of programs to reduce high-risk behavior in this high-risk population.

This report seeks to describe the degree to which gay and bisexual men have changed specific sexual practices that place them at risk for HIV infection, the degree to which these changes can be associated with specific educational or public health programs, and the costs of these specific programs. Methodological critiques of the research are also provided.

Risk factors for seroconversion in male-to-male sexual contact have been identified as number of male sexual partners and unprotected receptive or insertive anal intercourse. Estimates of the prevalence of infection vary from 750,000 to 2.5 million. Precise estimates are hampered because the size of the gay and bisexual population is not known, and estimates of infection are based largely on samples of convenience. When samples of convenience are compared to population-based samples in the same city, the latter produce lower estimates of the prevalence of infection. The best estimate would indicate that 37% of the homosexuals in the U.S. are seropositive. The current samples used to estimate incidence show that incidence is less than 1% (San Francisco, SF) or about 3.8% (Pittsburgh, Baltimore, Chicago, and Los Angeles). These samples, however, are highly sensitized and may not reflect incidence in the population.

The changes documented are impressive and important. Nonetheless, considerable proportions of gay men in these studies, especially from areas not at the epicenter of the epidemic, continue to engage in high-risk behavior. *Community-level risk reduction programs* appear to be the most efficacious available and are necessary for changing large populations. *Antibody testing*, when combined with counseling and completed with assurances of confidentiality and anonymity, can be effective in lowering rates of high-risk behavior. *Face-to-face group programs* may be effective in reaching some groups of men, especially those who have been recalcitrant to change. These strategies, however, reach considerably fewer people. *Contact tracing* has not been evaluated adequately to determine the efficacy of this approach.

Methodological problems in this research include: lack of data on the reliability and validity of various periods for assessing sexual behavior, data only on urban gay men, and data collected against the background of considerable information on AIDS. *Data collection and evaluation* needs include more studies to pinpoint the prevalence and incidence of disease and high-risk behaviors in specific communities. These data are essential for local and national planning efforts. *Specific groups have been neglected* in this research, including Black and Latino gay and bisexual men, low-income and low-education individuals, homosexual adolescents, bisexuals, and persons who use alcohol and drugs during sex. *Intervention strategies* showing promise, but needing evaluation, include community intervention approaches, focused counseling at STD clinics, health care providers, and condom distribution programs.

INTRODUCTION

The most important AIDS research and public health agenda is to prevent people who do not have HIV from getting infected with it. Because there is neither a cure nor a vaccine for AIDS, *only voluntary changes in behavior will stop the epidemic from spreading*. There are many statistics used in discussing AIDS, and they can be difficult to keep in mind. However, one statistic about

HIV stands out about all others: *100%! One hundred percent of those infected with the virus will suffer its consequences either in terms of early mortality or in terms of infections, cancers, or other consequences of weakened immunity.* AIDS is one of the most dangerous viruses affecting humans. There are few other viral infections that are as virulent as HIV (Francis & Chin, 1987).

The first line of treatment for HIV infection, AZT, has proven to be effective in treating some patients with AIDS and offers hope to everyone infected with HIV (Fischl et al., 1987; Yarchoan & Broder, 1987). Most encouraging are the reports of beneficial effects with patients with ARC. Not only were the death rates less (3.3% for those on drug vs. 27.5% for those taking placebo), but also the side effects were less for persons with ARC as well. However, it is important to note that after one year, the death rate among patients on AZT was 6%; 45% of all persons on the drug experienced bone marrow suppression resulting from anemia and neutropenia.

The drugs currently under investigation here in the U.S. and elsewhere offer additional hope and consolation. However, given the action of retroviruses, it is probable that a cure for AIDS will be very hard to find. *HIV infection will probably be a chronic infection. Those who have it will need to be treated for life.* The medical community has been struggling with many chronic diseases such as hypertension and diabetes for a long time, yet these conditions are still associated with premature morbidity and mortality.

AIDS was identified initially in gay and bisexual men; in fact, it was first named Gay-Related Immunodeficiency Syndrome, or "GRIDS." A total of 65% of the reported cases in the United States are among gay and bisexual men with no other risk factors; an additional 8% of cases have occurred among men who are homosexual and IV drug users. The Centers for Disease Control projects little change in these distributions through 1991. Thus, for good reasons, considerable attention has been devoted to identifying the risk factors (sexual and drug use) and describing the prevalence of specific activities related to transmission in these groups. Educational programs have been targeted at the gay and bisexual communities, and there has also been a focus on identifying what more can be done to contain the spread of infection in these risk groups.

THE EPIDEMIOLOGY OF HIV INFECTION BY MALE-TO-MALE SEXUAL CONTACT

This report of behavior change will focus on three outcomes of interest: number of male sexual partners, unprotected receptive and insertive anal intercourse, and condom use. Focus on these three outcomes is justified by current epidemiological studies, which have consistently reported an association between these variables and seropositivity (Friedland & Klein, 1987).

Epidemiological data on the transmission of HIV within homosexual men were limited, in the early research, to inferences drawn from cross-sectional and case-control studies. Several of these investigations showed that receptive anal intercourse, receptive manual-anal intercourse ("fisting"), and a large number of male sexual partners were the major risk factors for AIDS and seropositivity to HIV (Goedert et al., 1984; Jaffe et al., 1983; Melbye et al., 1984). These initial investigations also showed a low risk of exposure from oral-genital contact (Jeffries et al., 1985; Lyman, Ascher, & Levy, 1986; Scheuter et al., 1986).

These observations have been replicated and refined in the longitudinal analyses of the San Francisco Men's Health Study (SFMHS) and the Multi-center AIDS Cohort Studies (MACS). The SFMHS is a prospective study of a random sample of single men 25 to 54 years of age who live in the 19 census tracts of San Francisco where the AIDS epidemic has been the most intense. Subjects were interviewed semi-annually, and serologic and immuno-logic status and physical examination findings were documented at these semi-annual clinic visits. Winkelstein et al. (1987b) reported that a high number of sexual partners and the practice of anal receptive intercourse were associated with seropositivity. Those homosexual/bisexual men reporting no partners or a single partner during the two years before entry had relatively low levels of HIV seropositivity (18.1%) compared to those reporting two to nine partners (31.6%). For those reporting more that 50 partners in the two years before entry, the prevalence was increased by a factor of four (70.8%). Those practicing receptive anal intercourse (or both receptive and insertive) had an adjusted relative risk of 2.1 (p = .004) and 2.5 ($p < .001$, respectively), compared to 1.3 (p = .38) and 1.0 for those practicing only insertive or no anal intercourse, respectively. The relative risk for oral-genital contact only was 1.01 (p = .97; see also Lyman et al., 1986). Douche or enema before sexual contact contributed to risk of infection by receptive anal contact.

The MACS extended these finding by defining risk factors for seroconversion in a longitudinal study. This collaborative study recruited a cohort of homosexual and bisexual men from four locations (Los Angeles, Baltimore, Chicago, and Pittsburgh). Baseline examinations were obtained on 4,955 men. Receptive fisting, enema/douch use before intercourse, and perianal bleeding were strongly associated with prevalent HIV infection in the cross-sectional analysis (MACS, 1985). In a report dealing with 2,507 men who were seronegative at the beginning of the study and who completed the six-month follow-up examination, Kingsley et al. (1987) reported a seroconversion rate of 3.8% (N = 95). Receptive anal intercourse was the major mode of acquisition of HIV infection; discontinuation of this practice sharply reduced the likelihood of seroconversion in 6 to 12 months of follow-up. Receptive anal intercourse was the only sexual practice associated with a increased risk of seroconversion to HIV in this study and could account for nearly all new infections. The gradient of risk of seroconversion accelerated in proportion to the number of receptive anal partners, from about 3-fold for one partner to 18-fold for those with 5 or more partners during the observation period. Six of the 9 seroconverters who denied receptive anal intercourse in the 6-month longitudinal follow-up period practiced this activity within the 6 months before the initial evaluation. The remaining 3 seroconverters denying this activity practiced insertive anal intercourse during the pre-enrollment and followup period. Detels, Visscher, Kingsley, and Chmiel (1987) reported no seroconversions over 18 months for those not practicing receptive or insertive anal intercourse and 60% of those failing to seroconvert who engaged in sexual practices without anal intercourse.

None of the investigations are willing to rule out the risk associated with other sexual activities. The sizes of the subsamples under study for these practices generally have been insufficient to provide the necessary statistical power to reject the possibility of even the small relative risks demonstrated for these practices. However, further analyses and studies are needed to define more precisely the risk associated with these practices or to determine that they are, in fact, safe, even when with an infected individual.

Condom Use

Safer-sex guidelines list use of condoms during anal intercourse as "possibly safe (or unsafe)" rather than in the "unsafe" category. This strategy is supported by behavioral theory, which indicates that substitution of acceptable alternatives for proscribed behaviors is more likely to lead to a reduction in those behaviors than the proscription alone (Kelly & St. Lawrence, 1986). The transmission of HIV infection in the natural environment with the use of condoms is not known. Several studies have demonstrated the impermeability of condoms to STD agents. Conant, Hardy, Sematinger, Spicer, & Levy (1986) found that condoms were also effective barriers against HIV. A total of 12 varieties of latex and natural-membrane condoms were tested as barriers to HSV 1 and 2, CMV, and HIV. None of the viral agents passed through the latex, while there was occasional leakage with the latex condoms. Nonoxynol-9 was also found to be cytotoxic to HIV (Schesney, Gantz, & Sullivan, 1987). Studies designed to estimate the failure rate (and the reasons for these failures) using HIV infection as the dependent measures are under way.[1]

---

[1]We are aware of one such study funded by the National Institute of Child Health and Human Development currently beginning at UCLA; Roger Detels is the Principal Investigator.

TABLE 7.1
Description of Studies

Study	Sample N and Source	Age	% White	Income (> $20K)	Education (some college)
SAN FRANCISCO					
AIDS Behavioral Research Project (McKusick et al., 1985)	454, volunteers	M = 32	90%	—	67%
San Francisco Men's Health Study (Winkelstein et al., 1987a)	816, probability sample	Range = 25–55	87.4%	—	88%
Hepatitis B/AIDS Cohort (Doll, 1987)	126	M = 39	87%	—	M = 15.3 yrs.
Communication Technologies (1987)	500, random-digit dial	M = 37.6	87%	63%	—
NEW YORK					
Martin (1987)	745, volunteers	Range = 20–65	87%	$25,000 (Median)	—
Juran (1987)	108, volunteers	—	—	—	—
Siegel (1987)	162, volunteers	M = 37	—	30% > $35K	95%
OTHER AREAS					
MACS (Chicago, Baltimore, L.A., Pittsburgh)	4,955 volunteers	Median = 35	95%	—	87%
Klein et al. (1987) (L.A.)	132, university students and physicians	Range = 18–48	—	—	—
Communication Technologies (1987) (L.A.)	400, random-digit dial	Range = 21–60	86%	72%	89%
Joseph et al. (1987b) (Chicago)	465, Chicago	—	—	—	—
Kelly & St. Lawrence (1987a) (Mississippi)	100, response to ads and flyers	Range = 19–59	MACS 88%	35%	—
Calabrase (1987)	637, gay picnic and bars	Range = 17–67	90.1%	49.4%	74.5%
Jones et al. (1987)	166, gay paper and community AIDS or-ganization	M = 32	—	M = $16,000	M = 15

HOW MUCH BEHAVIOR CHANGE HAS OCCURRED?

Studies of Sexual Behavior in Gay and Bisexual Men

Table 7.1 presents the studies documenting change in sexual behavior among gay and bisexual men using cross-section, retrospective, or longitudinal designs. Four studies were available from San Francisco, three from New York, two from Los Angeles, and several from other cities in the middle to low prevalence ranges for AIDS.

San Francisco

The AIDS Behavioral Research Project (McKusick et al., 1984, 1985) recruited 824 volunteers from bars, baths, and advertisements, requesting men in relationships or who were celibate. *The Hepatitis B/AIDS Cohort* (Doll et al., 1987) was recruited to test the prevalence and prevention of hepatitis B. viruses. Two studies using population-based samples recruited through different methods have also been completed in San Francisco. *The San Francisco Men's Health Study* (Winkelstein, Samual, Padian, Wiley, & Lang, 1987b) cohort was selected using multi-stage household sampling techniques from the 19 census tracts in San Francisco with the highest cumulative incidence of AIDS. *Communication Technologies* (1987) conducted 30-minute telephone surveys in 1984 of 500 self-identified gay and bisexual men residing in the City and County of San Francisco. Households were selected according to a scheme weighting each census tract for the number of unmarried males in that tract. Random households were selected from listed telephones in the census tracts. In the fourth wave, 189 interviews were conducted with respondents interviewed at times one through three; an additional 201 cross-sectional interviews were completed to test sensitization effects. In each assessment, about 75% of the qualified contacted respondents completed an interview.

New York

Martin (1987) recruited 291 subjects through gay organizations, public health clinics, and a gay pride festival. An additional 454 were recruited through referrals to the study from the original 291 subjects. The major criteria for entry into the study were self-identification as gay, living in New York, and not diagnosed with AIDS. Juran (1987) studied 108 individuals recruited from gay bars in Greenwich Village; these people were compared with additional subjects recruited from heterosexual bars. Siegel, Mesagno, Chen, & Christ, (1987) studied 162 asymptomatic gay men recruited into a longitudinal study of patterns of change and stability in gay men's sexual practices.

TABLE 7.2
Behavior Changes

Study	Design and Assessment Period	Male Sexual Partners		Unprotected Anal Intercourse, Receptive		Unprotected Anal Intercourse, Insertive	
		Baseline	Last Assessment	Baseline	Last Assessment	Baseline	Last Assessment
AIDS Behavioral (SF)	longitudinal 30 days	1984 —	1986 —	1984 22.3%	1986 7.2%	1984 34.7%	1986 15.4%
SFMHS (SF)	longitudinal 6 mos	1984 —	1985 —	1984 14.4%[1]	1985 5.8%	1984 39.6%[2]	1985 13.3%
Hep B/ AIDS (SF)	longitudinal 4 mos	1978 Median = 16[3]	1985 Median = 1.5	1978 10.9[4]	1985 0.4	1978 12.9	1985 1.0
Comm. Tech. (SF)	longitudinal and cross sectional 30 days	1984 Mean = 1.8	1987 1.0	1984 Mean = 0.4[5]	1987 0.0	1984 —	1987 —
Martin (NYC)	retrospective annual	1980–81 Mean = 36	1984–85 8	1980–81 Mean = 70	1984–85 20	1980–81 Mean = 85	1984–85 25
Juran (NYC)	retrospective annual	1983 Median = 5	1986 3	1983 —	1986 —	1983 —	1986 —
Siegel (NYC)	prospective 30 days	1984–85 87.4%	1985–86 71.7%	1984–85 —	1985–86 —	1984–85 —	1985–86 —

Study	Design						
MACS	prospective / 6 mos	1984	1986	1984 71%	1986 51%	1984 80%	1986 55%
Klein (L.S.)	retrospective / 6 mos / MD's	—	—	79%	35.3%	90%	46.5%
	students	—	—	79%	60.9%	84%	67.3
Comm. Tech. (L.A.)	cross sectional / 30 days	—	1986 Mean = 1.8	—	1986 Mean = 1.6	—	1986
Joseph (Chicago)	longitudinal / 6 mos	1984	1985	1984 40%	1985 10%	1984	1985
Johnson & McGrath (Texas)	retrospective / 30 days	1984–85	1986–87 38.8% > 2	1984–85	1986–87 25.1%	1984–85	1986–87
Kelly (Miss.)	cross sectional / 12 mos	—	1986 Mean = 15	—	1986 Mean = 19.7	—	1986 Mean = 19.4
Hackert (Minn.)	cross sectional	—	—	—	—	—	—
Calabrese (Ohio)	cross sectional	—	—	—	—	—	—
Jones (New Mexico)	cross sectional	—	1985	—	1985 107	—	1985

[1] HIV negative only.
[2] HIV positive only.
[3] Non-steady partners (sexual contact only once or twice)
[4] N Partners x percent of time engaged in activity
[5] Mean receptive and insertive anal intercourse

Los Angeles

Communication Technologies (1986) completed a random telephone survey of listed households in 40 census tracts in Hollywood, West Hollywood, and Silver Lake (the areas with the presumed highest concentration of gay men) with a response rate of 59%. Klein et al. (1987) surveyed 132 gay-identified physicians and university students regarding their sexual practices.

Other Areas

The *MACS* recruited 4,955 volunteers from Chicago, Pittsburgh, Baltimore, and Los Angeles. Baseline assessments occurred between April 1984 and March 1985. The last assessment occurred between April 1986 and March 1987 and included 3,581 (73% of baseline) participants (Fox, Odaka, Brookmeyer, & Polk, 1987). Joseph et al. (1987) are completing intensive studies on MACS participants from the Chicago site. Volunteer samples have also been studied in *Mississippi* (Kelly et al., 1987), *Minnesota* (Hackert, 1987b), *Ohio* (Calabrese, 1987), *Texas* (Johnson & McGrath, et al., 1987) and *New Mexico* (Jones et al., 1987).

The majority of the subjects in these studies were white and college educated (see Table 7.1). Further limits on generalizability include the fact that most used volunteer samples. When probability samples were drawn, they occurred from defined areas (SFMHS) or used techniques that sampled only listed households. Longitudinal studies have been conducted only in San Francisco, New York, and the cities involved in the MACS (L.A., Chicago, Pittsburgh, and Baltimore).

Changes in Behavior

Table 7.2 presents changes in reported sexual behavior and the time periods for which these changes were documented. Dramatic behavior changes have occurred, and this accomplishment needs to be acknowledged. The amount and kinds of changes probably exceed anything documented to date in the public health education field or literature. In addition, it appears that these behavior changes are sustaining over time. Most behavior change efforts (e.g., in the areas of weight loss, tobacco use, drug and alcohol use, exercise) result in fairly high recidivism rates; relapse and maintenance are often perceived to be more difficult than the original change itself. Thus, in one sense, the overall AIDS risk-reduction campaign is working among gay and bisexual men, at least to the extent that these studies provide an accurate reflection of the degree of change in this risk group.

The San Francisco studies report the greatest magnitude of changes. The Hepatitis B/AIDS Cohort study reported, over a seven-year period of assessment, reductions of 91% in number of male sexual partners, and 96% and

92.2% reductions in unprotected anal intercourse, receptive and insertive respectively. The AIDS Behavioral Research Project documented reductions of 45.6% in unprotected anal intercourse from 1984 to 1986. The San Francisco Men's Health Study (Winkelstein et al., 1987a) reported reductions of 59.7% (receptive) and 66.4% (insertive) in unprotected anal intercourse. Communication Technologies (1987) reported 100% (receptive) and 80% (insertive) declines in these activities.

New York results are more variable. Martin (1987) reported 71 to 77% reductions in number of male sexual partners and number of incidents of anal intercourse in the previous year. Siegel et al. (1987), however, reported only an 18% reduction in the percentage of persons having multiple male sexual partners. Anal intercourse data were not reported.

The MACS (Fox et al., 1987) reported only a 28% decline in receptive anal intercourse (with 48% of the men still practicing this activity at the last assessment) and a 28% decline in insertive anal intercourse (with 55% of the men still practicing this activity at the last assessment). Joseph et al. (1987a) reported a 75% decline on this variable, but this was among a subset of the Chicago MACS subjects volunteering for their substudy. Fox et al. (1987) reported no differences in behavior changes among the four study sites. Thus, the changes reported by Joseph et al. (1987) are in excess of the entire cohort.

Current Levels of High-Risk Behaviors

Levels of high-risk behavior are lowest in San Francisco. The mean/median number of sexual partners for 1986 was estimated at 1 to 1.5; only 1 to 6% of the population were engaging in unprotected receptive anal intercourse (Communication Technologies, 1987; Winkelstein et al., 1987a). This low rate of high-risk behaviors probably accounts for the flattened rates of seroconversion reported by Winkelstein et al. (1987a) and the sharp decline in the incidence of rectal gonorrhea reported by the San Francisco Department of Health (see Pickering et al., 1986).

Reports from New York and the MACS raise serious concerns about continued levels of high-risk behaviors in other areas.

. Men in the Martin (1987) cohort reported a mean of 20 individuals with whom they had practiced receptive anal intercourse and 25 individuals with whom they had practiced insertive anal intercourse in the past 12 months.

. Forty-eight percent of the MACS participants reported engaging in receptive intercourse in 1986; 55% of the MACS participants engaged in insertive anal intercourse at the last visit. They reported using condoms with only 35% and 41% of partners.

. The mean number of partners with whom one had engaged in unprotected anal intercourse in Los Angeles in 1986 was 1.6, compared to 1.0 in San Francisco in 1986 (Communication Technologies, 1986, 1987).

. Participants in Mississippi reported a mean of 19.7 partners with whom they had practiced unprotected receptive anal intercourse during the past 12 months (Kelly, Lawrence, Hood, & Brasfield, 1987a).

. Of men at New Mexico STD clinics, 70% reported practicing receptive anal intercourse during the preceding 12 months; 87% stated that their partners used condoms in less than 10% of the receptive exposures (Jones et al., 1987). Thus, 67% of the participants practiced receptive anal intercourse without condoms.

. Of men in the Texas study, 25.1% reported practicing receptive anal intercourse (Johnson & McGrath, 1987).

. Of Men in a study in Boston, 35% reported practicing unprotected anal intercourse in the previous month (McKusker et al., 1987).

. In Vancouver, Canada, 35% of seronegatives and 7% of seropositives reported never using condoms during anal intercourse (Willoughby et al., 1987).

Table 7.3 presents available data on condom use, as the risk-reduction campaigns have stressed the importance of using condoms if a person chooses to engage in intercourse with anyone besides a steady partner with whom one has had a monogamous relationship for several years, or with whom one now has monogamous relationship and the HIV status of the partner is known. As can be seen in Table 7.3, very little is known and reported, regarding condom use at baseline, and condom use increases over time. While several reports have documented a decline in overall sexual activity, it is difficult to evaluate the degree to which these current levels of condom use are beneficial or not. Fox et al. (1987) reported that participants used condoms with 34% of partners, up from 14% at baseline. However, data were not presented on the percentage of persons who practiced any unprotected anal intercourse at each assessment. This assessment is necessary to determine the absolute level of risk reduction in these communities.

A report on condom use by Valdiserri, Lyter, Callahan, Kingsley, & Rinaldo, (1987) reinforces the concern that behavior changes are minimal outside of the major areas (San Francisco and, perhaps, New York). In a study of the men in the Pittsburgh site of the MACS, 65% (N = 328) reported at least one episode of anal intercourse during the six months prior to the period of 5-1-86 and 12-1-86. Sixty-two percent of these reported that they never or hardly ever used condoms during anal intercourse. A total of 91% identified receptive anal intercourse as the highest-risk sexual activity for AIDS transmission, and 90% endorsed the belief that condoms can "reduce the spread of AIDS." Reasons for not using condoms were that condoms spoil sex (22%), purchasing condoms is embarrassing (18%), using condoms turns partners off (16%), condoms are not readily available (22%), or condoms are used only by straights (26%).

TABLE 7.3
Condom Use

Study	Baseline	Last Assessment	% Change
New York			
Martin (1987)	1980–81	1984–85	
Insertive	1%	20%	11%
Receptive	2%	19%	85%
Juran (1987)	1983	1986	
	—	41%	
Siegel et al. (1987)	1985–85	1985–86	
	—	—	
San Francisco			
AIDS Behavioral	1982	1984	
Research Project	14.1%	23.8%	68.7%
SFMHS	1984	1985	
	—	—	
Hepatitis B/CDC	1978	1985	
	—	—	
Comm. Tech.	1984	1987	
	Mean = 0.03	0.3	0%
		23% always	
Other Areas			
MACS (Fox et al., 1987)	—	—	
	—	—	
Klein (L.A.)	—	—	
Comm. Tech.	—	1986	
	—	Mean = 1.5[1]	
Joseph (Chicago)	—	—	
Kelly (Mississippi)	—	1986	
Insertive	Mean = 3.0		
Receptive	Mean = 4.6		
Hackert (Minn.)	—	—	
Calabrase (Ohio)	—	—	
Jones (New Mexico)	—	1985	
	—	< 10%[2]	
Johnson and McGrath (Texas)	—	—	

[1]Excluding those in monogamous relationships.
[2]< of the 70% who engage in receptive anal intercourse.

TABLE 7.4
Prevalence of AIDS and Declines in Gonorrhea and Syphilis

City	AIDS Cases[1] (per 1,000 pop.)	Gonorrhea[2] (1980-85 change)	Syphilis[2] (1980-85 change)
San Francisco	1.25	-62.6%	-48.9%
New York	1.19	-10.0%	+1.6%
Jersey City	0.88	+7.1%	+1.2%
Miami	0.72	-50.4%	+57.4%
Newark, NJ	0.53	-10.0%	+5.3%
Houston	0.49	-49.0%	+13.9%
Los Angeles	0.48	+1.6%	-25.6%
Washington, DC	0.42	-8.2%	-33.9%
Atlanta	0.33	-21.0%	-18.2%
New Orleans	0.30	-14.9%	-26.4%
San Diego	0.29	-21.0%	-21.0%
Dallas	0.27	-21.0%	+31.6%
Seattle	0.25	-38.2%	-66.6%
Denver	0.24	-27.0%	-23.2%
Boston	0.24	-6.2%	+7.5%
U.S. Total	0.17	-13.4%	-13.0%

[1]Source: AIDS Weekly Surveillance Report—United States, October 12, 1987.
[2]Source: U.S. Department of Health and Human Services, Sexually Transmitted Disease Statistics, Calendar Year 1985 (1987).

Sexually Transmitted Diseases

Data on the incidence of gonorrhea have been cited as corroboration for remarkable behavioral changes made by gay men. Gonorrhea dropped by 32% in gay men in Denver (Judson, 1983), by 57% in Seattle (Hansfield, 1985), and by 63% in San Francisco (Zenilman, Cates, & Morse, 1986). Rectal and pharyngeal infections reported from males in New York City declined 59% during the years 1980 to 1983 (Hansfield, 1985). However, examination of declines in case rates per 100,000 population from 1980 to 1985 reveal uneven declines among cities in the high, middle, and low prevalence range for AIDS. Table 7.4 presents AIDS cases reported per 1,000 population, and the changes in cases of gonorrhea and syphilis from 1980 to 1985 (the latest data available as of this writing). Consistent and important changes have occurred in San Francisco and Seattle. Moderate, but still important, changes have occurred in Atlanta, New Orleans, San Diego, and Denver. The following cities cause concern because of increases in both gonorrhea and syphilis (e.g., Jersey City), or because one index has declined while the other has increased or remained stable: New York, Newark, Los Angeles, Washington, D.C., Boston, and Dallas.

Concern has been raised because of increases in primary and secondary syphilis in the United States. After a five-year trend of decreasing incidence, there was an increase of 23% over the cases reported in the first three months of 1986 (CDC, 1987). The three areas reporting the largest numerical increases were California, Florida, and New York City. Demographic data were available from these three areas. Primary and secondary syphilis declined by 47% in California and by 51% in New York among homosexual/bisexual males. However, cases increased by 108% in Florida among homosexual/ bisexual males.

Conclusions

Behavioral and STD data reveal that important behavior changes have occurred in many areas in the United States. However, some major metropolitan areas of the U.S. may be plagued by continuing levels of high-risk behaviors. In addition, it is possible that behavior has not changed substantially in this high-risk group in suburban or rural areas or those cities with low prevalence and incidence of AIDS.

Reliable data are not available for many areas. Knowledge of current levels of risk is essential if program planning is going to reflect the behavioral and attitudinal realities of high-risk groups. While rates of seroprevalence among gay and bisexual men may have leveled off in some cities, it is possible that windows of opportunity exist in other locales to prevent further infection in this high-risk group (see Friedland & Klein, 1987). Communities need to collect data on the behavior of high-risk groups, such as gay and bisexual men, and the CDC should be able to provide indicators of change using demographic data in STD surveillance.

The data collected by Communication Technologies provide an important and prime example of the importance of local data in reflecting changes in the community and indicating directions of research campaigns. Similar strategies have been used to great advantage by the British (British Market Research Bureau, Ltd., 1987). These data are essential to determine motivators of behaviors and to document accurately if risk-reduction programs are working in the groups that need to change.

THE IMPACT OF EDUCATIONAL PROGRAMS
ON HIGH-RISK BEHAVIORS

AIDS risk reduction depends on knowledge (of AIDS, how it is transmitted and how to reduce risk), a sense of personal susceptibility (the belief that I, too, can become infected with the AIDS virus), skills for changing (i.e., how to use prophylactics, how to negotiate safer-sex), a sense of personal efficacy (I can make the changes necessary to reduce risk for AIDS), and the perception that community norms support AIDS risk reduction (McKusick et al., 1985). Achieving these objectives requires maximizing opportunities for the transmission of knowledge, using specific methods for teaching skills, and devising and implementing strategies for changing and mobilizing community norms. These objectives are best reached through systematic, organized, and continuous community interventions which are multiple channels of communication to teach information, motivate through skill development, and modify community norms.

The changes observed in San Francisco, compared to those made in other cities, reflect the results that can be expected from concerted and systematic community organization and intervention. San Francisco's risk-reduction efforts have been quite successful; data converge from behavioral studies, from estimates of seroconversion, and from STD data to indicate that transmission among gay and bisexual men is quite low. Communication Technologies (1987) suggested that six elements contributed to the success of the San Francisco risk-reduction program:

(1) a community-based program including strong leadership from within the gay community;

(2) market research techniques to identify appropriate messages and communication channels for reaching the target audience;

(3) programs to inform and motivate target audiences;

(4) a focus on facilitating social and cultural change;

(5) reliance on multiple channels of communication including print, broadcast, and face-to-face channels of communication; and

(6) broad-scale grass-roots participation.

Community-Based AIDS Risk-Reduction Programs

Community-based approaches are aimed at providing individuals with information and skills for behavior change, and simultaneously providing a supportive social environment that supports engagement in behaviors to prevent the spread of AIDS. From the perspective of social learning theory, the commonly noted problem of sustaining health-related behaviors is well known (Bandura, 1977). While some individuals may be able to act on knowledge alone and others may be able to provide self-reinforcement for activity, many individuals have difficulty making and sustaining meaningful changes in behavior. However, when specific health-related behaviors become less socially acceptable in a community (and others are sanctioned to take their place); and when perceived social sanctions regarding unhealthy behaviors are persistent, inescapable, and concentrated on a sufficiently regular basis, the individual is much more likely to both initiate and maintain healthful behaviors. Thus, community-based programs are designed to channel interventions through major community structures and groups to provide information, skills, and ongoing support. The objective is to create a sum greater than the parts through synergistic action around community-wide AIDS prevention events and activities.

The Centers for Disease Control is sponsoring AIDS Community Demonstration Projects as flexible, community-based research centers in six locations across the country (Denver, Seattle—King County, Dallas County, Denver City and County, and New York State and City, Long Beach, and Chicago). The exact nature of the interventions differs from site to site, and the sites vary in the range of activities they employ. Generally, however, the interventions aim at three levels. At the broadest level, the interventions include public health communications to provide factual information about HIV infection and to create the impression that prevailing social norms support changes to lower risk behaviors. At a second level, the interventions include antibody testing to provide a cue to change behavior. Finally, the interventions include a variety of methods targeted to individuals resistant to change, individuals requiring additional help or skills to make changes, or individuals who have trouble maintaining the changed behaviors they have adopted.

The interventions will be evaluated by enrolling and following cohorts of homosexual or bisexual men (up to 1,000 per site). The men are screened for antibodies to HIV at entry, and then followed for behavioral changes and seroconversion every 6 months. The costs of the interventions for FY 1988 range from $382,430 (Dallas County) to $874,667 (Seattle—King County). Evaluations of these programs are under way and will be reported initially at the IV International Conference on AIDS in Stockholm. They should add significant and substantial data on the efficacy of concerted community-based programs on AIDS-related behavior change in the gay and bisexual community.

Adrien (1987) reported on a campaign to promote safe sexual practices among Montreal's homosexual population. The campaign included methods for disseminating the campaign slogan "Play Safe" (through advertisements in gay and regular media). Health education pamphlets on safe sex and condoms were distributed to 27 bars, clubs, and baths, representing the majority of the establishments serving the homosexual community. Condom vending machines were also installed in participating establishments. A survey was distributed one month following the campaign; 839 (77.9% response rate) respondents answered. Of these, 36.4% and 17.6% engaged in active and passive anal intercourse, respectively, without a condom. In addition, 34.3% used a condom in anal intercourse; 75.4% of these indicated that the campaign had influenced their behavior. There is no way to determine the ultimate impact of the campaign, due to lack of baseline data. However, the impact appears to be important and impressive.

Knowledge of Risk-Reduction Guidelines

Many of the organized efforts to prevent further HIV infection are focused on communication of health education messages regarding the risks of specific behaviors for acquiring or spreading HIV. Information is a necessary, but not a sufficient condition for change. Emmons, Joseph, Kessler, Montgomery, and Ostrow, (1986), using cross-sectional data from the Chicago MACS cohort, found that knowledge of AIDS risk was most strongly associated with reductions in risk behavior. The variables used for predicting change were perceived risk of AIDS, perceived efficacy of behavior change, barriers to behavior change, social network characteristics, and knowledge. Joseph et al. (1987) found that knowledge did not predict maintenance of behavior change in longitudinal analyses. McKusick et al. (1987) found five variables to be significantly related to sustained low-risk activity in a multiple regression analysis. Level of agreement with AIDS risk-reduction guidelines was significantly, but weakly, associated with the dependent variable.

Individuals must understand and believe the reasons for adapting pleasurable, intimate, and day-to-day activities before they are likely to attempt such changes. But, as in all areas of health education, information alone is not potent enough to change large segments of the population.

Antibody Testing

Antibody testing has been advocated as a method for encouraging behavior change. Testing should be accompanied by education and counseling for risk reduction, with appropriate referrals for follow-up medical and psychological care. Proponents have claimed that testing might motivate reductions in high-risk behavior. Opponents have claimed that the risks of discrimination or psychological distress far outweigh the benefits of mandatory testing and that high-risk persons have already been motivated to reduce risk of infection anyway. Data are available on the AIDS Behavioral Research Cohort beginning in 1984 before antibody testing was available; the most recent survey of the cohort occurred in November 1986. Testing for antibodies to HIV was done under the best conditions available, due to the California laws protecting confidentiality of results and mandating pre- and post-testing counseling and education.

Before testing was available, a majority (69%) indicated that they desired testing. Interestingly, by 6 to 8 months after testing had been available, only 23% had been tested and only 8% still desired testing. By November 1986, still less than a majority had been tested. This may well have changed, however, due to the increase in testing in the general population since that time. The majority (88%) were tested at the Alternative Testing Centers, and most received counseling (82%) and the results face to face. Most said that they would do it over again and learn the results again. Not surprisingly, this was more true of those who tested negative than those who tested positive.

Did the testing and counseling process make a difference in high-risk sexual behavior? Coates, Morin, and McKusick (1987) reported that significant and substantial changes occurred among those tested. However, the more striking result occurs among those who (unfortunately) found out that they were antibody positive in November 1986. Of those who were antibody positive, 12% reported practicing unprotected insertive anal intercourse in the past month, compared to 18% of those who were antibody negative and 27% of those who had not yet been tested ($X^2 = 7.04, p = .02$). All three groups reported significantly higher rates of unprotected insertive anal intercourse in November 1984 (before antibody testing was available and before they knew their status): 48% of those who ultimately tested positive versus 49% of those who had not been tested and 41% of those who ultimately tested negative ($X^2 = 1.34, p = .51$). These investigators also examined the proportion of protected to unprotected intercourse: Antibody positives practiced protected intercourse 80% of the time, while the other two groups practiced this behavior only 60% of the time.

Stempel and Moulton (1987), also in San Francisco, examined the knowledge of HIV antibody status on 126 subjects who were part of an ongoing epidemiological study of AIDS. Changes were found in levels of unsafe sexual practices. About 20% reported practicing unsafe sex before notification, and this was reduced to 10% at three months post-notification. There was a slight, but not significant, increase in distress among the seropositives, and a decrease in the same variable among seronegatives. Thus, it appears that antibody testing can contribute to additional change with minimal distress when counseling and education are adequate.

Fox et al. (1987) reported on 1,001 gay men from the Baltimore-Washington site of MACS who were offered the opportunity to learn their HIV antibody status; 670 (67%) elected to do so. Disclosure of results occurred during the third clinic visit (April to October 1985); participants were given results with individual counseling and education about the results, their meaning, and the importance of safer-sex practices. Follow-up data on sexual practices were obtained six months later at the next clinic visit. There were no differences between men electing and not electing to receive their results in terms of age, race, number of male partners in the six months before disclosure, and proportion with antibodies to HIV. Those ultimately finding out that they were seropositive were more likely at baseline to be more sexually active and to practice unprotected anal intercourse than those ultimately finding out that they were seronegative. There were striking results by HIV status.

Seropositives and negatives differed at baseline in mean level of sexual partners and activities; means at the final follow-up differed only slightly (although standard deviations appear to vary markedly among the four groups). For this reason, results were presented as percent change at follow-up from baseline in number of persons with whom an individual engaged in unprotected anal intercourse. Aware seropositives decreased unprotected insertive anal intercourse to 42% of baseline levels (compared to 59% for seronegatives and 52% for the uninformed group); aware seropositives decreased unprotected receptive intercourse to 42% of baseline (compared to 62% for the seronegative group and 57% for the uninformed group). All differences between informed and uninformed groups were statistically significant.

McCusker et al. (1988) reported the impact of antibody test results on 290 gay men in Boston. The level of all sexual activities of all study participants declined over time. There were no differences in receptive anal intercourse among those receiving versus not receiving their results with 58% (of 125) of those initially practicing unprotected intercourse still practicing unprotected receptive anal intercourse six months after initial assessment. Of those who received test results and who practiced insertive anal intercourse at baseline, 60% still practiced this activity six months later; this included 62% of those who found out that they were negative and 52% of those who found out that they were positive. Of those who practiced this activity at baseline, 80% who were positive, but who failed to receive their results, still practiced this activity.

Willoughby et al. (1987) followed a cohort of approximately 600 homosexual men recruited through general practitioners. An analysis of 430 men completing two visits revealed that 150 seropositives reduced their mean number of annual sexual partners from 9.2 to 5.8 ($p < .001$) as compared to 280 seronegatives (6.9 to 6.7, ns). Even when the analysis was restricted to those in the highest 50% of sexual behavior, the seropositives changed more than the seronegatives (16.2 to 7.7 partners, $p < .001$; compared to 15.6 to 10.9 partners, $p < .001$). In addition, 35% of the seronegatives, but only 7% of the seropositives reported never using condoms during receptive anal intercourse.

Not all studies report a positive effect of HIV antibody notification on behavior. Soucey (1986) reported on the participants in the Chicago MACS who elected to learn their HIV antibody results. As of that report, 200 of 800 men received their results; 74 of these men were in the Joseph et al. (1987a) cohort and were studied. Thirty-four were positive, and 40 were negative. Up to three months following disclosure, there was one significant difference between seropositives receiving and not receiving disclosure of results. Those who were positive and received their results increased receptive anal contact compared to those who were positive and did not receive their results. In addition, those who were positive and received their results increased in mental health symptoms compared to those who did not receive their results. Thus, the mental health consequences of disclosure and a possible adverse consequence in terms of risk were suggested. Larger samples and more follow-up are needed to confirm these findings.

The costs of antibody testing with appropriate counseling and education have been computed by the Coalition for AIDS Prevention and Education (1987). This group included in its costs the following necessary elements: (1) pre-test counseling for a minimum of 30 minutes (including individualized risk assessment, recommendations for behavior change, informed consent); (2) testing; (3) post-test counseling for a minimum of 30 minutes to assess reaction to the test result, risk behavior, and need for additional services; and (4) follow-up counseling in special cases where the individual's commitment to behavior change is unclear or where severe psychological distress is evident. The importance of this counseling is important to ensure that the opportunity for testing also provides an opportunity for education and to assess (and intervene, if necessary) the distress level of the client. Clients at alternative testing centers do not necessarily intend to share their test results with primary or secondary sexual partners (Kegeles, Catania, & Coates, in press). Emphasizing the importance of communication may be essential if the primary purpose of testing (namely, decreasing the spread of infection) is accomplished. The average costs are worked out to about $80.00 per person.

Testing can reduce levels of high-risk behavior by 50 to 75% in those studies which have found beneficial effects for testing. The ultimate level of high-risk behavior depends on several factors, including the baseline prevalence of high-risk activity, the prevalence of infection in the community, and other risk-reduction activities in the community.

Contact Tracing

Tracing sexual or needle-sharing contacts of those found to be HIV positive is designed to trace infection to its source. Ideally, appropriate education and counseling of the infected and susceptible contacts will prevent further transmission. While contact tracing would be impossible with individuals who have large numbers of sexual partners (and whose names or addresses might not be known), it might be useful even for high-risk seropositive individuals with few contacts in areas of low prevalence of infection. Contacts with the Colorado Department of Health revealed the following results between January 1986 and September 30, 1987. A total of 265 persons tested positive and were interviewed; about 66% were gay. From those tested, 453 partners were reported; 17% (77) could not be found. Of the 376 (83%) found, 334 had not been tested or had previously tested negative. Of the 334, 21% (70) would not be tested; 264 (79%) were tested and received counseling. Of the 264, 42 (9.3% of the total partners reported and 15.9% of those tested) were positive. The annual budget for contact tracing was reported to be $23,356.88 for salaries[2]; other costs are reportedly negligible. No behavioral follow-up has been conducted on these or the negative individuals, but this should be a high-priority research activity, as this method of disease prevention has important public policy implications.

Face-To-Face Programs

The STOP AIDS Project.

The STOP AIDS Project was begun in San Francisco as an innovative, community-based, peer-support AIDS prevention program. Initial analyses by the originators of this project (Larry Bye and Sam Puckett) indicated that gay men felt helplessly caught between the growing enormity of the AIDS epidemic and the sexual values and expectations of the gay community. The STOP AIDS program uses a focus group model to bring people together to engender a personal commitment to safer sex and personal participation toward ending the AIDS epidemic. More specifically, the program seeks to empower personal action toward stopping the AIDS virus, to hasten the adoption of safer sex as a community norm, to build peer support for safe activities, and to create peer pressure against activities that would spread the epidemic. The intent was to quickly change the social agreement about how gay men have sex, to make safer sex normatively and routinely expected behavior among San Francisco gay males, and to get gay men more personally involved in AIDS prevention.

There are some indications that STOP AIDS met some of its objectives. Communication Technologies (1987) reported in their fourth survey (in 1986) of gay men in San Francisco that 51% (up from 27% in 1985) of the sample had heard of the project; 20% had attended a meeting. STOP AIDS records show that over 7,000 men in San Francisco attended a meeting. No specific analyses were completed (nor, to our knowledge, have studies been done in San Francisco or elsewhere), however, to determine the specific impact of STOP AIDS on behavior.

The STOP AIDS budget in San Francisco for 1986–1987 was $217,864 to serve an estimated 3,500 individuals in groups. That translates to $62.24 per individual in a group. However, the ultimate impact of the program also needs to be estimated in relation to change in the community norms and behaviors of individuals not attending these meetings.

Multi-Session Interventions.

Face-to-face programs may be needed for certain kinds of individuals to change behaviors. Especially when individuals have a long-standing history of

---

[2]These data were provided by Nancy Spencer, Denver Department of Health, (303) 331–8318.

engaging in high-risk activities, when the immediate consequences of the risk behavior are reinforcing, and when the behavior is encouraged or expected by others, more potent behavior change programs may be needed to promote risk reduction. Kelley, Lawrence, Smith, Hood, and Cook, (1987b) recruited and randomized 104 homosexual men with a history of frequent high-risk behavior into experimental and wait-list control groups. The experimental intervention consisted of 12 weekly group sessions which provided AIDS risk education, cognitive behavioral self-management training to refuse coercions, and attention to the development of steady and self-affirming social supports. At four-month follow-ups, men in the experimental group reported only 0.2 episodes of unprotected anal intercourse (compared with 1.2 at baseline) in the previous month. The control group mean was 1.2 (compared to 0.9 at baseline). Experimental subjects reported using condoms in 70% of intercourse occasions at follow-up, compared to 40% at baseline. Comparable rates for control subjects were 20% at follow-up and 32% at baseline. Coates, McKusick, Kuno, and Stites (in press) recruited HIV antibody positive men into a study of the effects of stress management on behavior and immune function. The intervention was an 8-week program of weekly meetings and one retreat emphasizing meditation, relaxation, positive health habits, and coping with the stress of being seropositive. A total of 64 men participated; 32 in the experimental group and 32 in the wait-list control group. At posttreatment, the experimental subjects reported a mean of 0.50 ($\pm$ 0.50) partners in the previous month (1.37 $\pm$ 1.80 at baseline) compared to 2.29 ($\pm$ 3.79) for the control subjects (1.09 $\pm$ 2.44 at baseline; $F = 5.15$, $p = .027$).

Quadland, Shandis, Schuyman, and Jacobs, (1987) are conducting an evaluation of four different AIDS prevention education approaches in New York. These include: (1) informing participants about AIDS and how it is transmitted; (2) a program of eroticizing safer-sex alternatives; (3) the program described in #2 but without audiovisuals; and (4) a comparison group of individuals who simply received copies of safer-sex guidelines. Involved are 619 men being evaluated before and 3 months after the program. About 25% of the participants were still at risk, by virtue of having engaged in at-risk sexual activity in the previous 60 days. No further data were available as of this writing; more details are being requested from the investigators.

Multi-session interventions generally cost between $5,000 and $6,000 to mount. The upper limit of group members is usually set at 12 to 15. Thus, these interventions cost between $400 and $500 per person to conduct.

METHODOLOGICAL ISSUES IN
AIDS PREVENTION RESEARCH

Two methodological issues are paramount in evaluating this research on AIDS risk reduction: sampling and measurement of sexual behavior.

Sampling

Sampling issues have always been a primary methodological challenge in the study of male homosexuals (Morin, 1977; Weinberg, 1970). What we know of the behavioral responses to the AIDS crisis is based, almost without exception, on convenience samples of self-identified gay men living in large coastal cities. The question needs to be raised as to whether self-identified gay males who live in large urban centers and who have been exposed to innovative health-promotion campaigns are representative of all types of men who have sex with other men.

There are good reasons to believe that samples of self-identified gay men who live in large urban centers are not representative of the larger homosexual world. First, the communities of gay men which formed in large urban centers during the 1970s consisted of men who migrated primarily from other locales. Men came to these "magnet" cities (such as New York, San Francisco, and Los Angeles) to gain freedoms unknown in their hometowns and stayed to help build communities (Gorman, 1986). Thus, the gay male communities from which most of the behavior change samples have been drawn should be thought of as migrant or refugee populations. There is little reason to assume that gay men who feel compelled to migrate to large urban centers are the same as other men who also have sex with other men but who choose to stay at home.

Thus, researchers have concentrated their efforts among urban enclaves of openly homosexual men, both for the relatively easy availability of these respondents, and due to the fact that the prevalence and incidence of AIDS is so high within these populations. However, this concentration of research efforts has meant that we know little of the level of risk among homosexual men who live outside major urban settings and who may, or may not, be comfortable discussing the fact that they engage in homosexual behavior.

Although the circumstances under which individuals feel comfortable to "come out" varies considerably, it is almost certainly true that the proportion of men who are behaviorally homosexual and who feel comfortable admitting this fact to others is considerably higher in the magnet cities than in more traditional environments. In short, "gay" men have constructed a part of their social identity around their sexuality, while behaviorally homosexual men have not. The level of infection and high-risk behaviors among this latter group are not represented in any of the studies to date.

Measurement of Sexual Behavior

Attempts to measure sexual risk for HIV infection have relied on self-report. Despite the problems with reliability and validity inherent in these techniques, measures of sexual risk for HIV have demonstrated good construct validity in predicting the prevalence and incidence of HIV exposure. A dimension which is critical to the measurement of risk for HIV exposure has to do with the time period of measurement. One, 6, and 12 months represent the time periods chosen most often. The fact that there is no standardized window complicates efforts to synthesize this body of information. The use of a 1-month period presumably results in a more accurate respondent recall. The 6-month window is useful in measuring all sexual risk that occurs in long-term prospective studies (carried out in 6-month waves) and may also reduce individual variation in risk measurements that have to do with unique characteristics of the previous month. The 12-month window may suffer considerably from recall bias.

Reliability and validity studies are nonexistent in this literature. No one, to date, has determined whether a 1-, 6-, or 12-month period of assessment is best for assessing prevalence and incidence of infection, or for assessing the effects of interventions. It is possible, for example, that the failure to find risk associated with practices other than anal intercourse (e.g., oral sex), even when number of sexual partners remains a risk factor, could be due to the lack of reliability in the assessments of sexual behavior.

An additional issue influencing the evaluation of specific strategies involves the presence of disease in that community. One of the characteristics of the epidemic often noted by impressionistic observers has been that individuals sometimes respond to the threat of AIDS in stages, often involving denial and panic stages. These stages may occur on a community level. For example, Fitzgerald (1987) described the processes by which the gay community in San Francisco faced up to the threat of AIDS, and Des Jarlais (in press) has described stages in the adaptation of the drug addiction treatment community to the AIDS epidemic.

Whether or not such stages exist, it is likely that the time period of measurement of risk reduction within a particular community is likely to affect the outcome of the assessment. As the community response to AIDS becomes more widespread, specific programs are more or less likely to have greater impacts, depending on background strategies, campaigns, and normative beliefs. At this point in the epidemic, the majority of those who continue to engage in high-risk activities have had some contact with health education messages and are likely to be able to identify the sexual behaviors which transmit HIV infection. During the early days of the epidemic, before health education messages were widespread, it is likely that a proportion of those who engaged in high-risk activities had yet to understand that they were placing themselves and their partners at risk. Due to the increasing success (at least in some communities) of health education campaigns to communicate and motivate behavior change, any additional programs will be evaluated against this background of influence.

RESEARCH NEEDS

This report has revealed what is known about AIDS risk reduction among gay and bisexual men, but it is clear that the investigational needs are vast. The following provides an overview of the urgent problems.

Data Collection and Evaluation

Pinpointing Community Behavior.

This research was somewhat frustrating to complete because it revealed the lack of information that exists regarding the behavior of high-risk groups. We were able to locate data on prevalent sexual practices from only a handful of cities: San Francisco, Los Angeles, Chicago, Baltimore, Pittsburgh, and New York. All of the other studies are from small samples of volunteers. Many cities in the middle to high prevalence of ranges of AIDS cases could benefit enormously from better estimates of sexual behavior among gay and bisexual men. The example in San Francisco is clear. Data were collected and used systematically to design educational campaigns. Data were collected further to determine the efficacy of the programs and the pockets of individuals who were not responding to them. Low-prevalence cities might benefit from determining if the conclusions of this study are accurate; namely, that behavior may not be changing where the AIDS epidemic is not overwhelming. Documenting that behavior has not changed and using the information to facilitate program design should be an important priority for these cities.

Uniform Reporting Systems.

There is a clear need for a uniform system for reporting data. Studies need to determine which period of assessment provides the most accurate reflection of an individual's sexual activities. Studies use periods of 1, 3, 4, 6, and 12 months. It is not clear if science or custom dictates the interval. In addition, studies vary in the detail in which they gather and report behavior. At a minimum, it would be useful for each study to ask about the frequency of specific sexual activities that are known to be high risk, and to report both mean frequencies and percentages of individuals engaging in these activities. Comparison among studies is essential; this method of gathering and reporting data would facilitate such comparisons.

Specific Groups Needing Special Research Attention

Black and Latino Gay and Bisexual Men.

AIDS is a major problem for men who are both homosexual and members of ethnic minorities. Of all those at risk for AIDS, Black and Latino gay men may be the least studied. Given the extent of risk they face, this lack of research poses serious problems. This risk is underlined by the following observations: (1) gay men constitute the largest AIDS risk group among Black and Latino AIDS cases (46% and 55%, respectively); (2) 26% of gays with AIDS are Black and Latino gay men; and (3) recent reports suggest that the rate of HIV infection is higher in Black and Latino gays. While these figures suggest a high vulnerability to HIV infection, the reasons remain a mystery. There are almost no studies of the practices and lifestyles of minority gay men. Thus, there are few clues about how prevention strategies—aimed at alerting men to the dangers of certain behaviors—might be developed.

Bell and Weinberg (1978) studied the sexual practices of minority gay men ($N = 111$), compared to white gay men. The Black men in the sample did not differ from the white men in frequency of fellatio (53%), the most frequent sexual activity. However, there were racial differences in the second most frequently performed activity and in the preference for certain activities. While some form of hand-genital contact was the technique next most employed by white men, the Blacks were next most likely to engage in anal intercourse. A total of 75% of the Black men regularly performed insertive anal intercourse; 58% regularly performed receptive anal intercourse. About half of the white men most preferred either having fellatio performed on them or performing anal intercourse on their partners, while most of the Blacks preferred receptive anal intercourse. More Blacks (90%) than whites (78%) had received anal intercourse. The vast majority of the Black men in this study (75%) had greater than 250 lifetime sexual partners. This study was conducted in the 1960s, prior to the AIDS epidemic, and provides no information on such important issues as awareness of risk-reduction methods among Black gay men.

Samuel and Winkelstein (1987a, 1987b) studied a very small number of Black men ($N = 29$) in the SF men's Health Study cohort. They found a slightly elevated number of Blacks with two or more partners with whom they practiced receptive anal intercourse (65% vs. 57% for the whites) and more rectal douching among the Blacks (65% vs. 42% for whites). Even controlling for these differences, however, there was still a marginally significant increased risk for seroconversion for the Blacks compared to the whites. Even controlling for syphilis, there was still an independent contribution of race, and the interaction between race and syphilis was not significant. Thus, more research is needed to determine the higher rates of seropositivity among Blacks.

Awareness of such practices among minority gays is critical. One published report (Williams, 1986) described a community survey in Detroit which found that Black gays were less informed about the AIDS epidemic than Black IV drug users. Among the Black gay men surveyed, only 8 (13%) of the 62 respondents correctly identified that the AIDS virus was transmitted through blood and semen. Poor understanding of how the virus is transmitted could explain why only 12 (19%) of the respondents expressed that they were very worried that they might get AIDS. Approximately 37% reported that they were not worried about possible infection.

Persons Using Drugs and Alcohol During Sex.

A consistent literature has emerged to show that the combination of drugs and/or alcohol with sexual activity is associated with high-risk sex. Stall, Wiley, McKusick, Coates, and Strow (1986), in a cross-sectional analysis, showed that men who combine drugs or alcohol with sexual activity are consistently more likely to engage in high-risk sexual activity than men who do not. Communication Technologies (1987) have consistently found, in four waves of data collection, that those who continue to practice unsafe sex are more likely to combine drugs and/or alcohol with sexual activity. Further, men who combine drugs and/or alcohol with sex are "...the least likely to have changed the frequency of engaging in unsafe anal intercourse since 1984." In a comparative analysis of gay intravenous drug users, Stall and Wiley (1988) found that approximately 70% of all high-risk activity (sharing needles, dominant anal intercourse without a condom, dominant vaginal intercourse without a condom) by HIV seropositives was conducted by the group of men who combined drugs with sex but did not use needles. Finally, Siegel et al. (1987), in a multivariate discriminant analysis, found that the combination of drugs and sexual activity was the most powerful contributor to the discriminant function (the others being perception of emotional support, years engaged in sexual intercourse with males, and perception of difficulty in modifying sexual behavior). Thus creative strategies for dealing with persons who use drugs and alcohol excessively, especially during sex, are needed.

Low-Income and Low-Education Individuals.

Data are plentiful on individuals who are most likely to respond to educational programs: middle-income and college-educated persons. Ample data have determined that response to health education and health risk are correlated with these two variables. Data are needed on the prevalence of high-risk behaviors among other socioeconomic strata to describe current levels of high-risk behaviors and the impact of behavior change programs designed with these consumers in mind.

Homosexual Adolescents.

Little attention is given to the problems of homosexual adolescents. There are no specific data on the prevalence of HIV infection among homosexual youth. A study of homosexual/bisexual male teens found a mean of 7 sex partners annually, with 45% reporting a past history of sexually transmitted diseases. While relatively few AIDS cases have been reported among adolescents, approximately 20% of cases have occurred in individuals aged 20–29 years; since the incubation period of AIDS exists in the range of years, it is probable that HIV transmission is already occurring in the adolescent age group. Despite the proven efficacy of condoms, approximately 51% of adolescents fail to use any type of contraceptive at their first sexual intercourse experience, and 26% report never using contraception at all (Zelnick & Kantner, 1980). National data indicate that only 7% of adolescents ages 13–19 years) utilize condoms (Dryfoos, 1982). It is clearly desirable to assess the efficacy of AIDS prevention methods before HIV infection becomes highly prevalent in the group at risk. According to Remafedi (CDC, 1987), "... today's adolescents, who are not yet infected (by HIV) and who are newly exploring their homosexual lifestyles, are among those persons most likely to benefit from preventive effort" (p. 6).

Bisexuals.

There are not good data on the prevalence of bisexuality in the population, the prevalence of HIV infection in bisexuals, the degree to which this group has been influenced by AIDS risk-reduction education, and the potential for spread of infection to heterosexuals.

Gay and Bisexual Men
from Smaller Urban or Rural Settings.

The sampling procedures which form the basis of what we know of behavioral adaptations to the AIDS epidemic among gay men are almost entirely limited to self-identified gay men who live in large urban settings. Data from these studies have been invaluable in health education and prevention efforts designed to limit the further spread of HIV infection. Men who live outside of these large urban gay communities or men who do not live openly as gay men, but who nonetheless are behaviorally homosexual, have not been studied. The few studies in urban studies reveal relatively high levels of high-risk behavior. Studies of the prevalence and incidence of infection, and methods for intervening with these groups are essential. Homosexual activity remains the primary risk factor for HIV infection. It is conceivable that infection could (or could already have) spread easily from urban to suburban or rural areas.

Intervention Strategies

Data evaluating the efficacy of various interventions for AIDS risk reduction are sparse. Evaluations are needed to determine which approaches are efficacious for entire risk groups and for individuals in those risk groups which are resistant to change. We recommend the following priorities:

1. **Community Intervention Approaches.** The San Francisco model of AIDS risk reduction relies heavily on shifting community norms so that low-risk activities are practiced routinely by the community. To do otherwise violates norms. In addition, multiple channels of influence are used to inform, teach skills, and motivate. The CDC demonstration projects apparently are built on this model. Certainly, the model should be replicated in its entirety in middle- and high-prevalence cities; low-prevalence cities might be able to avoid the ravages already experienced in many places by instituting and implementing these kinds of broad-based interventions.

2. **Focused Counseling at STD Clinics.** STD clinics, family-planning clinics, and drug-abuse clinics reach an especially high-risk population. Attendance at these clinics implies that one is or is planning to become sexually active or has used intravenous drugs and, therefore, may be infected. Special techniques and procedures for mobilizing counseling, education, and motivation in these clinics should be implemented and evaluated so that theoretical and practical advances can be made in our ability to promote behavior change. Special attention should be given to the implementation and evaluation of strategies for shifting the norms of these groups so that low-risk activities are expected.

3. **Health Care Providers.** Every encounter with any health care provider should provide the opportunity for assessment of risk for AIDS, counseling for risk reducation, and follow-up as needed. Health care providers have been effective in promoting smoking cessation. They are looked upon as credible sources of health information. By placing AIDS risk reduction on their patients' agendas, providers can raise awareness of the motivation, assess specific practices that place patients at risk, and advise about risk reduction. This agenda item is even more compelling because of recent studies of the health care profession. Lewis and Freeman (1987) reported that the majority of physicians interviewed in a statewide survey of physicians lacked the AIDS-related knowledge and skills required to carry out their skills in dealing with AIDS. Kelly et al. (1987a), in studying random samples of physicians in Columbus, Phoenix, and Memphis, found that harsher attitude judgments and decreased willingness to engage even in routine conversations were associated with persons with AIDS as compared to persons with leukemia.

4. **Condom Distribution Programs.** Methods of making condoms more available to risk groups and evaluations of the efficacy of these programs should be undertaken.

CONCLUSIONS

Programs among gay and bisexual men for prevention of transmission of HIV may be vastly underfunded. Flynn et al. (1987) found great disparity between resources available for prevention of transmission and those for blood-transfusion testing. While $206,000 was spent to prevent an estimated 15 transmissions by transfusion, only $87,920 was spent to prevent transmission among individuals at high risk for HIV infection, in whom approximately 534 transmissions occurred. However, it is also essential to recognize that research is an essential component of program development. Good programs cannot do without it.

ACKNOWLEDGMENTS

Preparation of this report was supported in part by Office of Technology Assessment Contract No. H3-6695, by NIMH Grant No. MH39553, and by NIMH/NIDA AIDS Center Grant No. MH 42459.

REFERENCES

Adrien, A. (1987, January 24). A campaign to promote safe sexual practices in the Montreal homosexual population—Quebec. *Canada Diseases Weekly Report, 13,* 9-12.

Bandura, A. (1977). *Social learning theory.* Englewood Cliffs, NJ: Prentice-Hall.

Bell, A. P., & Weinberg, M. S. (1978). *Homosexualities: A study of diversity among men and women.* New York: Simon & Schuster.

British Market Research Bureau, Ltd. (1987). *AIDS advertising campaign: Report on four surveys during the first year of advertising, 1986-1987.* London: Author.

Centers for Disease Control. (1987). Public Health Service guidelines for counseling and anti-body testing to prevent HIV infection and AIDS. *Morbidity and Mortality Weekly Reports, 36,* 509-515.

Cleary, P. D., Barry, M. J., Mayer, K. H., Brant, A. M., Costin, L., Fineberg, H. V. (1987). Compulsory premarital screening for the human immunodeficiency virus. *Journal of the American Medical Association, 258,* 1758-1762.

Coalition for AIDS Prevention and Education. (1987). *AIDS counseling and HIV-antibody testing: A position paper.* Washington, DC: Author.

Coates, T. J., McKusick, L., Kuno, R., & Stites, D. P. (in press). *Stress management training reduces number of sexual partners but does not enhance immune function in men infected with human immunodeficiency virus (HIV). American Journal of Public Health.*

Coates, T. J., Morin, S. F., & McKusick, L. (1987). Behavioral consequences of AIDS antibody testing among gay men. *Journal of the American Medical Association, 258,* 1889.

Communication Technologies. (1986). *Designing an effective AIDS prevention campaign strategy for Los Angeles County.* San Francisco: Author.

Communication Technologies. (1987). *A report on designing an effective AIDS prevention campaign strategy for San Francisco: Results from the fourth probability sample of an urban gay male community*. San Francisco: Author.

Conant, M., Hardy, D., Sernatinger, J., Spicer, D., Levy, J. A. (1986). Condoms prevent transmission of AIDS-associated retroviruses. *Journal of American Medical Association, 255*, 1706.

Darrow, W. W., Echenberg, D. F., Jaffe, H. W., O'Malley, P. M., Byers, R. H., Getchell, J. P., Curran, J. W. (1987). Risk factors for human immunodeficiency virus (HIV) infections in homosexual men. *American Journal of Public Health, 77*, 479–483.

Des Jarlais, D. C. (in press). Stages in the response of the drug abuse treatment system to the AIDS epidemic in New York City. *Journal of Drug Issues*.

Detels, R., Visscher, B., Kingsley, L., Chmiel, J. (1987, June 1–5). *No HIV seroconversion among men refraining from anal-genital intercourse*. Paper presented at the IIIrd International Conference on AIDS, Washington, DC.

Doll, L., Darrow, W. W., O'Malley, P., Bodecker, T., Jaffe, H., (1987, June 1–5). *Self-reported changes in sexual behaviors in gay and bisexual men from the San Francisco City Clinic Cohort*. Paper presented at the IIIrd International Conference on AIDS, Washington, DC.

Dryfoos, J. G. (1982). Contraceptive use, pregnancy intentions and pregnancy outcome among U.S. women. *Family Planning Perspectives, 14*, 81–91.

Emmons, C., Joseph, J. G., Kessler, R. C., Montgomery, S., & Ostrow, D. (1986). Psychosocial predictors of reported behavior change of homosexual men at risk for AIDS. *Health Education Quarterly, 13*, 331–345.

Fischl, M. A., Tichman, D. D., Griego, M. H., Gottlieb, M. S., Volberding, P. A., Laskin, O. L., Leedon, J. M., Groopman, J. E., Mildran, D., Schooley, R. T., Jackson, G. G., Durack, D. T., King, D. (1987). The efficacy of azidothymidine (AZT) in the treatment of patients with AIDS and AIDS-related complex. *New England Journal of Medicine, 317*, 185–191.

Fitzgerald, F. (1987a, July 21). The Castro–I. *The New Yorker*, 34–70.

Fitzgerald, F. (1987b, July 28). The Castro–II. *The New Yorker*, 44–63.

Fleming, D. W., Cochi, S. L., Steece, R. S., Hull, H. S. (1987). Acquired immunodeficiency syndrome in low incidence areas: How safe is unsafe sex? *Journal of the American Medical Association, 258*, 785–787.

Flynn, N., Harper, S., Jain, S., Holland, P., Fernando, L., Baily, V. (1987, June 1–5). *Underemphasis on publicly funded programs for prevention of transmission of HIV among gay men and intravenous drug users*. Paper presented at the IIIrd International Conference on AIDS, Washington, DC.

Fox, R., Odaka, N. J., Brookmeyer, R., & Polk, B. F. (1987). Effect of HIV antibody disclosure on subsequent sexual activity in homosexual men. *AIDS, 1*, 241–246.

Fox, R., Ostrow, D., Valdisseri, R., VanReiden, B., Polk, B. F. (1987, June 1–5). *Changes in sexual activities among participants in the Multicenter AIDS Cohort Study*. Paper presented at the IIIrd International Conference on AIDS, Washington, DC.

Francis, D. P., & Chi, J. (1987). The prevention of acquired immunodeficiency syndrome in the United States. *Journal of the American Medical Association, 257*, 1357–1366.

Friedland, G. H., & Klein, R. S. (1987). Transmission of the human immunodeficiency virus. *New England Journal of Medicine, 317*, 1125–1135.

Goedert, J. J. (1987). What is safe sex? *New England Journal of Medicine, 316*, 1339–1342.

Goedert, J. J., Sarngadharan, M. G., Biggar, R. J., Weiss, S. H., Winn, D., Grossman, R. J., Greene, M. H., Bodner, A., Mann, D. L., Strong, D. M., Gallo, R. C., Blattner, W. A. (1984). Determinants of retrovirus (HTLV-III) antibody and immunodeficiency conditions in homosexual men. *Lancet, 2*, 711–716.

Gorman, E. M. (1986). The AIDS epidemic in San Francisco: Epidemiological and anthropological perspectives. In D. Janes, R. Stall, & S. Gifford (Eds.), *Anthropology and epidemiology* (pp. 57–172). Boston: Reidel.

Hansfield, H. H. (1985). Decreasing incidence of gonorrhea in homosexually active men—minimal effect on risk of AIDS. *Western Journal of Medicine, 143*, 469-470.

Jaffe, H., Choi, K., Thomas, P., Haverkos, H. W., Auerbach DM., Guinds, ME., Rogert MF., Spira TJ., Dorrow WW., Kramer, MA., Friedman, SM., Monroe JM., Friedman-Kien, AE., Laubenstein L. J., Marmor M., Safai, B., Dritz SK., Crispi SJ., Fannin SL., Orkwis JP., Kieter A., Rushing WR., Thacker SB., Curran J. W. (1983). National case control study of Kaposi's sarcoma and *Pneumocystis carinii* pneumonia in homosexual men: Part I, epidemiological results. *Annals of Internal Medicine, 99*, 145-151.

Jeffries, E., Willoughby, B., Boyko, W. J., Schechter, M. T., Wigg, B., Foy, S., O'Shaughnessy, M. (1987). Persistence of high-risk sexual activity among homosexual men in an area of low incidence of the acquired immunodeficiency syndrome. *Sexually Transmitted Diseases, 14*, 79-82.

Joseph, G. G., Montgomery, S., Kessler, R. C., Ostrow, D. G., Emmons, C. A., & Phair, J. P. (1987a, June 1-5). *Behavioral risk reduction in a cohort of homosexual men: Two-year follow-up*. Paper presented at the IIIrd International Conference on AIDS, Washington, DC.

Joseph, J. G., Montgomery, C., Kirsch, J., Kessler, R. C., Ostraw, D., Wortman, C., Brian, K., Eller, M., Estrlems, S. (1987b). Perceived risk of AIDS: Assessing the behavioral and psychological consequences in a cohort of gay men. *Journal of Applied Social Psychology, 17*, 231-250.

Judson, F. N. (1983). Fear of AIDS and gonorrhea rates in homosexual men. *Lancet, 2*, 159.

Juran, S. (1987, April 3). *Sexual concern and behavioral changes as a result of a fear of AIDS*. Paper presented at the Society for the Scientific Study of Sex, Eastern Region Conference, Philadelphia.

Kegeles, S., Catania, J. A., & Coates, T. J. (in press). Intentions to communicate positive HIV antibody status to sex partners. *Journal of the American Medical Association*.

Kelly, J. A., & St. Lawrence, J. S. (1986). Behavioral intervention and AIDS. *The Behavior Therapist, 6*, 121-125.

Kelly, J. A., St. Lawrence, J. S., Hood, H. V., Brasfield, T. L. (1987a). *Behavioral intentions to reduce AIDS risk activities*. Unpublished manuscript, University of Mississippi, Jackson.

Kelly, J. A., St. Lawrence, J. S., Smith, S., Hood, H. V., Cook, D. J. (1987b). Stigmatization of AIDS patients by physicians. *American Journal of Public Health, 77*, 789-791.

Kingsley, L. A., Detels, R., Kaslow, R., Polk, B. F., Rinaldo, C. R., Chmiel, J., Detre, K., Kelsey, S. F., Odaka, N., Ostrow, D., Van Ruden, M., Visscher, B. (1987). Risk factors for seroconversion to human immunodeficiency virus among male homosexuals. *Lancet, 1*, 345-347.

Kinsey, A. C., Pomeroy, W. B., & Martin, C. R. (1948). *Sexual behavior in the human male*. Philadelphia: W. B. Saunders.

Klein, D. E., Greer, S., Wolcott, D. L., Landesverk, U., Namir, S., Fawzy, F. I. (1987). Changes in AIDS risk behaviors among homosexual male physicians and university students. *American Journal of Psychiatry, 144*, 742-747.

Koop, C. E., (1986). *Surgeon General's report on acquired immune deficiency syndrome*. Washington, DC: U.S. Department of Health and Human Services.

Lewis, C. E, Freeman, H. E. (1987) The sexual history-taking in counseling practices of primary care physicians. *Western Journal of Med., 147*, 165-167.

Lyman, D., Ascher, M., & Levy, J. A. (1986). Minimal risk of transmission of AIDS-associated retrovirus infection by oral-genital contact. *Journal of the American Medical Association, 255*, 1703.

Lyter, D. W., Valdisseri, D. O., Kingsley, L. A., Ameros, W. P., Rinaldo, C. R. (1987). The HIV antibody test: Why gay and bisexual men want or do not want to know their results. *Public Health Reports, 102*, 468-474.

Martin, J. L. (1987). The impact of AIDS on gay male sexual behavior patterns in New York City. *American Journal of Public Health, 77*, 578-581.

McCusker, J., Stoddard, A. M., Mayer, K. H., Zapka, J., Morussen, C., Saltzman, M. S. (1988).

Effects of HIV antibody test knowledge on subsequent sexual behaviors in a cohort of homosexual men. *American Journal of Public Health, 18,* 462-467.

McKusick, L., et al. (1985). Reported changes in the sexual behavior of men at risk for AIDS, San Francisco, 1982-1984—the AIDS Behavioral Research Project. *Public Health Reports, 100,* 622-628.

McKusick, L., Coates, T. J., Wiley, J., Morin, S., Stall, R. (1987, June 1-5). *Prevention of HIV infection among gay and bisexual men: Analysis of two longitudinal studies.* Paper presented at the IIIrd International Conference on AIDS, Washington, DC.

McKusick, L., Conant, M., & Coates, T. J. (1985). The AIDS epidemic: A model for developing intervention strategies for reducing high-risk behavior in gay men. *Sexually transmitted Diseases, 2,* 229-234.

Melbye, M., Biggar, R. J. Ebbesen, P., Sarngadharan, M. G., Wiess, S. H., Gallo, R. C., Blattner, W. A. (1984). Seroepidemiology of HTLV-III antibody in Danish homosexual men: Prevalence, transmission, and disease outcome. *British Medical Journal, 289,* 573-575.

Morin, S. F. (1977). Heterosexual bias in psychological research on lesbianism and male homosexuality. *American Psychologist, 32,* 629-637.

Multicenter AIDS Cohort Study (MACS). (1985, October). Prevalence and correlates of HTLV-III antibodies among 5,000 gay men in four cities. *Interscience Conference on Antimicrobial Agents and Chemotherapy* (abstract).

Pickering, J., Wiley, J. A., Padian, N. S., Lieb, L., Ekenberg D., Walker, J. (1986). Modeling the incidence of acquired immunodeficiency syndrome (AIDS) in San Francisco, Los Angeles, and New York. *Mathematical Modeling, 7,* 661-688.

Quadland, M. C., Shandis, W. D., Schuyman, R., & Jacobs, K. (1987, June 1-5). *The 800-Men Study: A controlled study of an AIDS prevention program in New York City.* Paper presented at the IIIrd International Conference on AIDS, Washington, DC.

Rees, M. (1987). The sombre view of AIDS. *Nature, 326,* 343-345.

Samuel, M. C., & Winkelstein, W. (1987a). In reply. *Journal of the American Medical Association, 258,* 473-474.

Samuel, M. C., & Winkelstein, W. (1987b). Prevalence of human immunodeficiency virus infection in ethnic minority homosexual/bisexual men. *Journal of the American Medical Association, 257,* 1901-1092.

Schesney, S., Gantz, W. M., & Sullivan, J. L. (1987, June 1-5). *Impermeability of condoms to HIV and inactivation of HIV by the spermicide Nonoxynol-9.* Paper presented at the IIIrd International Conference on AIDS, Washington, DC.

Scheuter, M. T., Boyko, W. J., Douglas, B., Maynard, M., Willoughby, B., McLeod, H., Craib, K. J. (1986). Can HTLV-III be transmitted orally? *Lancet, 1,* 379.

Siegel, K., Mesagno, F. P., Chen, J. Y., Christ, G. (1987, June 1-5). *Factors distinguishing homosexual males practicing safe and risky sex.* Paper presented at the IIIrd International Conference on AIDS, Washington, DC.

Sivak, S. L., & Wormser, G. P. (1952). How common is HTLV-III infection in the United States? *New England Journal of Medicine, 313,* 1352.

Soucey, J. (1986, June). *Human immunodeficiency virus antibody disclosure and behavior change.* Paper presented at the meetings of the American Psychiatric Association, Chicago.

Soucey, J. (1987, May). *The impact of HIV antibody disclosure on behavior and mental health.* Paper presented at the meetings of the American Psychiatric Association, Atlanta.

Stall, R., & Wiley, J. (1988). *A comparison of homosexual and heterosexual drug and alcohol use practices.* Manuscript submitted for publication.

Stall, R., Wiley, J., McKusick, L., Coaks, T. J., Ostrow, D. (1986). Alcohol and drug use and risk for AIDS. *Health Education Quarterly, 13,* 1-13.

Stempel, R., & Moulton, J. (1987, June 1-5). *The psychological and behavioral responses to HIV antibody testing.* Paper presented at the IIIrd International Conference on AIDS, Washington, DC.

Valdiserri, R. O., Lyter, D., Callahan, C., Kingsley, L., Rinaldo, C. (1987, June 1-5). *Condom use in a cohort of gay and bisexual men.* Paper presented at the IIIrd International Conference on AIDS, Washington, DC.

Weinberg, M. S. (1970). Homosexual samples: Differences and similarities. *The Journal of Sex Research, 6,* 312-325.

Williams, L. S. (1986). AIDS risk reduction: A community health education intervention for minority high-risk group members. *Health Education Quarterly, 13,* 407-421.

Winkelstein, W., Lyman, D. M., Padian, N., Grant, R., Samuel, M., Wiley, J., Anderson, R. E., Lang, W., Riggs, J., Levy, J. A. (1987a). Sexual practices and risk of infection by the human immunodeficiency virus. *Journal of the American Medical Association, 257,* 321-325.

Winkelstein, W., Samuel, M., Padian, N., Wiley, J. A., Lang, W. (1987b). Reduction in human immunodeficiency virus transmission among homosexual/bisexual men: 1982-1986. *American Journal of Public Health, 76,* 685-689.

Yarchoan, R., & Broder, S. (1987). Development of antiretroviral therapy for the acquired immunodeficiency syndrome and related disorders. *New England Journal of Medicine, 316,* 557-564.

Zelnick, M., & Kantner J. F. (1980). Sexual activity, contraceptive use and pregnancy among metropolitan-area teenagers: 1971-1979. *Family Planning Perspectives, 12,* 230-237.

Zenilman, J. M., Cates, W., & Morse, S. A. (1986). *Neisseria gonorrhoeae:* An old enemy rearms. *Infectious Diseases Medical Letter of Obstetrics and Gynecology, 7,* 2ff.

A Cross-Cultural Comparison of Psychosocial Responses To Having AIDS and Related Conditions in London and San Francisco

8

Kristy Straits
Lydia Temoshok
Jane Zich
School of Medicine
University of California, San Francisco

The psychosocial ramifications of acquired immunodeficiency syndrome (AIDS) have only recently begun to be quantified, although biomedical research has been ongoing since the appearance of AIDS in the United States in 1979. In interviews with people with AIDS, Morin, Charles, and Malyon (1984) found that, although their medical needs were addressed, their psychological needs were not. Themes of uncertainty, isolation, self-blame (illness as retribution), and general fears of life-threatening illness, such as fears of disability, loss of body control, pain, and death, have been reported in consultations with people with AIDS (Dilley, Ochitill, Perl, & Volberding, 1985; Gorman, 1986).

In addition to dealing with a progressively degenerating illness, people infected with HIV-1 (Human Immunodeficiency Virus, Type 1, previously referred to as HTLV-III, ARV, or LAV) too often must confront the stigma attached to culturally deviant behavior, especially homosexuality. Some gay men find that, while in the midst of coming to terms with an HIV infection, they must take on the added burden of coping with the reactions of friends and family, who often were not aware of the patient's sexual orientation until diagnosis. Additionally, the phenomenal expenses incurred with HIV disease, including medical expenses and income loss, place a devastating financial burden on people with AIDS (Martin & Vance, 1984). These psychosocial factors may combine to create a potentially overwhelming effect on HIV-related illness. As one might expect, parallel themes have emerged in the British literature on psychosocial aspects of AIDS (Green, 1986; Madeley, 1987; Miller, 1986, 1987). Yet, cultural differences might also be present, which would be especially important to consider when designing health-education programs or psychosocial interventions.

There is an extensive literature in medical sociology and medical anthropology which has analyzed ways in which different societies, as well as different societal sectors, define, treat, and explain ill health (Helman, 1985; Kleinman, 1980). People become ethnically enculturated within a group and share explanatory concepts and attitudes toward health and illness (Harwood, 1981). The Malawi people in Africa, for example, link illness to taboos and witchcraft, as well as social behavior outside of clearly prescribed rules governing behavior (Chilivumbo, 1973). The Navajo Indians traditionally explain illness as due to a "breach of taboo," such as incest or coming in contact with a dangerous object. Illness is also believed to be contracted by "soul loss," as well as spirit intrusion (possession) and wizardry (Kunitz & Levy, 1981). Mexican Americans employ folk concepts of disequilibrium between hot and cold exposure (both internally and externally), as well as beliefs in the "evil eye" and "fright," which can result in soul loss following such trauma (Schreiber & Homiak, 1981). Haitian Americans are likely to speculate about their diagnosis, rather than describe symptoms, and tend to attribute illness to poor diet and personal hygiene, as well as supernatural causes such as voodoo (Laguerre, 1981). Even among similar Caucasion urban dwellers, Zola (1983) found that Americans of Italian heritage complained of more symptoms, more bodily areas affected, and more kinds of dysfunction than Americans of Irish descent with the same diagnosis.

Although the United Kingdom and the United States are Western societies with many cultural and political similarities, they have distinct cultural traditions, different economic and class systems, and, most importantly for our present considerations, different ways of organizing medical care. In the United Kingdom, for instance, all residents, as well as visitors of more than 24 hours, are entitled to free access to sexually transmitted disease clinics (Forster, 1986). Such free services are provided by the National Health Service in Britain (Ham, 1985) and are not uniformly available in the United States.

The impact of cross-cultural factors in defining health, illness, and treatment is important in considering the psychosocial aspects of having AIDS or ARC in these two societies. Although an in-depth analysis of health concepts in the United States and the United Kingdom is beyond the scope of this chapter, this study examines attributions for health and disease, self-blame, treatment-seeking behavior, social support, and optimism in groups of gay men with AIDS and AIDS-related complex (ARC) in London and San Francisco.

EPIDEMIOLOGICAL IMPACT OF AIDS
IN THE UNITED STATES AND BRITAIN

AIDS is currently recognized as an international pendemic (Panos Institute, 1987). As of January 1, 1988, a total of 75,768 AIDS cases had been reported to the Centers for Disease Control (CDC) in the U.S., while in Great Britain, the Communicable Disease Surveillance Center (CDSC) had reported 1,794 AIDS cases (WHO, 1988). At the time of our study in May–June 1985, San Francisco had reported 1,235 cases of AIDS. Only 150 cases of AIDS had been reported in Britain at that time. These figures represent only the diagnosed cases of frank AIDS and do not represent the much higher estimated numbers of people with ARC or those who had been exposed to the AIDS virus but had not yet developed symptoms that met fairly stringent criteria for an AIDS diagnosis.

In England, the rise in prevalence of HIV has been documented by routine testing of all blood specimens collected at sexually transmitted disease (STD) clinics. In March 1982, only 3.7% of all blood samples collected at one large London STD clinic were antibody positive (Carne, Sutherland, Ferns, et al., 1985). In June 1984, two years later, 21% of the same clinic's blood samples were antibody positive. Another epidemiologic study conducted during 1984–1985 found that 17% of the blood specimens collected at all British STD clinics were antibody positive, and one central London STD clinic reported 35% of their samples tested antibody positive (Jesson, Thorp, Mortimer, & Oates, 1986). These statistics indicate a sizeable increase in prevalence of the AIDS virus in England and suggest that AIDS will have a major impact on public health in England.

IMPACT OF AIDS ON HOMOSEXUAL COMMUNITIES
IN SIMILAR URBAN CENTERS

London is within the Thames region, where 77% of the AIDS cases have been reported in England. This clustering of AIDS cases in a large metropolitan center may be related to the existence of a large gay community in the London area, as 87% of the AIDS cases reported in England are among homosexual or bisexual men (Report from PHLS, 1987). Similarly, the largest proportion of cases in the U.S. have occurred among homosexual or bisexual men, originally clustering around the large gay communities in New York City and San Francisco.

The existence of a gay community or subculture in both London and San Francisco makes the two cities ideal for a cross-cultural comparison of a similarly defined group. In an earlier comparison of European and American attitudes about homosexuality, Weinberg and Williams (1974) surveyed the public in the U.S., the Netherlands, and Denmark. They found the Dutch public to be the most tolerant and the Dutch government to be the most liberal regarding laws impacting homosexuality, whereas the U.S. public was the most negative and U.S. laws were the most discriminatory toward homosexuality. In addition to indicating that homosexuals are less threatened by the heterosexual community in certain European countries than in the U.S., the authors also suggested that gay subcultures in all societies may neutralize the negative effects of societal reaction by providing support and acceptance to their members. Gorman (1986) suggested that this emergence of gay culture in urban centers may be attributed to migration of gay people to "magnet cities" where nontraditional lifestyles are better tolerated. The men with AIDS and ARC in London and San Francisco may, therefore, be part of similar "magnet" communities, within the context of differing cultures.

INFLUENCE OF THE MEDIA

Another sociocultural factor that may influence the experience of coping with a diagnosis of AIDS is the impact of the media. In a survey of the general public in London, New York, and San Francisco during May and June 1985, Temoshok, Sweet, and Zich (1987) found the London public to rank significantly higher in fear and lower in knowledge of AIDS than the San Francisco public. Further, low knowledge of AIDS and antigay attitudes were more highly correlated in London, as compared to New York and San Francisco. Several hypotheses were proposed to explain the differences between London and San Francisco, the cities with the most extreme differences in knowledge and attitudes: (1) the lower absolute and per-capita number of AIDS cases in London than in San Francisco; (2) more negative cultural attitudes about homosexuality in London than in San Francisco; and (3) more hysteria-producing reporting of AIDS in London than in San Francisco.

At roughly the same time, in a content analysis of newspaper articles during May 1 to June 15, 1985, in London and the San Francisco Bay area, London reports were found to be more alarmist, sensationalizing, and fear-promoting than the San Francisco articles (Temoshok, Grade, & Zich, 1989). Sensational London headlines and media coverage of "the Gay Plague" probably exacerbated blame and hatred of homosexuals. At that time, portrayals of individual victims with AIDS in London were generally shadowy descriptions of foreigners and/or drug addicts, unaccompanied by photographs or names of the individuals. In contrast, San Francisco articles were more sympathetic in their descriptions of life histories of people with AIDS and were often accompanied by names and photographs, which humanized and normalized these portraits. Such differences in media coverage of people with AIDS must be considered in comparing the psychosocial responses to having AIDS in London and in San Francisco.

Since the time of these surveys and media content analysis, the British government, through the Department of Health and Human Services, has made a concerted effort to educate the public and dispel some of the myths and stigmas surrounding AIDS (Beck, Cunningham, Moss, et al., 1987; Sherr, 1987; Sonnex, Petherick, Adler, & Miller, 1987). These efforts included a massive multi-media, public-education campaign and the mailing of an AIDS information pamphlet. The media launched its own campaign and helped to humanize the problem by publishing photographs such as Princess Diana shaking hands with hospitalized AIDS patients in the spring of 1987. However, in the summer of 1985, when the present study was conducted, the media focus and public attitudes were reflective of the community response to the AIDS crisis at that time and may have helped to form that community's response. Temoshok, Sweet, and Zich (1987) proposed that the London public was in a less evolved stage of coping with the crisis, whereas San Francisco had been dealing with the epidemic for a longer period of time and had reached a generally more informed, less fearful stage of coping.

INFLUENCE OF PSYCHOSOCIAL FACTORS

In addition to these sociocultural factors that may affect people with AIDS, psychosocial factors such as stressful life events, amount and quality of social support, bereavement, and coping styles may affect responses to having AIDS and ARC. Biopsychosocial research may suggest factors that influence health outcome beyond what is known through biomedical research (Coates, Temoshok, & Mandel, 1984; Temoshok, Mandel, Solomon, Zich, Moulton, & Mead, 1986). Such information could have considerable impact in shaping interventions for people with AIDS and may be applicable to interventions for people with other serious conditions as well.

Disease Progression

Although AIDS and ARC are often viewed as the same disease at different points along a continuum, with ARC sometimes referred to as "prodromal AIDS," the experience of having ARC and the "not knowing" whether or not one will subsequently develop AIDS has been associated with higher self-reported distress (Temoshok, Mandel, Moulton, Zich, & Solomon, 1986). The authors also found differences in the number of symptoms reported and the number of alternative therapies and new ways of managing life used in groups of AIDS and ARC patients. In a related study, Moulton, Sweet, Temoshok, and Mandel (1987) found that distress was positively correlated with attributing cause of illness to self for persons with AIDS only, whereas distress was negatively correlated with attributing cause of health improvement to self for persons with ARC only. These results suggest that an evaluation of psychosocial variables and HIV disease must be interpreted within the context of disease progression along the AIDS/ARC continuum (Temoshok, Sweet, Moulton, & Zich, 1987).

Holland and Tross (1985) pointed out that the normal stress reactions to a diagnosis of AIDS are similar to the reactions that occur with any life-threatening disease, such as cancer. These reactions may include anxiety, depression, sense of isolation, and anger, and may change over time. Due to the process involved in dealing with such a diagnosis, time elapsed since diagnosis is also a factor that must be considered when evaluating coping strategies or attributions made regarding one's health improvement or cause of health problems.

Influence of Individual Characteristics

An individual's personality or characteristic coping style may influence his capacity to deal with AIDS. Some people tend to expect better outcomes than others, and there is some speculation that optimism is a personality trait that may be stable across time and situation (Scheier & Carver, 1985). Optimistic people (as defined by a self-report responses) were found by Scheier and Carver (1985) to be subsequently less likely to report being bothered by physical symptoms than those less optimistic. Further, they suggested that optimism acts as a buffer against stress and is associated with active coping, such as seeking social support. Although optimism may be a personality trait, it is apt to be modified by the realities of the situation one faces. For example, optimism has been found to be influenced by prior life event history and the frequency of self-initiated activities performed (Reich & Zautra, 1981). Perhaps optimism in persons with AIDS is influenced by the psychosocial aspects of the situation they face.

TOWARD A CROSS-CULTURAL, PSYCHOSOCIAL UNDERSTANDING

From a consideration of these complex cultural, subcultural, social, and psychological issues, the following hypotheses were proposed to provide the focus of this study:

1. Within the context of sensationalizing media reports and relatively low public knowledge about AIDS, London men with AIDS and ARC will be more likely to blame themselves for their health problems than San Francisco men with AIDS and ARC.

2. Because London men may be as highly distressed upon receiving a diagnosis of AIDS and ARC but have fewer resources at their disposal than San Francisco men, London men may feel more helpless. As a consequence, they may attribute less health improvement to self than do their San Francisco counterparts.

3. Because of stigmas and fears, as well as fewer AIDS resources available in England, London men with AIDS and ARC will report seeking fewer alternative therapies.

4. Additionally, perhaps due to the same reasons, London men with AIDS and ARC will report trying fewer new ways of managing their lives than do San Francisco men.

5. London men with AIDS and ARC will report spending less time with friends and family since diagnosis than will their San Francisco counterparts, perhaps due to lower public knowledge of AIDS and fear of rejection or stigmas associated with anti-gay attitudes.

6. Because AIDS was and still is more prevalent in San Francisco than in London, fewer London men with AIDS and ARC will include people with their same diagnosis among their circle of social support.

7. London men with AIDS and ARC will report knowing fewer people who have died of AIDS than San Francisco men, due to the lower prevalence of AIDS in London.

8. Because optimism is associated with active coping and self-initiated activity, the more option-limited London men will be less optimistic in the way they see the future than San Francisco men with AIDS and ARC.

In addition to differences between San Francisco and London, there may be psychosocial differences within these cities between those with AIDS and ARC, as we have found in our studies (Moulton et al., 1987; Temoshok et al., 1986a, 1986b, 1987).

SUBJECTS

London

Twenty-three people with a diagnosis of AIDS and ARC were referred to the study during the period from May 1 to June 15, 1985. Referrals were made by physicians in STD clinics, which originally diagnosed and followed all AIDS cases in London at that time. All eligible referrals agreed to participate in a structured interview. Of the 23 audiotaped interviews, one interview tape was inaudible and was removed from the sample due to insufficient codable data. One participant was a female AIDS patient who had married a man of African descent and had lived in Zaire, where heterosexual transmission of AIDS is more prevalent. This interview was also excluded from the final analysis, as her concerns and experiences with AIDS were very different from the rest of the all-male sample. The remaining 21 subjects were homosexual men who were being treated in London for their health problems and who lived in London or nearby communities. Thirteen men were recruited from St. Stephen's Hospital (62%), seven from St. Mary's Hospital (33%), and one from St. James' Hospital (5%).

The Centers for Disease Control's 1985 diagnostic criteria for a diagnosis of AIDS were used to operationally define an AIDS diagnosis. Therefore, the sample included men with *Pneumocystis carinii* pneumonia (PCP) only, men with Kaposi's sarcoma (KS) only, men with both PCP and KS, and men with KS/PCP and other opportunistic infections. The definition of ARC proposed by Bay Area Physicians for Human Rights (BAPHR) was used to define the ARC participants. These subjects experienced two or more of the following symptoms: unexplained lymphadenopathy for at least 6 months, oral thrush, hairy leukoplakia, herpes zoster (shingles), fever for 3 months or more, weight loss of 10% of body weight, central or peripheral neurologic deficit, diarrhea for 3 months or more, night sweats for 3 months or more, fatigue, pruritis (itching), extensive dermatitis, sinusitis, or persistent skin fungal/bacterial infections (Haverkos, Gottlieb, Killen, & Edelman, 1985).

It is important to note that an ARC diagnosis was inferred from the subject's description of symptoms, as the subject had rarely received this specific diagnosis, especially in London. At this time in 1985, AIDS was just emerging in London, and physicians were adhering to strict exclusionary diagnostic criteria of AIDS. Therefore, "date of diagnosis" referred to date of diagnosis of current health problems for ARC patients and date of diagnosis of AIDS for AIDS patients.

In this study's London sample, 11 men were diagnosed with AIDS and 10 men with ARC. Among the AIDS subjects, 3 had KS, 7 had PCP, and 1 had both KS and PCP. The London sample ranged in age from 24 to 48 years of age ($M = 34.1$). There was no significant difference found for mean time elapsed since date of diagnosis to time of interview between AIDS patients ($M = 29.1$ wks.) and ARC patients ($M = 17.8$ wks.). For the entire group of London subjects, the mean time elapsed from date of diagnosis to time of interview was 23.7 weeks.

San Francisco

Twenty-one subjects were drawn from a larger San Francisco sample of 130 homosexual men with AIDS and ARC who were participating in a longitudinal psychosocial study (Temoshok, 1983–1988). These subjects had been re-cruited from San Francisco General Hospital (SFGH) during May through August 1985. These 21 subjects were matched with the London sample according to: (1) AIDS/ARC diagnosis; (2) KS, PCP, or KS and PCP diagno-sis; (3) total number of symptoms reported; (4) time elapsed since diagnosis; and (5) age. There was no significant difference found for mean time elapsed since date of diagnosis between AIDS subjects (M = 17.8 wks.) and ARC subjects (M = 22.0 wks.). The mean time elapsed from date of diagnosis to time of interview for the entire group was 20.0 weeks. Age ranged from 23 to 43 years (M = 34.3) in this matched San Francisco sample.

PROCEDURE

In June 1985, two of the authors (Temoshok and Zich) supervised the inter-viewing of a large proportion of all persons with AIDS currently being treated in London. A structured interview[1] was administered and audiotaped by a pool of nine trained volunteers who were participating in a research project on AIDS in London sponsored by the University Research Expeditions Program (UREP), University of California, Berkeley.

At roughly the same time, audiotaped interviews were conducted in San Francisco with 130 men with AIDS and ARC, utilizing the same structured interview as was used in part of the study mentioned above (Temoshok, 1983–1988).

THE STRUCTURED INTERVIEW

The psychosocial interview was developed in 1983–1984 in a cooperative effort by members of the Biopsychosocial AIDS Project (BAP) at the Univer-sity of California, San Francisco, and by consultants in the community dealing directly with AIDS-/ARC-related problems. The interview protocol included.

1. *History of health problems and reactions to health changes and medical treatment.*

2. *Attributions of cause of health problems and improvement in health prob-lems.* This section required the subject to determine how much (what percent) he attributed the cause of his health problems to each of four categories: self,

---

[1]In the present study, only some of the archival data collected in 1985 were analyzed. Those interested in the complete version of the structured interview may contact Dr. Lydia Temoshok, Henry M. Jackson Foundation/Walter Reed Army Medical Center, 6825 16th St., N.W., Washington, D.C. 20307–5001.

environment, chance, and someone else. The same ratings were made for a possible improvement in health. The subject was then asked to respond to a question about self-blame ("Do you blame yourself for your health problems? Yes, no, or maybe?"). Due to the distinction between this question and the attribution ratings, and the clear presentation of the concept of self-blame, men who responded "yes" and "maybe" were combined and coded for analysis as "self-blamers."

3. *Life changes made subsequent to onset of health problems.* This section inquired about changes in ways of managing life, including areas such as improving diet/more rest, relying more on others, opening up more and discussing feelings and problems, or trying assertiveness training or support groups. Seeking of alternative health care, such as acupuncture, megavitamins, visualization, herbal treatments, and so forth were also inquired about in this section.

4. *Social support.* Subjects reported whether they were spending more or less time with friends and family since their diagnosis, whether or not they included people with their same diagnosis in their social support circle, what helped the most in dealing with their illness, and how many people they knew who had died of AIDS or other causes in the last year.

5. *Optimism and scope of future.* In this section, the interviewer rated the subject for optimism on a five-point Likert scale from very pessimistic to very optimistic. The subject was then asked whether he thought of the future in terms of a few days, weeks, months, 1–2 years, or more than 2 years.

RESULTS

In order to prevent diagnosis from becoming a confounding variable in the statistical results, all analyses were run separately for AIDS and ARC groups, although no hypotheses regarding specific AIDS and ARC differences were postulated. Fisher's exact probability test, rather than chi-square, was used to determine significance for two-dimensional variables such as self-blame because of this study's small sample size (expected frequency of less than 5 in some cells) and the reliance of chi-square on the assumption of a normal distribution (Rosenthal & Rosnow, 1984). A summary of group differences for all psychosocial variables according to city is provided in Table 8.1. Table 8.2 contains a summary of group differences for all psychosocial variables according to diagnosis.

As predicted by hypothesis #1, London men with AIDS and ARC blamed themselves for their health problems more frequently than did their San Francisco counterparts (Fisher's exact test, $p < .03$, one-tailed). Only 4 out of 21 San Franciso men blamed themselves for their health problems, whereas

TABLE 8.1
Group Differences According to City

Variable	Means[a]		TEST	p
	London Men	San Francisco Men		
Self-blame	11 (52%)	4 (19%)	Fisher's exact[b]	.03
Attributed improvement to self	38.8	47.7	$F = $ .806	NS
Number of alternative therapies	1.0	2.4	$F = 6.155$	.02
Number of new ways of managing life	2.7	1.95	$F = 2.164$	NS
Time spent with friends/family since diagnosis	2.14	2.05	$F = $ .124	NS
Most supportive circle includes men with same diagnosis	11 (52%)	8 (38%)	Fisher's exact[b]	NS
Number of people personally known who died of AIDS	1.48	6.52	$F = 3.003$	.09
Optimism	2.0	2.1	$F = $ .013	NS
Scope	3.5	4.0	$F = 1.078$	NS

[a]All values listed are means, except for "Self-blame" and "Most supportive circle...," which are reported by frequencies.

[b]One-tailed, Fisher's exact test.

nearly three times as many London men (11 out of 21) blamed themselves. No significant effect was found for self-blame according to diagnosis. Among the 15 "self-blamers," 8 had AIDS and 7 had ARC.

Hypothesis #2 predicted that London men with AIDS and ARC would attribute less health improvement to themselves than would San Francisco men. Analysis of variance was performed on the percentage of health improvement attributed to self. Although the San Francisco men attributed health improvement to themselves slightly more ($M = 47.71$) than did the London men ($M = 38.81$), this difference was not found to be statistically significant. Therefore, hypothesis #2 was not supported by the data. Additionally, no significant difference was found for health improvement attribution according to diagnosis. Men with AIDS attributed almost the same amount of health improvement to themselves ($M = 41.43$) as did men with ARC ($M = 45.10$).

As predicted by hypothesis #3, London men with AIDS and ARC sought fewer alternative therapies than did the San Francisco men [$F(1,38) = 6.155$,

TABLE 8.2
Group Differences According to Diagnosis

Variable	Means[a]		TEST	p
	AIDS	ARC		
Self-blame	8 (38%)	7 (33%)	Fisher's exact[b]	.03
Attributed improvement to self	41.43	45.10	$F = .107$	NS
Number of alternative therapies	1.86	1.52	$F = .515$	.02
Number of new ways of managing life	1.81	2.86	$F = 4.389$	NS
Time spent with friends/family since diagnosis	2.19	2.00	$F = .475$	NS
Most supportive circle includes men with same diagnosis	7 (33%)	12 (57%)	Fisher's exact[b]	NS
Number of people personally known who died of AIDS	3.1	4.9	$F = .291$	.09
Optimism	2.25	1.86	$F = .683$	NS
Scope	4.07	3.53	$F = 1.315$	NS

[a]All values listed are means, except for "Self-blame" and "Most supportive circle...," which are reported by frequencies.
[b]One-tailed, Fisher's exact test.

$p < .05$]. In fact, San Francisco men used over twice as many alternative therapies ($M = 2.38$) as did the London men ($M = 1.00$). There was no significant difference found for the mean number of alternative therapies used by people with AIDS ($M = 1.86$) as compared to people with ARC ($M = 1.52$).

Hypothesis #4 predicted that London men with AIDS and ARC would report trying fewer new ways of managing their lives since their diagnosis than would San Francisco men with AIDS and ARC. The difference between the two groups was in the opposite direction of that hypothesized, although this difference was not significant. However, an unpredicted main effect for diagnosis was found [$F(1,38) = 4.389, p < .05$]. Across cities, men with ARC tried more new ways of managing their lives ($M = 2.86$) than did those with AIDS ($M = 1.81$).

No support was found for hypothesis #5, which predicted that London men with AIDS and ARC would report spending less time with friends and family since their diagnosis than would San Francisco men. No significant difference was found between those with AIDS or those with ARC in the amount of time spent with friends and family.

Hypothesis #6 predicted that fewer London men with AIDS and ARC would include people with their same diagnosis in their circle of social support than would San Francisco men. About half of the men with AIDS and ARC in London included people with their same diagnosis in their circle of social support; only 38% of the San Francisco men did so. This difference between cities was not significant. Almost twice as many men with ARC included same-diagnosis people in their social support circle as did men with AIDS, but this difference also failed to reach significance.

As predicted by hypothesis #7, London men with AIDS and ARC reported knowing fewer people who had died of AIDS (M = 1.48) than San Francisco men (M = 6.52). Analysis of variance showed that the difference between the two cities approached significance [$F(1,38)$ = 3.003, $p < .10$], lending some support to hypothesis #7. No significant difference was found according to diagnosis for the number of people known personally who had died of AIDS (M for men with AIDS = 3.10; M for men with ARC = 4.91).

Hypothesis #8 predicted that London men with AIDS and ARC would be less optimistic than their San Francisco counterparts. However, analysis of variance showed no significant difference between cities for interviewer-rated optimism. There was also no significant difference found for optimism by diagnosis.

A second measure of optimism approximated the scope of time the subject encompassed in describing his foreseeable future, ranging from a few days to more than two years. This measure was highly correlated with the optimism rating (r = .57, $p < .01$). Analysis of variance showed no significant difference in this measure according to city or diagnosis.

In summary, hypotheses #1, #3, and #7 were supported by the data on group differences according to city. An unpredicted main effect was found for number of new ways of managing life according to diagnosis, as ARC patients reported having tried more new ways of managing their lives than did AIDS patients.

In looking more closely at the group differences between cities, further analyses were indicated. To clarify the findings for the composite indices "number of alternative therapies" and "number of new ways of managing life," Fisher's exact tests were performed for their component variables. Table 8.3 lists the frequencies for types of alternative therapies used by the London and San Francisco groups. The San Francisco men with AIDS and ARC used megavitamins ($p < .05$, two-tailed test) and meditation ($p < .001$, two-tailed test) significantly more frequently than did the London men. The San Francisco men also used acupressure, massage, herbal treatments, psychic healing, yoga, hypnosis, and visualization more frequently than did the London men, but these differences were not statistically significant. Both city groups reported the same frequency for use of acupuncture, and neither group reported using biofeedback techniques.

TABLE 8.3
Frequency of Alternative Therapies Used

Therapy Type	Frequencies London		San Francisco		p^a
Acupuncture	2	(10%)	2	(10%)	NS
Acupressure	0		1	(5%)	NS
Biofeedback	0		0		—
Herbal treatment	2	(10%)	6	(29%)	NS
Massage	0		4	(19%)	NS
Megativamins	3	(14%)	10	(48%)	.04
Meditation	0		9	(43%)	.001
Psychic healing	1	(5%)	3	(14%)	NS
Yoga	0		1	(5%)	NS
Hypnosis	0		1	(5%)	NS
Chiropractics	1	(5%)	0		NS
Special diets	5	(24%)	4	(19%)	NS
Visualization	2	(10%)	4	(19%)	NS
Other	5	(24%)	5	(24%)	NS

[a]Two-tailed, Fisher's exact test.

TABLE 8.4
Frequency of Use of New Ways of Managing Life

New Ways of Managing	Frequencies London		San Francisco		p^a
Assertiveness training	0		1	(5%)	NS
Support group	6	(29)	5	(24%)	NS
Stress management	1	(5%)	4	(19%)	NS
Psychotherapy	3	(14%)	4	(19%)	NS
Increased reliance on others	7	(33%)	5	(24%)	NS
More health information	6	(29%)	2	(10%)	NS
Opened up more/discussed feelings	7	(33%)	0		.01
Psychologist/psychiatrist	3	(14%)	4	(19%)	NS
Social worker	0		0		——
Therapy group	0		1	(5%)	NS
Improved diet/more rest	13	(62%)	2	(10%)	.001
Other ways	11	(52%)	10	(48%)	NS

[a]Two-tailed, Fisher's exact test.

Table 8.4 lists the frequencies for new ways of managing life used by the San Francisco and London groups. London men with AIDS and ARC reported opening up more with friends "to discuss feelings, thoughts, and problems" since the onset of their health problems significantly more than did San Francisco men ($p < .01$, two-tailed test).

Additionally, the London men also reported improving their diets and getting more rest significantly more frequently than did the San Francisco group ($p < .01$, two-tailed test). The London group reported using support groups, increased reliance on others, and seeking health information more frequently than the San Francisco group, but these differences were not statistically significant. The San Francisco group reported using assertiveness training, stress management, psychotherapy groups, and psychologists or psychiatrists more often than did the London group, but these differences were also not found to be statistically significant.

Differences between cities were examined among variables rated as most helpful in coping since onset of health problems. No significant differences between the city groups were found, although the London men listed "close relationship with physician" nearly three times as frequently as did the San Francisco group. Social support was most frequently reported as being helpful by men with AIDS and ARC in both cities, as indicated in Table 8.5.

Across cities, a significant difference between AIDS and ARC groups was found for a factor rated as helpful in coping with illness. Men with AIDS indicated that they found their own inner resources to be helpful in coping more frequently than did men with ARC ($p < .05$, two-tailed test). As shown in Table 8.6, no significant differences were found for the other "most helpful" variables by diagnosis.

TABLE 8.5
Frequency of Variables Cited as Most Helpful
Since Onset of Health Problems by City

	Frequencies		
Most Helpful Variable	London	San Francisco	p[a]
Social support	11 (52%)	10 (48%)	NS
Close relationship with M.D.	8 (38%)	3 (14%)	NS
Mental health assistance	2 (10%)	1 (5%)	NS
Nothing	0	3 (14%)	NS
Myself, inner resources	4 (19%)	4 (19%)	NS
Other	9 (43%)	12 (57%)	NS

[a]Two-tailed, Fisher's exact test.

TABLE 8.6
Frequency of Variables Cited as Most Helpful
Since Onset of Health Problems by Diagnosis

| Most Helpful Variable | Frequencies | | p^a |
	AIDS	ARC	
Social support	9 (43%)	12 (57%)	NS
Close relationship with M.D.	8 (38%)	3 (14%)	NS
Mental health assistance	1 (5%)	2 (10%)	NS
Nothing	0	3 (14%)	NS
Myself, inner resources	7 (33%)	1 (5%)	NS
Other	9 (43%)	12 (57%)	NS

[a]Two-tailed, Fisher's exact test.

DISCUSSION

Self-blame

None of the differences found between cities can be attributed to differences in age, number of symptoms, or length of time since diagnosis because of the specific matching of the two samples of these variables. Thus, the finding that men with AIDS and ARC in London blamed themselves for their health problems significantly more frequently than did men in San Francisco with the same diagnosis is particularly noteworthy, even more so because of the relatively small sample size ($N = 42$).

However, other characteristics of the London sample may have influenced their blaming themselves for their health problems more often than did the San Francisco men. They were among the first AIDS cases ever diagnosed in England, and all of the 21 subjects had traveled extensively, including several trips to the U.S. Perhaps knowledge of the advancing AIDS epidemic in the U.S. and/or their sexual behavior while traveling caused the London men to blame themselves for their health problems.

Although objective data were not collected on level of income or education for the London group, the interview content revealed that these men often held positions that afforded travel and financial benefits. In contrast, the San Francisco subjects' annual mean income was within the $12,001 to $15,000 range—an income unlikely to afford opportunities such as those often described by the London subjects. The San Francisco sample may have been drawn from a less-privileged group, as they were recruited from a large county hospital (San Francisco General Hospital) serving the indigent population, as well as people with health insurance. In San Francisco, some men with AIDS who could afford to seek health care through another facility or private physician may have done so, but in London all AIDS cases were handled through the STD clinics within the socialized medicine system. Therefore, recruitment of London subjects may have included all levels of income and social status, while the San Francisco recruiting may not have included men with high incomes who may have sought health care outside the county hospital. This possible sample bias may have influenced the reporting of self-blame if upper-income men with AIDS were not adequately represented in the San Francisco sample.

Pill and Stott (1982) found that among working-class mothers in the United Kingdom, women who had more education or who were buying their own homes stressed internal factors or individual behaviors when explaining reasons for illness, whereas less-educated women stressed external factors and held fatalistic views about reasons for illness. Perhaps the London men in our study were accustomed to being able to influence their own lives because of their experiences with power and responsibility in the work setting, and felt influential in determining their own health outcomes.

AIDS was also more widespread and several times more dense among the gay population in San Francisco than in London during 1985 (Carne et al., 1985; Report from PHLS, 1986). It is possible that the San Francisco men with AIDS and ARC in our sample represented a general cross-section of the gay population, whereas the London men with AIDS and ARC may have represented a somewhat elite group that was initially infected with the virus.

Another possible reason for the higher prevalence of self-blame among the London men is that they may have internalized some of the homophobia and negative AIDS hysteria that was then prevalent in London. The level of knowledge about AIDS was much lower in London at that time (Temoshok, Sweet, & Zich, 1987). Further, as Temoshok, Grade, and Zich (1989) noted in their content analysis of newspaper articles covering AIDS in May–June 1985, the London papers were initially highly sensational and fear promoting, while neglecting to report new research. More recently, the British media has participated in a massive AIDS information campaign, but this difference in media coverage of AIDS at that time may have contributed to the self-blame experienced by the London men.

Dr. Anthony Pinching (1987), of St. Mary's Hospital and Medical School in London, spoke of his frustration in dealing with the British media at the onset of the AIDS epidemic in England. During a roundtable discussion on AIDS and the media at the Third International AIDS Conference in Washington, DC (June 1, 1987), Dr. Pinching described how he repeatedly contacted the tabloids in an effort to get information to the public:

> ...but I was told, "Don't tell me about homosexuals, give me blood!" And the headlines read, "Hospitals Using Killer Blood!"

Such resistance to printing information provided by medical professionals may have led to more self-blame by people with AIDS and ARC in London. With an extremely limited amount of information to draw from, people with AIDS may have adopted the widespread attitude that they "brought this on themselves" and blamed themselves for their health problems. Michela and Wood (1986), in their review of the literature on attributions in health and illness, suggested that one's medical knowledge of an illness influences the causal attributions one makes. Naive patients tend to adopt the most simple attributional explanations. Patients may also look to a single major cause to explain a major illness, such as cancer. Perhaps the men with AIDS and ARC in London were more medically naive than the San Francisco men, due partially to the relative novelty of AIDS in London and to the generally biased media coverage at that time. The London men may, therefore, have adopted a simple and socially reinforced explanation for their illness by blaming themselves.

British health care professionals in mid-1985 may have inadvertently contributed to patient self-blame by assuming a position similar to the one promulgated by the sensational early news headlines. As one London AIDS patient stated:

> I resented being told I was promiscuous and would have to change. It was just not true. Some doctor read it in a book...but that's what we're told in this country.

Although the patients who felt that they had not been particularly promiscuous reacted to such assumptions with anger, others seemed to adopt the explanation almost at face value, citing their "indiscretions" or "excessiveness" as the explanation for their illness. However, there were qualitative differences in the responses to the self-blame question. For example, two London men made the following statements:

> . There's a lot of abuse in the gay scene...did we really have to get this (AIDS) to realize it?

> . I pushed my body to the limit and eventually it gave out!

In the first statement, contracting AIDS is linked to the whole "gay scene"; the implication is that "abuse" connected with the gay lifestyle is the source of AIDS, which comes as retribution for such abuse. The second statement reflects a less judgmental approach, and offers a more behavioral, even mechanistic explanation for why the person contracted AIDS. This important distinction between punitive self-blame for being gay and behavioral accountability was not tapped by the self-blame question. Both men simply responded "yes" to the self-blame inquiry.

Janoff-Bulman and Wortman (1977) differentiated behavioral self-blame (involving past behavior) from characterological self-blame (involving personality traits). In their work with accident victims, they found that assigning blame for misfortune to controllable factors, such as past behavior, was actually adaptive and afforded a more optimistic view of the future. In a related study of women who had been raped, Janoff-Bulman (1979) found that only characterological self-blame was associated with depression; behavioral blame was not. This pattern has been replicated in subsequent research with a different population (Peterson, Schwartz, & Seligman, 1981). Perhaps because of the relatively new onset of the AIDS epidemic in England and the paucity of information available to the public through the press or other media, some London men with AIDS and ARC assumed self-blame for their illness as an adaptive effort to maintain control.

The London men may have felt that they could continue to influence their health in the same way they felt they had influenced the onset of their health problems. Consistent with the adaptive interpretation of self-blame, we found that in some ways the London men made more changes in managing their lives than did the San Francisco men, perhaps acting on the belief that they could influence (improve) their health themselves.

Ways of Coping

As hypothesized, San Francisco men with AIDS and ARC tried more alternative therapies than did the London men with AIDS and ARC. It is widely thought that Americans, especially Californians, are likely to use nontraditional therapies, such as megavitamins and herbal treatments. Such treatments are, in fact, widely available in San Francisco and were commonly being used by people with AIDS and ARC in 1985. San Francisco has long been known for its tolerance of nontraditional lifestyles, and nontraditional therapies may be more prevalent as a result. It is quite possible that if we had compared a different U.S. city than San Francisco to London, there may have been less difference in number of alternative therapies used.

Another factor influencing use of alternative therapies may be what appears to be a cultural "trait." In a national comparison of personality characteristics, Skinner and Peters (1984) found that British respondents scored significantly lower than did Americans or Canadians for "extraversion" on Eysenck's Personality Inventory. The British have a reputation for keeping a "stiff upper lip," and, at least in the stereotype, look with amused disdain on America's fascination for various therapies ("You Americans consult your therapist before peeling an orange!"). As another London subject responded, "I've always been independent...I'm not relying on a therapist to face things."

Another possible factor affecting the London men's choice not to seek alternative therapies could be fear of contagion or stigmatization. Most alternative therapies involved physical contact with an alternative health care provider, as in acupuncture and massage. It was our impression that London men in our sample feared transmitting the disease inadvertently through casual contact, perhaps based on misconceptions about AIDS transmission that were prevalent in London at that time (Temoshok, Sweet, & Zich, 1987). London men could also have been fearful of a negative response (stigmatization) in telling an alternative health care provider about health problems because of the anti-gay attitudes that were also prevalent in the London public at that time.

The total number of new ways of managing one's life since diagnosis was not found to be significantly different between the San Francisco and London samples. However, two specific new ways of managing life were used significantly more frequently by the London group. "Opening up more with friends to discuss feelings, thoughts, and problems" was often cited by London men with AIDS and ARC, although not one of the 21 San Francisco men endorsed that response. Such openness is apparently a deviation from the stereotypical British "stiff upper lip" approach, and may be viewed by the London men as a *new* way of managing, whereas the San Francisco men may have been communicating in such a manner all along.

There is an alternative explanation: During the time of this study (and currently) co-counseling with peers (not professional therapists) was a prominent movement in London among health care workers providing services to persons with AIDS and HIV infection. Support groups for STD clinic patients often employed co-counseling principles, and it has become the philosophical foundation of more than one AIDS-oriented community resource. Some of those health care workers most familiar with the co-counseling movement have explained the appeal of it as a way to get help without becoming a patient or seeing oneself as needing help in order to cope. Instead, within co-counseling, everyone is the helper as well as the helped. Within this context, emotional disclosure runs less risk of seeming pathological or being seen by the discloser as a sign of weakness or inability to cope. Shifting the roles of helper and helped is believed to minimize a sense of being "one down" and needy.

Another possible explanation for the London subjects' more reported openness with friends and family may be that the San Francisco men were *objectively* not opening up and discussing their feelings and problems as often as the London men. Although this possibility seems unlikely, considering the more reserved British personality, further analysis of types of disclosure patterns and openness after diagnosis of a serious illness is necessary to clarify any cultural differences.

London men also indicated "improving diet, getting more rest" as a new way used to manage life significantly more frequently than did the San Francisco men. This response is consistent with the British tendency to not disclose problems to an outsider, since no therapist is necessary to improve one's diet and rest. Also, this rest/diet recommendation is consistent with the medical advice most often cited as having been received by the London subjects. In dealing with a disease considered terminal, which has no known effective treatment, such advice is probably common, but was frequently mentioned in the course of the London interviews, for example: "He (the doctor) told me to get plenty of rest, sleep, and don't burn the candle at both ends."

Besides "seeking more health information," which was indicated more frequently by the London men, although not significantly so, the remaining "new ways of managing life" inquired about involved contact with persons outside the medical profession. For instance, assertiveness training, psychotherapy, and stress management all involved seeking outside help and potentially disclosing health status. These options may not have been selected by the London men for the reasons suggested previously to explain selection of alternative therapies, as they would have involved the same type of risk taking.

An unpredicted main effect was found for total number of new ways of managing life by diagnosis. Men with ARC in both London and San Francisco reported trying more new ways of managing their lives than did those with AIDS in either city. This may be partially explained by the increased anxiety and distress reported by ARC patients, as noted by Temoshok et al. (1986a). If ARC patients were more distressed than AIDS patients, they may have attempted to cope actively with that distress by trying other ways of managing their lives. Also, men with ARC may have felt that they had a better chance to influence their health outcome, in that ARC did not carry the "death sentence" connotation to the degree that AIDS did, particularly in 1985 (Moulton et al., 1987). Thus, men with ARC may have tried more new ways of managing their lives because they felt that they could effect a change in their health outcome or because they viewed the outcome of ARC as more malleable than that of AIDS.

Additionally, it is possible that men with ARC had been experiencing health problems for a shorter amount of time than men with AIDS. Although there was no significant difference in time elapsed from diagnosis to interview for the AIDS and ARC groups, it is likely that the men with AIDS were experiencing health problems for some time before receiving a formal AIDS diagnosis. Shortly after developing symptoms of illness, people may attempt to take action in dealing with the newly recognized life threat of HIV, such as trying new ways of managing their lives. As the disease progresses, men with AIDS may rely more heavily on resources known to them to be effective, as part of an effort to economize energy and disengage from extraneous relationships, as noted in other serious illnesses (Kalish, 1985).

Social Support

This study found that social support was more frequently cited as "most helpful in coping" by men in both London and San Francisco. Responses coded as "other" for this question were often specific references to individuals or organizations that provided social support. The importance of social support among people with AIDS and ARC has been documented previously (Dilley, et al., 1985; Holland & Tross, 1985; Temoshok et al., 1986a; Zich & Temoshok, 1987).

Although social support was indicated as most important by both men with AIDS and ARC, the AIDS respondents also reported that their own inner resources were most helpful in dealing with their health problems. The reliance of men with AIDS on their own inner resources may be related to the higher mortality rate among those with AIDS as compared with those with ARC (Barnes, 1986). If men with AIDS perceive their illness as more life-threatening than those with ARC, they may be more likely to experience the stages of dying described by Kubler-Ross, Wessler, and Avioli (1972). In the fifth, or final, stage—acceptance, the seriously ill patient is likely to separate himself from what he may leave in the near future and concentrate on concluding unfinished business. This behavior or attitude implies an increasing reliance on the self, accompanied by a decreased reliance on others.

Another possible reason for self-reliance being more helpful in coping for people with AIDS may be that they are relying on their inner resources out of necessity, because of increased isolation. Several authors have reported isolation as an issue articulated by people with AIDS during in-depth interviews (Dilley et al., 1985; Holland & Tross, 1985; Miller, 1987). Zich and Temoshok (1987) found that persons with AIDS who reported more physical symptoms also perceived social support to be less available. People with AIDS may also experience a decrease in available support from others. Wortman and Lehman (in press) pointed out that support providers may respond to victims of a life crisis in an unsupportive manner because of: (1) their own feelings of vulnerability; (2) inexperience or uncertainty as to what to say or do; or (3) misconceptions about how to react or deal with people in a life crisis. Such inappropriate attempts to provide support may result in the seriously ill person relying more on the self, in order to prevent caregivers from feeling uncomfortable, as well as to buffer oneself from distress. A clearer picture of what is most helpful in dealing with AIDS will have important clinical implications.

The finding that London men with AIDS and ARC reported opening up more with friends may be related to the finding that London men did not spend less time with friends and family than did men in San Francisco. Even though the general public was found to be more fearful and less knowledgeable about AIDS in London than in San Francisco at that time (Temoshok, Sweet, & Zich, 1987), the London men still spent the same amount of time (or more) with their friends and family as did men in San Francisco. It has been observed that patients with a serious illness often disengage from attachments and relationships, while maintaining only those relationships most important to them (Kalish, 1985). Future studies may find that this is true for AIDS patients specifically; but in this study, only time spent with family and friends was investigated.

If the London men withdrew socially at all due to the prevalent homophobia or fear of stigmatization, they did not isolate themselves from friends and family. This does not necessarily mean that the London men were entirely candid about their health problems with friends and family, however. Several of the London men reported telling family that they had cancer or leukemia rather than AIDS or ARC. One subject remarked that he had a brother still in school, and it would be hard on him at school if news got out about AIDS in his family. It seems that one way the London men coped was by maintaining their alliances with their social-support system (friends and family) and monitoring what they disclosed about their health condition.

In addition to maintaining contact with friends and family, it appears that London men also were in communication with people with their same diagnosis. It was hypothesized that the London men with AIDS and ARC would not include people with their same diagnosis in their most supportive circle as frequently as did the San Francisco men, but this was not true. One possible explanation is that the gay subculture had already moved toward organizing support for people with AIDS/ARC, along the line of Shanti in San Francisco. The Terrence Higgins Trust, established after Terrence Higgins died in 1982, has been a major influence in providing support groups. Self-help groups such as "Body Positive" were cited by several London ARC patients as helpful in their coping. Occasionally, London subjects described how well-meaning health professionals would discourage them from socializing with same-diagnosis people, although such suggestions were not necessarily heeded:

> The hospital discourages AIDS patients from mingling…because it's so depressing, I suppose. I met a fellow here just yesterday…I hear he died this morning.

Finding no difference between the two cities for same-diagnosis support is especially interesting in view of the much smaller numbers of AIDS and ARC patients in London. It seems that the London men were just as likely as the San Francisco men to include other men diagnosed with AIDS or ARC in their support circle, despite the possible influence of fewer total AIDS/ARC cases in London, knowing fewer people personally who had dies of AIDS, and occasional discouragement from health professionals regarding socializing with the same-diagnosis people. The existence of these apparant circles of same-diagnosis support may have facilitated networking of support services as the AIDS epidemic progressed in the United Kingdom.

Optimism

The hypothesis that London men with AIDS and ARC would be less optimistic than San Francisco men was not supported by the data. The finding that London men did not isolate themselves from friends and family, and often used the gay support network noted in references to Body Positive groups and the Terrence Higgins Trust, may have influenced the optimism rating for the London men. Perhaps facing AIDS with an intact social system offsets the negative influences of the stigmatizing headlines and public homophobia. This explanation is partially supported by Scheier and Carver (1985), who found optimism to be associated with seeking of social support.

It is also possible that the interviewer optimism rating was not a valid measure. Because all interviewers were American, the London subjects may have been hesitant to disclose their more pessimistic thoughts about the future to foreign strangers. Such reluctance would be consistent with Skinner and Peters' (1984) findings regarding lower extraversion among British nationals. Possible interviewer bias may also have influenced the optimism ratings, as this was one of the few interview questions that required the interviewer to interpret and code a response based on the interviewer's own judgment. Perhaps the optimism measure would be more accurate if determined by self-report, to avoid interviewer bias and to avoid the possibility of obtaining a socially desirable response in the presence of an interviewer.

IMPLICATIONS AND CONCLUSIONS

It should be emphasized that this study was conducted at a particular point in the AIDS epidemic—mid-1985. Public perceptions of AIDS, including the perceptions of those with AIDS and ARC, have changed considerably as knowledge of AIDS has increased and more effective treatments have become available. It should also be stressed that this is a tale of two specific cities and that the findings are probably not directly generalizable to Minneapolis or Kampala.

One of the goals of our study was to underline the culturally specific nature of coping with AIDS. It will be important to conduct parallel studies with other groups who have AIDS and ARC, including women, minorities, intravenous drug users, and hemophiliacs. Future research must investigate any qualitative differences in coping means found to be most helpful to people with AIDS and ARC over time and across cities and nations. Any differences noted in needs, means of coping, and patterns of health attributions made may be helpful in shaping the direction of AIDS interventions. Additionally, an international attempt should be made to use similar measures in this research. A consistency in methodology would make generalizing across cultures a more viable possibility, as well as indicating more clearly where reasons for differences lie.

There is an urgent need for collaborative efforts between nations and disciplines, as not only the spread of AIDS is at stake, but also the longevity and quality of life of those afflicted.

In conclusion, this study highlights the need to make comparative investigations of how people respond to having AIDS and ARC in various cities, nations, and cultures. A better understanding of these different responses could lead to more effective and compassionate medical and mental health interventions that are appropriate for the values, proclivities, and perspectives of the populations targeted for care.

ACKNOWLEDGMENTS

Special thanks are extended to Marcelle Kardush, Ph.D., whose support and guidance were deeply appreciated in reviewing an earlier version of this study submitted by the first author as a Master's thesis to San Francisco State University. Thesis advisors Virginia Saunders, Ph.D., and Sheila Zipf, Ph.D., also contributed helpful editorial suggestions. We would like to express our gratitude to the individual members of the Biopsychosicial AIDS Project and participants in Dr. Temoshok's Clinical Health Psychology seminar (both at UCSF), who were extremely helpful in providing comments and insights throughout the development of this study.

Funding for the London portion of the study was provided through the University Research Expeditions Program, Berkeley. The San Francisco component was supported by National Institute of Mental Health Grant #MH 39344 (Lydia Temoshok, Ph.D., Principal Investigator). Dr. Zich's involvement in this research was supported by National Research Service Award #1F 32 MH09046 and by Clinical Investigator Award #1 K08 MH00608, both from the National Institute of Mental Health.

We are indebted to Anthony Pinching, M.D., and John Green, Ph.D., at St. Mary's Hospital in London, who generously agreed to allow us to interview persons with AIDS there and helped with logistical arrangements. We also thank Dr. Jackie Parkins and Dr. Jonathon Weber for referring their patients to the study. At St. Stephen's Hospital, Charles Farthing, M.D., and John Shine were extremely helpful in allowing us to interview patients and arranging interviews. David Miller, now Principal Psychologist at James Pringle House, Middlesex Hospital, provided invaluable information and insights about psychological aspects of AIDS in London.

We wish to acknowledge, in particular, the participants in the 1985 UREP Program in London who conducted the London interviews along with Drs. Temoshok and Zich: Cisca Arndt, B.A., Julia Gregg, R.N., Carl Hopkins, Ph.D., Joy Key, R.N., Steve Marson, M.S.W., June Mathwich, L.P.N., Mary Merwin, Ph.D., Karla Necessary, M.A., and Marilyn Nichols, R.N. In San Francisco, the interviews were conducted by Jeffrey M. Moulton, Ph.D.,

Christopher Mead, Ph.D., and Thomas Irish, Ph.D. Finally, we wish to express our appreciation to the study participants for sharing their time and their personal experiences.

REFERENCES

Barnes, D. (1986). Grim projections for AIDS epidemic. *Science, 232,* 1589-1590.

Beck, E. J., Cunningham, D., Moss, V., Harris, J., Pinching, A., & Jeffries, D. (1987). HIV testing: Changing trends at a clinic for sexually transmitted diseases in London. *British Medical Journal, 295,* 191-193.

Carne, C., Sutherland, S., Ferns, R., Mindel, A., Weller, I., Cheingsong-Popov, R., Williams, P., Tedder, R., & Adler, M. (1985). Rising prevalence of Human T-Lymphotrophic Virus Type III (HTLV-III) infection in homosexual men in London. *Lancet, 1,* 1261.

Centers for Disease Control (1987). Update: AIDS—United States. *Mortality and Morbidity Report, 36,* 522-526.

Chilivumbo, A. B. (1973). Social basis of illness: A search for therapeutic meaning. In F. Grolig & H. Haley (Eds.), *Medical anthropology* (pp. 67-79). Paris: Mouton Publishers.

Coates, T., Temoshok, L., & Mandel, J. (1984). Psychosocial research is essential to understanding and treating AIDS. *American Psychologist, 39,* 1309-1314.

Dilley, J., Ochitill, H., Perl, M., & Volberding, P. (1985). Findings in psychiatric consultations with patients with acquired immune deficiency syndrome. *American Journal of Psychiatry, 142,* 82-85.

Forster, G. (1986). Venereology. In D. Miller, J. Weber, & J. Green (Eds.), *The management of AIDS patients* (pp. 65-80). London: The Macmillan Press.

Gorman, E. M. (1986). The AIDS epidemic in San Francisco: Epidemiological and anthropological perspectives. In C. R. Jones, R. Stall, & S. M. Gifford (Eds.), *Anthropology and epidemiology* (pp. 157-172). Voorstrat, Holland: D. Reidel Publishing Company.

Green, J. (1986). Counselling HTLV-III seropositives. In D. Miller, J. Weber, & J. Green (Eds.), *The management of AIDS patients* (pp. 151-168). London: The Macmillan Press.

Ham, C. (1985). *Health policy in Britian.* Second Edition. Farmingdale, NY: Baywood Publishing Co.

Harwood, A. (Ed.), (1981). *Ethnicity and medical care.* Cambridge, MA: Harvard University Press.

Haverkos, H. W., Gottlieb, M. S., Killen, J. Y., & Edelman, R. (1985). Classification of HTLV-III/LAV-related diseases. *Journal of Infectious Diseases, 152,* 1095.

Helman, C. (1985). *Culture, health and illness.* Bristol: John Wright & Sons.

Holland, J., & Tross, S. (1985). The psychosocial and neuropsychiatric sequelae of the acquired immunodeficiency syndrome and related disorders. *Annals of Internal Medicine, 103,* 760-764.

Janoff-Bulman, R. (1979). Characterological vs. behavioral self-blame: Inquiries into depression and rape. *Journal of Personality and Social Psychology, 37,* 1798-1809.

Janoff-Bulman, R., & Wortman, C. (1977). Attributions of blame and coping in the "real world": Severe accident victims react to their lot. *Journal of Personality and Social Psychology, 35,* 351-363.

Jesson, W., Thorp, R., Mortimer, P., & Oates, J. (1986). Prevalence of anti-HTLV-III in UK risk groups 1984/85. *Lancet, 1,* 155.

Kalish, R. (1985). Coping with death. In R. Kalish (Ed.), *The final transition* (pp. 11-24). Farmingdale, NY: Baywood Publishing Co.

Kleinman, A. (Ed.). (1980). *Patients and healers in the context of culture.* Berkeley: University of California Press.

Kubler-Ross, E., Wessler, S., & Avioli, L. V. (1972). Therapeutic grand rounds, number 36: On death and dying. *Journal of the American Medical Association, 221,* 174–179.

Kunitz, S. J., & Levy, J. E. (1981). Navajos. In A. Harwood (Ed.), *Ethnicity and medical care* (pp. 1–36). Cambridge, MA: Harvard University Press.

Laguerre, M. (1981). Haitian Americans. In A. Harwood (Ed.), *Ethnicity and medical care* (pp. 172–210). Cambridge, MA: Harvard University Press.

Madeley, T. (1987). ABC of AIDS: Having AIDS. *British Medical Journal, 295,* 320–321.

Martin, J., & Vance, C. (1984). Behavioral and psychosocial factors in AIDS. *American Psychologist, 39,* 1303–1308.

Michela, J. L., & Wood, J. V. (1986). Casual attributions in health and illness. In D. C. Kendall (Ed.), *Advances in cognitive-behavioral research and therapy* (Vol. 5, pp. 179–235). New York: Academic Press.

Miller, D. (1986). Psychology, AIDS, ARC, and PGL. In D. Miller, J. Weber, & J. Green (Eds.), *The management of AIDS patients* (pp. 131–150), London: The Macmillan Press.

Miller, D. (1987). ABC of AIDS: Counselling. *British Medical Journal, 294,* 1671–1674.

Morin, S., Charles, K., & Malyon, A. (1984). The psychological impact of AIDS on gay men. *American Psychologist, 39,* 1288–1293.

Moulton, J., Sweet, D., Temoshok, L., & Mandel, J. (1987). Attributions of blame and responsibility in relation to distress and health behavior change in people with AIDS and AIDS-related complex. *Journal of Applied Social Psychology, 17,* 493–506.

Panos Institute (1987). *AIDS and the Third World.* London: The Panos Institute, in association with the Norwegian Red Cross.

Peterson, C., Schwartz, S. M., & Seligman, M. E. P. (1981). Self-blame and depressive symptoms. *Journal of Personality and Social Psychology, 41,* 253–259.

Pill, R., & Stott, N. (1982). Concepts of illness causation and responsibility: Some preliminary data from a sample of working class mothers. *Social Science & Medicine, 16,* 43–52.

Pinching, A. (1987, June). *AIDS and the media.* Roundtable discussion held during Third International AIDS Conference. Washington, DC.

Reich, J. W., & Zautra, A. (1981). Life events and personal causation: Some relationships with satisfaction and distress. *Journal of Personality and Social Psychology, 41,* 1002–1012.

Report from PHLS. (1986). A report from the PHLS Communicable Disease Surveillance Centre. *British Medical Journal, 293,* 326–327.

Report from PHLS. (1987). A report from the PHLS Communicable Disease Surveillance Centre. *British Medical Journal, 294,* 1402.

Rosenthal, R., & Rosnow, R. (1984). *Essentials of behavioral research.* New York: McGraw-Hill.

Scheier, M., & Carver, C. (1985). Optimism, coping and health: Assessment and implications of generalized outcome expectancies. *Health Psychology, 4,* 219–247.

Schreiber, J. M., & Homiak, J. P. (1981). Mexican Americans. In A. Harwood (Ed.), *Ethnicity and medical care* (pp. 265–282). Cambridge, MA: Harvard University Press.

Sherr, L. (1987). An evaluation of the UK government health education campaign on AIDS. *Psychology and Health, 1,* 61–72.

Skinner, N., & Peters, P. (1984). National personality characteristics: Comparison of Canadian, American and British samples. *Psychological Reports, 54,* 121–122.

Sonnex, C., Petherick, A., Adler, M., & Miller, D. (1987). HIV infection: Increase in public awareness and anxiety. *British Medical Journal, 295,* 193–195.

Temoshok, L. (1983–1988). *A longitudinal psychoimmunologic study of ARC patients.* NIMH grant award #MH 39344.

Temoshok, L., Grade, M., & Zich, J. (1989). Public health, the press, and AIDS: An analysis of newspaper articles in London and San Francisco. In I. Corliss & M. Pittman-Lideman (Eds.), *AIDS: Principles, practices and politics* (pp. 525–542). New York: Harper & Row.

Temoshok, L., Mandel, J., Moulton, J., Zich, J., & Solomon, G. (1986a, May). *A longitudinal* psychosocial study of AIDS and ARC in San Francisco: *Preliminary results*. Paper presented at annual meeting of the American Psychiatric Association. Washington, D.C.

Temoshok, L., Mandel, J., Solomon, G. Zich, J., Moulton, J.M., & Mead, C. (1986b, June). *Applying a biopsychosocial perspective to research on AIDS*. Paper presented at the Second International Conference on AIDS. Paris, France.

Temoshok, L., Sweet, D.M., Moulton, J.M., & Zich, J. (1987, June). *A longitudinal study of distress and coping in men and with AIDS and AIDS-related complex*. Paper presented at the Third International Conference on AIDS. Washington, D.C.

Temoshok, L., Sweet, D.M., & Zich, J. (1987). A three-city comparison of the public's attitudes about AIDS. *Psychology and Health, 1*, 43-60.

Weinberg, M., & Williams, C. (1974). *Male homosexuals: Their problems and adaptions*. New York: Oxford University Press.

World Health Organization. (1988). Statistics from the World Health Organization and the Centers for Disease Control. *AIDS, 2*, 487-490.

Wortman, C.B., & Lehman, D.R. (in press). Reactions to victims of life crises: Support attempts that fail. In I.B. Sarason & B.R. Sarason (Eds.), *Social support: Theory, research and application*. The Hague: Martinus Nijof.

Zich, J., & Temoshok, L. (1987). Perceptions of social support in men with AIDS and ARC: Relationships with distress and hardiness. *Journal of Applied Social Psychology, 17*, 193-215.

Zola, I. (1983). *Social-medical inquiries*. Philadelphia: Temple University Press.

The Behavioral Aspects of AIDS: An International Perspective

9

Peter G. Bourne
Department of Psychiatry
St. Georges Medical School, Grenada
President, American Association for World Health

From the days when an infective agent was first suspected as being the causative factor in the sudden appearance of Kaposi's sarcoma and *Pneumocystis carinii* pneumonia, our thinking has been dominated by historical concepts based on our past experience with infectious epidemics. Smallpox, measles, and typhoid rushed to mind as comparable earlier examples of what we faced in dealing with the human immune deficiency virus. With the early conceptual thinking dominated by immunologists, virologists, and medical epidemiologists, the nature of the virus and the hunt for a vaccine that could be made universally available skewed the dialogue and became the central focus both for trying to understand the epidemic and in defining the shape of our response. Such thinking was also highly consistent with our cultural tendency to look for quick technological solutions to any problem confronting modern society. That the disease should have emerged first in this country among homosexuals caused speculation, no matter how irrational it may now seem, that this group might have some particular susceptibility to the virus rather than suggesting that we might be learning something fundamental about the behavioral ecology of the disease in a larger human context.

Now we are finally beginning to understand that the AIDS epidemic is not like bubonic plague spreading willy-nilly through the population as a whole. Rather, it is far better understood from the perspective of a behavioral model than an infectious disease model. It is also clear that, at least for the moment, a thorough understanding of such a behavioral paradigm offers the best basis for a strategy to control the epidemic. This becomes particularly clear if one looks at the disease on a global basis, examining both the demographic and the social patterns of who became involved as it has emerged in different countries.

Early reports from Africa suggested that there was a one-to-one male/ female ratio among those infected, occasioning sudden hysteria in this country that the entire global heterosexual population might be at risk. Looked at more closely, it became evident that the picture in Africa was not only complex, but involved a range of social and individual behaviors that clearly explained why the profile of those becoming infected was different from that in the United States. For instance, in Ghana, six times as many women are infected as men (Neequaye, Osei, & Asamoah-Adu, 1988). However, they are nearly all from the Krobo tribe in the Eastern part of the country that was devastated by the economic crisis in the early 1980s. These women left Ghana and went else-where in Africa, especially to the Ivory Coast, where, to make ends meet, they had engaged in prostitution and became infected with HIV. Returning to Ghana as the economy improved, they have since infected a certain number of Ghanaian men.

In Zimbabwe, there is a relatively high prevalence of HIV positivity, with men outnumbering women. It is, however, overwhelmingly present among members of the Zimbabwe African Peoples Union (ZAPU) forces who fought under Joshua Nkomo during the war for independence, and only minimally so among the Zimbabwe African National Union (ZANU) forces of Prime Minister Robert Mugabe. The reason is that during the independence struggle, the ZAPU forces were based primarily in Zambia where they had access to a heavily infected Zambian prostitute population. The ZANU force was based in Mozambique where the disease was, for all practical purposes, nonexistent at the time (Gloyd, personal communication, April 22, 1988).

In Uganda, the building of roads to increase commerce into an area of apparent longstanding endemic HIV infectivity has led to the spread of the disease into the cities. Truck stops along the route attracted permanent populations of prostitutes, and the progressive spread of the disease transmitted by truck drivers from one stop to the next until it eventually reached the capital, Kampala, has been clearly demonstrated.

In Zaire, studies comparing seropositivity in rural areas in 1986 demonstrated no change from the level of under two percent in blood samples drawn in 1976. However, in the capital, Kinshasa, seropositivity had risen from less than one percent to more than 25 percent, and higher in select populations, during the same period of time (Tinker, 1987). Among employees of the Central Bank in Kinshasa, more than 50 percent were seropositive in 1986 (Tinker & Sabatier, 1987). A similar pattern appears to exist in Zambia and Kenya. The dramatic increase in the AIDS problem in Africa is a product of the urbanization process during the last 20 years and the change in lifestyle that accompanied it. In each instance, it is primarily the better-educated and more affluent men, together with female prostitutes, who are the most frequent victims. It is apparent that having multiple sex partners had become a relatively socially accepted symbol of male success among the new urban elite in many African countries.

An additional factor is the frequency of anal intercourse among prostitutes as a recreation of choice among their clients, including expatriates. In Moslem regions of the continent, even among nonprostitutes, anal intercourse is practiced as a way of preventing pregnancy and preserving virginity. Whatever the reason, the behavior has helped to foster the spread of the disease.

In Brazil, the AIDS epidemic can be considered not as one, but as three separate and distinct epidemics. The first is among an educated affluent gay population which has long had close connections with New York's gay community. The second is among a small but growing population of needle-sharing intravenous drug users, which did not exist a few years ago, but which has emerged recently as part of a growing urban addiction problem across Latin America. The third is among the largely impoverished urban population that is dependent for health care on trained and untrained practitioners who re-use needles and other equipment without proper sterilization, and a private blood-products industry involving many small-scale entrepreneurs that is largely outside government supervision or regulation.

What is evident from all of the data that have been gathered around the world is that AIDS is, under ordinary circumstances, a poorly transmitted disease of low infectivity. What is vital for its evolutionary success are what might be called "augmenting behavioral scenarios." These are sociocultural events which are in some ways out of the ordinary and which allow the virus to burst out of an endemic situation, where it may have been relatively well contained, and mushroom forth into an epidemic crisis in a new population. These events that allow this to happen are characterized by the fact that they lead to behavior which will break or traumatize the human integument (or they may involve tissue that, through the prior existence of other sexually transmitted disease or for other reasons, is already damaged) and are carried out in conjunction with someone already infected with the virus. The clearest example is the sharing of needles by IV drug users where one of the users is infected. In sexual transmission, the sex of the partners is fundamentally irrelevant to the disease process. What is crucial is the extent to which the sexual act is traumatic to the tissues of the genitalia involved. The production of micro-fissures, especially if accompanied by inflammation that attracts crucial T cells to the area, is the most vital outcome of the behavior to enable the virus to cross from one individual to another. Anal intercourse, whether male/male or male/female, is clearly more conducive than vaginal intercourse to this process, and repetition with multiple partners in a short period of time compounds the likelihood of injury. In addition, of course, the larger the number of partners, the greater the statistical probability of exposure. It is perhaps analagous to the athlete training for a marathon who, if he overdoes his miles, will inevitably end up with an injury. No matter which organs of the body are involved, overuse leads to physical breakdown. In a recent brief report,

Konotey-Ahula (1987) described the extensive perineal trauma encountered in a study of 88 prostitutes in West, East, and Central Africa, many of whom engaged in both vaginal and anal intercourse. While it is hard to generalize, a low emphasis on foreplay and a high frequency of unlubricated, "dry" sex seems also to be a factor.

There are, of course, other medical factors which have a catalytic effect in facilitating the transfer of the virus, such as the presence of intercurrent venereal disease and the use of birth-control pills.

While a breach of the human integument is a physiological requirement for the spread of AIDS, one can look at these "augmenting behavioral scenarios" as the social equivalent, representing a break in the normal social fabric which becomes equally vital for the spread of the disease. There is every reason to believe that HIV has existed for a long time in isolated locations. What has changed is that in the last 20 years, as a result of social, technological, economic, and political developments, there has been a historical confluence of the necessary "augmenting behavioral scenarios" in the right number, with the right connections to allow the virus to jump from one situation to another in which the right behaviors allowed it to flourish.

The report of the finding of HIV in preserved tissue specimens from an individual who died in St. Louis in the late 1960s is particularly instructive (Kolata, 1987). One can speculate that this individual acquired the virus from an international traveler who apparently infected no one else, and who may have been in this country for only a brief period of time. It may or may not be significant that St. Louis is the base of a major international air carrier. The individual who acquired the virus apparently passed it on to no one else. Because the correct "augmenting behavioral scenario" was not present, the virus had to wait another 10 years to establish itself in North America. Had the individual involved lived in another city and led a different lifestyle, the result could have been today's AIDS epidemic 10 years earlier rather than one isolated case. Indeed, it may be true that the AIDS virus was brought to the United Stated several times and died out before it finally connected with the right behavioral environment and was able to establish a foothold.

Perhaps far more frequently than we have appreciated up until now, the trail of viral transmission has, like the St. Louis case, resulted in a dead end with regard to the perpetuation of the virus. This is particularly true when the disease has been passed to someone outside of the population directly involved in an "augmenting behavioral scenario." As there is now more public education about AIDS, this is likely to become even more true. Trails of transmission in a linear fashion from one individual to another to another will be highly atypical and, therefore, of relatively little significance. The crucial feature will be the major disseminators, infected individuals who spread the disease to an array of other contacts, especially if any of those contacts constitute entry points in new and distinct "augmenting behavioral scenarios."

A special situation exists with regard to the spread of the HIV virus when it exists in a closed or quasi-closed society. Prison populations are one example. Another is small island nations. We tend to think of AIDS as being first and foremost a U.S. problem, and, indeed, more than half of the reported cases so far have been from the United States. However, the prevalence of AIDS cases per capita is by far the highest in the Caribbean. In Bermuda, as of the end of 1987, there were 1,107 cases per million; in the Bahamas, 536; and in Haiti, Trinidad, and Barbados, approximately 145 cases per million. This compares with 172 cases per million in the US, and 40 per million in Switzerland, the European country with the highest prevalence. The most affected African countries report between 120 and 150 cases per million (Tinker, 1987).

While the Caribbean islands with high prevalence levels rely heavily on tourism and may have been disproportionately affected by virus-carrying visitors, they now face a situation where the risk for any individual of having sex with an infected individual would seem to be dramatically higher than in the U.S. and Europe. What remains as yet unknown, however, is the extent to which the cases are restricted to narrow segments of the society; for instance, those who have multiple sex partners, many of whom may be foreign visitors.

Understanding in detail these behavioral processes will be vital in determining whether we can control this epidemic. Resources need to be skillfully targeted to ensure the most potent interventions in the natural history of the disease. A rifle shot rather than a shotgun blast is what is required. The biggest struggle we are likely to face, both nationally and internationally, will be against a relenting pressure to spend funds aimed at calming an alarmed and frightened public which faces a minimal threat from the disease, rather than on programs to reduce spread among high-risk groups who are also, for the most part, highly stigmatized. There is perhaps no phrase more offensive in connection with the AIDS epidemic than the term, "innocent victims," as though there is anyone with the disease who is not an innocent victim. Massive public-education campaigns directed at the population as a whole may be desirable in helping to allay public alarm and in engendering a more healthy attitude about sex in general, but they should not be seen as a cost effective way of controlling the epidemic.

Effective control, in many instances, will involve carrying out policies that are unpopular. It is clear that the spread of AIDS in the IV-drug-using community in the United States is largely a product of disastrous national drug policies over the last seven years which have sought to emphasize criminalization of the drug user rather than treatment. The resulting atmosphere of fear has helped to spawn the "shooting galleries" and the quick sharing of intravenous needles among desperate addicts fearful of detection. The situation has been severely compounded by treatment waiting lists of three months or longer, periods during which infected addicts are likely to be spreading the virus to others.

The relatively modest spread of AIDS in Britain, which has a significant IV-drug-using population, is clearly due to the more responsible policies toward the handling of drug addicts. Studies show that the provision of clean needles in Amsterdam and in Birmingham, England has reduced the incidence of AIDS (Van den Hoek, Van Zadelhof, Goudsmit, & Coutinho, 1986). This has also clearly been true with regard to patients in Europe who were put in methadone maintenance programs (Tidone, Sileo, Goglio, & Borra, 1987). The cutting of drug-treatment budgets and the closing of such programs in this country has clearly contributed to the magnitude of the AIDS epidemic.

While constituting a difficult social and political problem, prostitution is clearly a central element in the spread of AIDS in Africa, which education alone is unlikely to change. Stringent measures also need to be taken against the failure to screen blood and the re-use of needles and other medical equipment in several developing countries.

We should not underestimate the magnitude of the threat that the AIDS epidemic poses, especially in Africa. However, a strategy for controlling it based on a carefully researched and thorough understanding of the behavioral aspects of the disease offers the potential for drastically limiting its spread, regardless of whether an effective cure or a vaccine is developed in the foreseeable future. If we are capable of overcoming the emotional and political pressures that tend to distort the translation of scientific studies into public policy, then it appears that we have the tools already to minimize the real threat which this disease poses for the world.

REFERENCES

Kolata, G. (1987, October 28). Boy's 1969 death suggests AIDS invaded U.S. several times. *The New York Times*, A15.

Konotey-Ahulu, F. I. D. (1987). AIDS: Origin, transmission, and moral dilemmas. Letter to the editor. *Journal of the Royal Society of Medicine, 80*, 720.

Neequaye, A., Osei, L., & Asamoah-Adu, A. (1988, March 8–10). *Dynamics of HIV epidemic: The Ghanaian experience*. Paper presented at the First International Conference on the Global Aspect of AIDS, London.

Tidone, L., Sileo, F., Goglio, G., & Borra, G. C. (1987). AIDS in Italy. *American Journal of Drug and Alcohol Abuse, 13*, 485–486.

Tinker, J. (1987). *AIDS and the Third World*. London: Panos Institute.

Tinker, J., & Sabatier, R. (1987). AIDS and the hidden enemy. *Development International, 1*, 22–27.

Van den Hoek, J. A., Van Zadelhof, A. W., Goudsmit, J., & Coutinho, R. A. (1986, June 23–25). *Risk factors for LAV/HTLV-III infection among drug users in Amsterdam*. Paper presented at the International Conference on AIDS, Paris.

Implications of Different Strategies for Coping with AIDS

10

Sheila Namir
Deane L. Wolcott
Fawzy I. Fawzy
Mary Jane Alumbaugh
University of California, Los Angeles
Department of Psychiatry and Biobehavioral Sciences

AIDS creates a multifaceted group of stressors that often exceed the coping abilities people have developed before becoming ill. The disease frequently has an adverse impact on vocational and social functioning, self-esteem, mood states, physical abilities, family and other relationships, and sexual functioning (Christ & Weiner, 1985; Fornstein, 1984). Successful coping might have an impact on the length and course of survival, the functioning of the immune system, physical symptoms, mood, role and social functioning, and one's self-concept.

Coping with the AIDS crisis is a topic that is important for our society as a whole. Although this chapter will focus on coping with a diagnosis of AIDS and living with AIDS in a way that may diminish emotional problems associated with a life-threatening illness, coping also has preventive aspects. We need to develop strategies to help people who are worried about AIDS, who are seeking to change their behaviors in ways that will prevent contracting the virus responsible for AIDS, who are positive for HIV-antibodies, and who are bereaved. These coping strategies will have to address traditional issues of people with a life-threatening illness; the vast literature on stress, coping, and adaptation; the psychological knowledge about behavior change; and issues of prejudice and social discrimination.

The current study explored the relationship of coping to both psychological and health parameters in gay men with AIDS. Coping has been defined in a variety of ways, including Lazarus and Folkman's (1984) process-oriented definition of coping as "constantly changing cognitive and behavioral efforts to manage specific external and/or internal demands that are appraised as taxing or exceeding the resources of the person" (p. 141). The tasks of coping with illness have also been described, including three major adaptive tasks involved in coping with illness described by Taylor (1983): the search for meaning in the event, attempting to master the situation and efforts to enhance self-esteem, or the responses described by Pearlin and Schooler (1978) in terms of the functions of three major types of coping.

Coping with a life-threatening illness, such as AIDS, demands coping skills that may involve a reassessment of the situation in more positive terms or active involvement in confronting the realities of the situation and taking appropriate actions. Weisman (1979), based on his study of people with cancer, found that "good copers" with cancer are resourceful, optimistic, and "avoid avoidance; do not deny" (p. 42).

We explored the attempts made by people to cope with a diagnosis of AIDS and developed an instrument based on Billings and Moos' (1981) descriptions of three methods of coping: active-cognitive coping, active-behavioral coping, and avoidance coping. The items in the instrument were selected from Amerikan's (1985) 25-item "Dealing with Illness" coping instrument used as part of the Epidemiology Catchment Area Study, which, in turn, was based on Lazarus' Ways of Coping Checklist (Lazarus & Folkman, 1984). The Health and Daily Living Form (Moos, Cronkite, Billings, & Finney, 1984) was also used in developing additional items.

The relationships of these coping strategies to psychological and physical functioning were explored in this study, with the purpose of understanding more about how best to intervene with people who have AIDS and to help them cope more effectively with the stressors imposed by their illness.

METHOD

Participants

The subjects were recruited from the population of individuals diagnosed with AIDS being treated in the Departments of Immunology and Hematology/ Oncology at the University of California, Los Angeles Medical Center. All participants were within three months of diagnosis, with 72% being diagnosed with Kaposi's sarcoma and 28% with opportunistic infections. They were ambulatory outpatients at the time of recruitment (although some may have been inpatients at a prior time).

The sample consisted of 50 self-identified homosexual or bisexual males who resided in the Los Angeles area. The participants were between the ages of 26 and 57, with a mean age of 36. The majority of the subjects were Caucasian (94%), with only 4% Hispanics, 2% Afro-Americans, and no Asians.

Procedure

Eligible subjects were given written and/or oral information about the study by one of their treating physicians and the study director. Upon agreeing to participate, each subject was given a packet of instruments to complete. Some of the instruments were collected at the time of initial contact, the remainder were returned by mail following completion. A follow-up letter was sent approximately two weeks after the initial contact to those subjects who had not returned the completed packets. Eighty-five percent of those approached (N = 70) gave written informed consent to participate in the study. Fifty of the 70 (71.5%) actually completed the initial data-point instrument package and provided the basis of this study.

Measures

Dealing with Illness.

A 47-item coping inventory was developed, as described above. The inventory assesses cognitive and behavioral responses made in efforts to cope with the illness, with subjects responding on a five-point scale (1 = never and 5 = always) to the question "Which of these things have you used to help you deal with your illness?" Table 10.1 lists the items for each category of coping response: *active-cognitive* efforts that deal with the appraisal of the stressfulness of the illness and include one's beliefs, attitudes, and thoughts about the illness; *active-behavioral* efforts that deal directly with problem and its events and relying on others for emotional, informational, and instrumental support; and *avoidance* efforts that attempt to avoid thinking about or behaving in direct response to the illness and include self-medication with alcohol and drugs. These three coping methods were then analyzed as eight more-specific coping strategies. Table 10.2 gives the items contributing to each strategy and the internal consistency of the strategy as measured by Cronbach's alpha.

Inventory of Current Concerns.

This is a 72-item questionnaire which measures subjects' life concerns in seven areas, including health, work/finances, religion, family, friends, self-appraisal, and existential issues. A summary Total Concerns scores is generated from the subscale scores. The Inventory of Current Concerns was developed by Weisman, Worden, and Sobel (1980) and used in their study of cancer patients (Project Omega). Higher scores indicate higher levels of concern in each area.

TABLE 10.1
Coping Methods

Active-Cognitive

Tried to keep it from bothering or upsetting me

Prayed hard for a good ending to the situation

Thought about one day at a time

Accepted the situation, since nothing could be done

Thought about the positive changes in me since the illness

Formed a plan of action in my mind

Thought more about the meaning of life

Trusted my belief in God

Prepared for the worst

Tried to understand what brought on my illness

Tried to understand how other people in the same situation were thinking or feeling

Believed that time would make the difference and the best thing to do was wait

Went over the situation again and again in my mind

Thought about how I could have done things differently

Thought a lot more about what is really important in my life

Trusted my doctors to know the best treatments for me

Active-Behavioral

Went out more socially

Talked to people, just to be able to talk about it

Went to a friend, or a professional, for advice on how to change things in the situation

Tried to get someone, like a doctor, to do something about it

Took more vitamins and ate healthy food

Went to a friend or a professional to help me feel better

Talked with others in the same situation

Turned to work or other activities to keep my mind off things

Enjoyed everyday things, events, and experiences more than I used to

Developed myself as a person

Exercised more

Depended on others to cheer me up and make me feel better

Used meditation, self-hypnosis, or imagery

Got involved in political activities related to my illness

Stood firm and fought for what I wanted

Cried, yelled, or laughed more to express my feelings

Tried to find out more about my illness

Worked on reaching a bargain or compromise to change things

Bought something or did something special for myself

Avoidance

Tried to keep others from knowing how I was feeling

Avoided being with people

Refused to think about it

Tried to reduce tension by:
    drinking more than usual

eating more than usual

taking drugs more than usual

sleeping more than usual

Increased my sexual activity alone

Joked about it, refused to get too serious about it

Daydreamed about better times

176

TABLE 10.2
Coping Strategies

	Cronbach's Alpha
Active-Positive Involvement	.90
Took more vitamins and ate healthy food	
Formed a plan of action in my mind	
Enjoyed everyday things more than I used to	
Developed myself as a person	
Used meditation, self-hypnosis or imagery	
Got involved in political activities related to my illness	
Stood firm and fought for what I wanted	
Active-Expressive/Information Seeking	.88
Talked to people, just to be able to talk about it	
Talked with others in the same situation	
Tried to find out more about my illness	
Active-Reliance on Others	.86
Went to a friend or professional for advice on how to change things in this situation	
Tried to get someone, like a doctor, to do something about it	
Went to a friend or professional to help me feel better	
Cognitive-Positive Understanding/Create Meaning	.66
Prayed hard for a good ending to the situation	
Thought about it one day at a time	
Thought about the positive changes in me since the illness	
Thought more about the meaning of life	
Trusted my belief in God	
Tried to understand how other people in this situation were thinking or feeling	
Thought about what is really important in my life	
Cognitive-Passive/Ruminative	.63
Believed that time would make a difference and the best thing to do was to wait	
Daydreamed about better times	
Thought about how I could have done things differently	
Distraction	.66
Tried to keep it from bothering or upsetting me	
Went out more socially	
Refused to think about it	
Worked on trying to solve problems that my illness brought	
Joked about it, refused to get too serious about it	
Bought or did something special for myself	

(Continued)

TABLE 10.2 (Continued)

	Cronbach's Alpha
Passive Resignation	.81
Tried to keep others from knowing how I was feeling	
Prepared for the worst	
Trusted my doctors to know the best treatment for me	
Avoidance-Solitary/Passive Behaviors	.80
Avoided being with people	
Smoked more than usual	
Took drugs more than usual	

People Around You.

An extensive social-support questionnaire was developed, which assessed multiple factors of the subjects' social network and resources. This instrument is based on the empirical literature on social support and its measurement (Donald & Ware, 1983; Myers, in press) and has been used extensively with cancer patients and kidney transplant patients. This measure assesses quantitative and qualitative aspects of an individual's support system, and yields scales measuring social support needs; satisfaction with support; perceived availability of emotional and instrumental support; and indices of the number of people in one's support network; number of people one can expect real help from in times of trouble; and the composition of the support network. Reliability on satisfaction with support scale is Cronbach's alpha = .87, emotional support = .90, and instrumental support = .81 (Wolcott, Namir, Fawzy, Gottlieb, & Mitsuyasu, 1986).

Profile of Mood States (POMS).

This 65-item self-report instrument measures current mood. Six factor-analytically derived subscales for anxiety, anger, depression, confusion, fatigue, and vigor are summed to generate a total mood disturbance (TMD) score. The POMS has scoring and reference group norms and has been previously used in studies of cancer and AIDS patients (Donlou, Wolcott, Gottlieb, & Landsverk, 1985; McNair, Lorr, & Droppleman, 1971; Wolcott, Fawzy, Wellisch, & Landsverk, 1986).

Simmons Scale.

This is a nine-item measure of self-esteem previously used in studies of transplant recipients, cancer patients, and AIDS patients (Donlou et al., 1985; Wolcott et al., 1986a; Simmons, Klein, & Simmons, 1977).

Feelings About Your Health.

This is a 15-item self-report instrument which consists of five subscales measuring self-perceptions of current health status. These items assess physical health in terms of functioning or illness-caused limitations on activities, pain severity in the past month, general physical symptoms, rating of quality of life during the past month on a visual analogue scale, and perceived current global health status. The Health Aggregate score was a summed score from patients' numerically scored global health perceptions, pain level, physical symptoms, and illness-caused limitations of physical activities. Higher health aggregate scores indicate better subjectively reported current health status.

RESULTS

Descriptive Statistics

The mean scores of the three coping methods and the eight coping strategies are presented in Table 10.3 with the ranges of the scores. For comparision purposes, the means (sums of items weighted by the number of items for each scale) for each method show that active-cognitive coping was used most frequently (item means = 3.4, range = 2.78-4.04), with active-behavioral coping employed next (item means = 2.97, range = 1.19-4.22) and avoidance coping used least frequently (item means = 2.48, range = 1.41-3.48).

TABLE 8.3
Means, Standard Deviations, and Range of Scores
for Coping Methods and Strategies

Coping Method	Item Means	S.D.	Range
Active-Cognitive	3.40	1.08	2.77-4.04
Active-Behavioral	2.97	1.01	1.18-4.22
Avoidance	2.48	1.09	1.41-3.48
Coping Strategy			
Cognitive-Positive	3.97	0.99	3.40-4.80
Active-Expressive	3.53	1.27	2.80-4.40
Active Reliance	3.47	1.18	3.20-3.80
Active-Positive	3.23	1.33	2.00-4.40
Distraction	3.17	0.87	2.40-3.80
Cognitive-Passive	3.13	1.24	2.80-3.60
Passive/Resignation	3.07	1.02	2.20-3.80
Avoidance	1.86	1.57	1.80-2.20

Item means are the grand means for the scale items, with a possible score of 5 and a range from 1 to 5.

TABLE 10.4
Highest and Lowest Item Means and Frequencies

Item	Mean	Always/Often (percentage)
Tried to find out more about my illness	4.4	85.36
Took more vitamins and ate healthy food	4.4	80.50
Thought about what is really important in my life	4.8	78.04
Trusted my doctors to know the best treatment for me	3.8	63.41
Thought more about the meaning of life	4.4	63.40
Trusted my belief in God	3.8	62.50
Tried to keep it from bothering or upsetting me	3.8	58.50
Thought about it one day at a time	4.2	53.66
Went to a friend or professional to help me feel better	3.8	48.78
Tried to understand how other people in this situation were thinking or feeling	3.8	46.50
Stood firm and fought for what I wanted	3.8	43.59
Smoked more	1.2	2.56
Took drugs more	1.4	5.00
Got involved in political activities	2.0	5.00

Exploration of the coping strategies indicated that cognitive-positive understanding/create meaning was used most frequently, followed by active-expressive/information seeking, active-reliance on others, and active-positive involvement.

Table 10.4 presents the individual items that scored the highest from the coping measure, with the percentage of people who used each one "often or always." Over 85% of the participants in this study "tried to find out more about my illness" and 80.5% "took more vitamins and ate healthy foods." The lowest scoring items are also presented, with 92.5% "never or rarely" getting involved in political activities and 92.31% never or rarely smoking more. It is interesting that 32.5% of people stated that they "often or always" prepared for the worst, and an equal percentage stated that they "never or rarely" prepared for the worst. Cognitive strategies were clearly used most frequently by people in this study to attempt to cope with AIDS.

Psychological Correlates of Coping Methods

Men with AIDS who were using *avoidance* of thinking about or dealing directly with their problems experienced greater distress than those who used coping methods related to relying on others for emotional and tangible support or active-behavioral approaches to their problems (including taking vitamins, getting involved in political activities related to AIDS, developing themselves as people) or those who used active-cognitive methods (such as praying, forming a plan of action in their minds, gaining information and understanding about the illness). Avoidance coping was related to greater depression, $r = .43$, $p < .01$; more anxiety, $r = .31, p < .05$; and lower self-esteem, $r = -.47, p < .01$. Active-behavioral coping was inversely correlated with total mood disturbance $(r = -.45, p < .01)$ and depression $(r = -.31, p < .05)$ and positively correlated with self-esteem $(r = .36, p < .05)$. Active-cognitive coping was inversely correlated, without reaching statistical significance, with total mood disturbance, depression, and anxiety; and positively correlated with self-esteem.

Avoidance coping was strongly correlated with statistically significant increased concerns in the areas of health, existential issues, friends, self, and total concerns; whereas active-behavioral coping was inversely related to these concerns. However, the only correlation to reach statistical significance was with existential concerns, $r = -.34, p < .05$. Clearly, avoidant coping was not protecting these people from distressful feelings and concerns. The correlations between active-cognitive coping and concerns were not statistically significant.

There were significant relationships between avoidant coping and people's support networks. As shown in Table 10.5, the higher the use of avoidant coping, the fewer close friends in one's support network and the fewer people they could expect help from in times of need. On the other hand, the use of active-behavioral coping was related to a greater number of close friends and more people available to help in times of need. Active-behavioral coping was also related to the likelihood that people were more satisfied with the support they received from others in their networks.

A stepwise regression was conducted of coping methods and support variables on the total mood disturbance score from the POMS. As shown in Table 10.6, satisfaction with support, instrumental support, avoidance coping, and

TABLE 10.5
Correlations Between Coping Strategies and Support Network

	Number of close friends	Number of people to help	Satisfaction with support
Active-Behavioral	.38*	.35*	.51*
Active-Cognitive	.19	−.05	.06
Avoidance	−.33*	−.32*	−.24

*$p < .05$
**$p < .001$

TABLE 10.6
Stepwise Regression of Coping Methods and Support Variables
on Profile of Mood States Total

Variables	F	r	R^2	R Change	Beta
Satisfaction with support	.75	-.54	.28	.28	-.15
Instrumental support	1.45	-.56	.39	.11	-.20
Avoidance	6.69**	.27	.46	.07	.50
Active-Behavioral	4.08*	-.16	.54	.08	-.45

*$p < .05$
**$p < .01$

active coping explained 54% of the variance in TMD scores. However, avoidance and active coping were the only variables that were statistically significant.

Physical Health Correlates of Coping

We wondered whether or not active-behavioral coping was related to health status; that is, if one's health were worse, it would be difficult to use active-behavioral coping. However, five different self-report health indices (limits on health, global health, activities of daily living, amount of pain, and quality of life) did not correlate with coping methods, except for self-ratings of global health ("In general, would you say your health right now is excellent, good, fair, or poor?"). Active-behavioral coping was correlated strongly with better self-report of health, $r = .53$, $p < .001$. Avoidance coping was negatively related to all of the criteria health measures. Although none of these reached significance, the direction of the relationships is noteworthy. Active-cognitive coping was related to the health measures in an inverse direction, though none of these reached significance. Active-behavioral coping showed consistently positive associations to health.

Physicians' ratings of their patients' physical performance capacity did not correlate significantly with any of the three methods of coping: active-behavioral, $r = .01$, $p > .05$; active-cognitive, $r = .22$, $p > .05$; and avoidance, $r = .10$, $p > .05$.

The total number of medical symptoms did not correlate with coping methods: active-behavioral, $r = -.24$, $p > .05$; active-cognitive, $r = .19$, $p > .05$; and avoidance, $r = .19$, $p > .05$.

A stepwise regression was conducted of coping methods and support variables on the total aggregate health score. Coping methods did not predict physical health ($F = 3.22$, $p > .05$), with only avoidance coping meeting criteria for entrance into the model.

TABLE 10.7
Correlations Between Coping Strategies and Mood States

Strategy	TMD	Anxiety	Depression	Lack of vigor	Confusion	Fatigue
Active-Positive	-.58***	-.34*	-.50***	-.69****	-.54***	-.59****
Active-Expressive	-.30	-.27	-.16	-.30	-.30	-.08
Active-Reliance	-.11	-.01	-.02	-.18	-.08	-.11
Distraction	-.38*	-.31*	-.37*	-.46**	-.24	-.43**
Cognitive-Positive	-.27	-.16	-.17	-.29	-.32*	-.35*
Cognitive-Passive/ Ruminative	.40**	.39**	.46**	.17	.35*	.32*
Passive/Resignation	.16	.12	.11	.28	.11	.26
Avoidance	.42**	.43**	.56***	.21	.33*	.14

$*p < .05$
$**p < .01$
$***p < .001$
$****p < .0001$

Psychological Correlates of Specific Coping Strategies

Eight different types of coping strategies were explored in relationship to psychological distress to understand more about specific strategies that might be helpful in coping with AIDS. Table 10.7 presents these strategies, with the active-behavioral ones first (active-positive involvement, active-expressive/ information seeking, and active-reliance on others), followed by distraction (both cognitive and behavioral attempts to distract oneself). The cognitive strategies are presented next, including positive understanding/create meaning, and a ruminative or passive cognitive strategy. The last two strategies are passive resignation and avoidance activities.

As can be seen in Table 10.7, active-positive involvement was strongly associated with lower mood disturbance, including anxiety, depression, lack of vigor, confusion, and fatigue. The other two active strategies were negatively correlated with mood disturbance, but did not reach statistical significance. A positive approach in an attempt to cognitively understand one's illness and to create meaning were also negatively correlated with mood disturbance, although the only two correlations that reached significance were lowered levels of confusion and fatigue.

Distraction activities were moderately associated with lowered levels of mood disturbance, whereas as ruminative/passive cognitive strategy was positively associated with mood disturbance. Avoidance activities were also associated with increased levels of mood disturbance, including a strong relationship with depression.

Self-esteem was positively correlated with positive involvement and positive understanding, while inverse correlations between self-esteem, ruminative

TABLE 10.8
Correlations Between Concerns, Self-Esteem, and Coping Strategies

		Concerns				
Strategy	Self-Esteem	Total	Health	Existential Issues	Friends	Self
Active-Positive	.58****	-.35*	-.16	-.45**	-.42**	-.39**
Active-Expressive	.20	-.12	-.12	-.19	-.17	-.02
Active-Reliance	.09	.15	.24	-.05	-.01	.19
Distraction	.11	-.33*	-.22	-.21	-.30	-.32*
Cognitive-Positive	.34*	.03	.05	-.26	.06	-.06
Cognitive-Passive/ Ruminative	-.39**	.60****	.54***	.36*	.46**	.65****
Passive/Resignation	-.19	.17	.17	.12	.20	.21
Avoidance	-.40**	.48**	.55***	.35*	.51***	.47**

*p < .05
**p < .01
***p < .001
****p < .0001

cognitions, and avoidance were found (see Table 10.8). People who used an active-positive coping strategy experienced fewer total concerns and, in particular, fewer existential, friend, and self concerns. Distraction was also negatively associated with the number of total concerns. Those who used a ruminative cognitive strategy experienced a high level of total concerns, health concerns, and self concerns, as did those who used an avoidance strategy.

Social-Support Correlates of Specific Coping Strategies

Satisfaction with total support was strongly associated with an active-positive involvement coping strategy, and there was a moderate association between the strategy of expressive/information seeking and satisfaction with one's total support. There was a moderate relationship between avoidance and dis-satisfaction with one's support, as well as with perceptions regarding the availability of emotional and instrumental support.

Positive involvement and expressive/information seeking coping were associated with perceptions of instrumental support being available, as was the strategy of distraction. Table 10.9 illustrates these relationships.

Physical Health Correlates of Specific Coping Strategies

Seven indices of physical health were explored and included: perception of overall health (global health ratings), activities of daily living, pain, limits

TABLE 10.9
Correlations Between Social-Support Variables and Coping Strategies

Strategy	Satisfaction	Emotional	Instrumental
Active-Positive	.50**	.24	.45**
Active-Expressive	.32*	.24	.34*
Active-Reliance	.21	.02	-.05
Distraction	.25	.13	.52***
Cognitive-Positive	.18	-.20	-.11
Cognitive-Passive/Ruminative	-.20	.14	-.09
Passive/Resignation	-.09	.07	-.18
Avoidance	-.41**	-.40*	-.47**

*$p < .05$
**$p < .01$
***$p < .001$

imposed on activities by one's health, perceived quality of life, physicians' ratings of patients' performance, and number of medical symptoms.

Positive involvement and distraction were strongly associated with self-ratings of good health (as shown in Table 10.10), whereas ruminative cognitions, passive resignation about one's illness, and avoidance coping were negatively associated with global perception of health. It is interesting to note that reported pain level was significantly associated only with the cognitive-ruminative coping strategy, and this is an inverse direction (reported more pain).

Activities of daily living were positively correlated with positive involvement and negatively correlated with ruminative coping, and perceived limits

TABLE 10.10
Correlations Between Physical Health Indices and Coping Strategies

Strategy	Global	ADL	Pain	Limit	Quality	Symptoms
Active-Positive	.57***	.37*	.10	.20	.26	.30
Active-Expressive	.29	.09	.24	-.08	-.09	-.44*
Active-Reliance	.03	.22	.01	.11	.02	-.14
Distraction	.39*	.38*	.05	.34*	.31*	-.48**
Cognitive-Positive	.27	-.11	.08	.26	.09	.02
Cognitive-Passive/ Ruminative	-.41**	-.42**	-.43**	-.31*	-.30	.06
Passive/Resignation	-.39**	-.25	-.11	-.34*	-.20	.09
Avoidance	-.36*	-.06	-.29	-.09	-.45**	.39

*$p < .05$
**$p < .01$
***$p < .001$

on activities were associated with both passive resignation and ruminative coping strategies. Distraction activities and cognitions were associated with fewer limits on activities and a higher perception of quality of life, while avoidance coping was associated with a lower perception of quality of life.

It is important to note that on the two indices of physical health that did not involve participants' perceptions of their health, the only correlations that reached statistical significance were a lower number of physical symptoms in those using expressive/information seeking and distraction coping strategies.

DISCUSSION

The current study explored three coping methods (active-behavioral, active-cognitive, and avoidance) and eight coping strategies (active-positive involvement, active-expressive/information seeking, active-reliance on others, distraction, cognitive-positive understanding/create meaning, cognitive-passive/ruminative, passive resignation, and avoidance) employed by men with AIDS who were recently diagnosed with the illness.

What becomes clear from the pattern of relationships between coping methods and mood disturbance, self-esteem, and expressed concerns is that avoidance coping did not protect these people from distressful feelings, mood disturbances, and concerns. Those who were using avoidance coping had the highest levels of concerns regarding one's health, existential issues, friends, and self. They also had the highest levels of depression and the lowest scores on a measure of self-esteem. Previous research has also found a positive association between avoidance coping and psychological distress in people who have physical illnesses (Bloom, 1982; Holahan & Moos, 1983; Moos, 1983).

The three coping methods evidenced distinctly different associations. An active-behavioral coping method is clearly associated with a more positive affective state and self-esteem level. Those who are mobilized to deal with the illness in positive and behavioral ways are functioning much better than those who are not. The active-cognitive coping method consists of attempts to achieve a mind set to defend against concerns or to create meaning in light of the dismal prognosis. However, it appears that cognitive attempts at coping can lead to thoughts and attitudes of an obsessional and ruminative nature. If an individual attempts to master the illness by "positive thinking" solely, what emerges is a pattern of ruminations and obsessive thinking which is not entirely successful. The strategy labeled cognitive-positive/create meaning had the highest mean score across items when compared to the seven other coping strategies and was used most frequently by participants in our study.

Following the use of the cognitive strategy called positive/create meaning, individuals in this study reported the use of active-behavioral coping strategies, including positive involvement in activities, expression of thoughts and feelings, information seeking, and reliance on others. Only 32.5% avoided being with people, and the lowest means for items were avoidant coping strategies of smoking more than usual and taking drugs more than usual.

Attempts at distracting oneself, both cognitively and behaviorally, were also related to better mood states, fewer concerns, and a higher level of perceived quality of life.

It should be noted that avoidance coping is not a consequence of poor health. There was no significant association between avoidance coping, activities of daily living, health limits, or number of medical symptoms. Avoidance coping is not an illness-imposed inability to respond more actively.

There is evidence that the ability to copy effectively may influence the availability of support (Wortman, 1984). Those who indicate that they are coping well with a crisis are regarded as more attractive and less likely to be avoided than those who indicate that they are having difficulty. The result is that "poor copers" who are in the greatest need of support are least likely to receive it. Considering the correlations between coping strategies and social-support variables, we conducted a stepwise multiple-regression analysis, entering the coping variables last. It was the coping responses that were predictive of psychological well being, as measured by the Profile of Mood States.

It is clear from the specificity of the coping strategies and their associations with psychological mood states, self-esteem, and concerns that individuals who are engaged in attempting to master the illness through positive and active behaviors and attitudes are faring better than individuals who are not. Therefore, interventions that encourage problem solving, participation in decision making, and active coping strategies rather than passive acceptance of the illness, especially in the early stages of the illness, may be more helpful. This is consistent with the literature which has found a "fighting spirit" to be associated with longer survival time (Derogatis, Abeloff, & Melisaratos, 1979; Greer, Morris, & Pettingale, 1979). Self-efficacy is a sense that a person can have control over one's life and behavior that will reduce stress reactions and increase one's sense of being in control. Given the helplessness and powerlessness that may be inherent in the diagnosis of a life-threatening illness, it is important that we work with people to increase their involvement in treatment decisions, their efforts to change their behaviors, and involvement in activities that will enhance the quality of their lives.

It also appears that the use of distractions—including going out more socially, treating oneself in special ways, and not obsessing about the illness—may protect people from mood disturbances. We do not know, as yet, whether or not this "fighting spirit" is associated with longer survival time for persons with AIDS.

The importance of self-esteem and its association with positive measures suggests that strategies that focus on the maintenance of self-worth will increase feelings of control and combat passive, helpless feelings and despair. This is also consistent with literature which has found that education and behaviorally oriented group interventions are more effective than emotional support group interventions (Jacobs, Ross, Walker, & Stockdale, 1983; Fawzy, Namir, & Wolcott, 1989; Weisman et al., 1980). Strategies for increasing verbal and behavioral self-assertion, learning to express one's feelings and beliefs as an affirmation of self, seeking information and help, and learning problem-solving skills are important here.

An area that is not often addressed in working with people to cope with AIDS is the issue of time. There may be a tendency to ruminate about the past and what one could have done differently. If too much emphasis is placed on the past, one can become trapped in feelings of blame and loss. If there is too much focus on the present ("live for today"), people may engage in risky behaviors and not pay enough attention to health-promoting ones. If there is too much attention on the future, anxiety over uncertainty may be created, and attention to immediate planning and control over one's health and quality of life may be ignored. Interventions with people who have AIDS should include seeking a balance in one's sense of past, present, and future time.

This study is one of the first to explore the relationships between different coping methods and strategies and their relationships to the psychological and health status of people with AIDS. Additionally, longitudinal studies that consider these relationships are needed; but to be effective, these studies should be initiated before the illness is present. Once the illness is diagnosed, changes may occur in people's support networks, ways of coping, and psychological states. By studying individuals at risk, but not ill, variables that presage successful coping may be identified and may help us to understand more about coping with a life-threatening illness, changes that occur after diagnosis in people's coping strategies, and how best to intervene to help people cope more effectively.

Several factors limit the generalizability of our results. This study explored coping in only 50 men with AIDS, three months or less after diagnosis, and who self-selected to participate in the study. They were also being seen in medical clinics of a university. The use of self-report inventories almost exclusively represents a subjective bias that may be operative across all the measures. However, as an initial exploration of coping with AIDS, the information obtained by this study may be helpful to those who are attempting to intervene with people who have both AIDS and AIDS-related conditions, and to implement preventive efforts for changing behaviors thay may put one at risk for AIDS. A careful consideration of the types of interventions and the goals of these interventions is needed, rather than assuming that supportive psychotherapy or group interventions are sufficient.

ACKNOWLEDGMENTS

This research was supported by NIAID Grants #AI-15332 and AI-20672. Please address correspondence to Sheila Namir, Ph.D., California School of Professional Psychology, 2235 Beverly Blvd., Los Angeles, CA 90057.

REFERENCES

Amerikan, J. (1985) *Stress, perceived control, and coping in a community sample*. Unpublished doctoral dissertation, University of California, Los Angeles.

Billings, A. G., & Moos, R. (1981). The role of coping responsess and social resources in attenuating the stress of life events. *Journal of Behavioral Medicine, 4*, 139-157.

Bloom, J. R. (1982). Social support, accommodation to stress and adjustment to breast cancer. *Social Science Medicine, 16*, 1329-1338.

Christ, G. H., & Weiner, L. S. (1985). Psychosocial issues in AIDS. In V. T. DeVita, S. Hellman, & S. A. Rosenberg (Eds.), *AIDS: Etiology, diagnosis, treatment, and prevention* (pp. 275-297). Philadelphia: J. B. Lippincott.

Derogatis, L. R., Abeloff, M. D., & Melisaratas, N. (1979). Psychological coping mechanisms and survival times in metastatic breast cancer. *Journal of the American Medical Association, 242*, 1504-1508.

Donald, C. A., & Ware, J. E. (1983). *The measurement of social support*. Washington, DC: U.S. Department of Health and Human Services (Publication Number WD-1839-HHS).

Donlou, J. N., Wolcott, D. L., Gottlieb, M. S., & Landsverk, J. (1985). Psychosocial aspects of AIDS: A pilot study. *Journal of Psychosocial Oncology, 3*, 39-55.

Fawzy, F. I., Namir, S., & Wolcott, D. L. (1989). A structured group intervention model for AIDS patients. *Psychiatric Medicine, 7*, 35-46.

Fornstein, M. (1984). The psychosocial impact of the acquired immunodeficiency syndrome. *Seminars in Oncology, 11*, 77-82.

Greer, S., Morris, T. E., & Pettingale, K. W. (1979). Psychological responses to breast cancer: Effect on outcome. *Lancet, 2*, 785-787.

Holahan, C. J., & Moos, R. H. (1983). *Life stress and health: Personality, coping and family support in stress resistance*. Palo Alto, CA: Stanford University, Social Ecology Laboratory.

Jacobs, C., Ross, R. D., Walker, I. M., & Stockdale, F. E. (1983). Behavior of cancer patients: A longitudinal study of the effects of educational and support groups. *American Journal of Clinical Oncology, 6*, 347-352.

Lazarus, R. S., & Folkman, S. (1984). *Stress, appraisal and coping*. New York: Springer Publishing Company.

McNair, D., Lorr, M., & Dropplemann, L. (1971). *Manual for the Profile of Mood States*. San Diego: Educational and Industrial Testing Service.

Moos, R. (1983, August). *Context and coping: Toward a unifying conceptual framework*. Address presented to the American Psychological Association Annual Convention. Anaheim, CA.

Moos, R. H., Cronkite, R. C., Billings, A. G., & Finney, J. W. (1984). *The health and daily living form*. Palo Alto, CA: Stanford University, Social Ecology Laboratory.

Myers, H. F. (in press). Social support and social network scales: A multidimensional scale. In R. Jones (Ed.), *Handbook of tests and measures for black populations*. New York: Holt, Rinehard & Winston.

Pearlin, L. I., & Schooler, C. (1978). The structure of coping. *Journal of Health and Social Behavior, 19*, 2-21.

Simmons, R. G., Klein, S. D., & Simmons, R. L. (1977). *Gifts of life: The social and psychological impact of organ transplantation.* New York: John Wiley and Sons.

Taylor, S. E. (1983). Adjustment to threatening events: A theory of cognitive adaptation. *American Psychologist, 11,* 1161–1173.

Weisman, A. D. (1979). *Coping with cancer.* New York: McGraw Hill.

Weisman, A. D., Worden, J. W., & Sorbel, H. J. (1980). *Psychosocial screening and intervention with cancer patients.* Washington D. C.: National Cancer Institute (Publication No. 19797).

Wolcott, D. L., Fawzy, F. I., Wellisch, D., & Landsverk, J. (1986a). Adaptation of adult bone marrow transplant long-term survivors. *Transplantation, 41,* 478–483.

Wolcott, D. L., Namir, S., Fawzy, F. I., Gottlieb, M. S., & Mitsuyasu, R. T. (1986). Illness concerns, attitudes towards homosexuality and social support in gay men with AIDS. *General Hospital Psychiatry, 8,* 395–403.

Wortman, C. B. (1984). Social support and the cancer patient: Conceptual and methodologic issues. *Cancer, 53* (Supplement), 2339–2359.

Understanding Attributions and Health Behavior Changes in AIDS and ARC: Implications for Interventions

11

Jeffrey M. Moulton
David M. Sweet
Lydia Temoshok
School of Medicine
University of California, San Francisco

Distress experienced by people with AIDS (PWA) and people with ARC (PWARC) transcends the medical dimensions of the disease. This distress negatively affects their ability to function, health behaviors, social behaviors, and possibly the trajectory of disease. Understanding the sources and consequences of this distress and the means to ameliorate it are paramount as the AIDS epidemic widens and a cure or vacinne is still nowhere in sight.

With the current AIDS situation in San Francisco as our guide and with an eye toward the future, we present the following considerations about the relationships of attributions of blame, responsibility, and perceived control over one's health to psychosocial distress in a general review, and in a specific study of 103 gay men with AIDS and ARC. In addition, we offer some suggestions for clinical interventions.

ATTRIBUTIONS OF BLAME, RESPONSIBILITY, AND CONTROL IN RELATION TO PSYCHOSOCIAL DISTRESS

As in other diseases in which casual links to personal behavior are assumed, such as lung cancer, contracting AIDS and ARC has been associated with factors of personal responsibility and blame since it was first labled as "gay-related immunodeficiency (GRID)" in the early 1980s. In the search for casual responsibility in AIDS, the moral connotations associated with homosexuality and venereal disease have been applied (Fletcher, 1984; Forstein, 1984), at times with vehemence.

When discussing other diseases not as closely linked to health behavior, several authors have cautioned against suggesting that patients are responsible for contracting their disease or are responsible for the course of their illness. Negative emotions, such as guilt or despair, may be aroused if people believe that their lifestyle has caused or influenced the course of their disease (Cassileth, Lusk, Miller, Brown, Miller, 1985). Having to accept personal responsibility for health outcome in a disease state may create an unnecessary burden for the patient (Angell, 1985). Self-blame for outcomes such as cancer associated with such negative emotions as guilt, shame, and feelings of inferiority often lead to poorer emotional adjustment (Abrams & Finesinger, 1953; Bard & Dyk, 1956; Mastrovito, 1974; Weisman, 1976). In addition, Mastrovito (1974) indicated that attributions of cause assigned to external factors such as the environment or another person tended to leave self-esteem intact. Similarly, Bard and Dyk (1956) found that attributions of cause assigned to external factors helped guard against guilt, self-criticism, and feelings of powerlessness.

In a study of quadriplegic and paraplegic victims of accidents, Janoff-Bulman and Wortman (1977) reported that self-blame was associated with superior coping, while blaming another for the accident was associated with great difficulty in coping. Despite the fact that few of these victims could be considered in any way "at fault" for their accidents, the "self-blamers" conducted an attributional search to find some aspect of their accidents to which they could assign personal responsibility.

In contrast to the above studies, Taylor, Lichtman, and Wood (1984) reported that blaming another person was significantly related to poor adjustment, although they also found that most causal attributions were not associated with better or worse adjustment among their breast-cancer patient cohort. These researchers believe that it may be premature to conclude that attributional explanations are functionally interchangeable. However, they do propose that the process of creating meaning through the assignment of cause may be the goal of the attributional search, rather than trying to find a particular factor on which to blame a negative outcome (Taylor, 1984).

Although it is difficult to generalize from these studies of patients with different medical problems to PWA and PWARC, one common denominator appears to be that more effective coping is associated with the process of creating meaning. In order to evaluate the psychological impact of attributions, it is essential to differentiate concepts of *blame, responsibility*, and *control*, which have been used interchangeably in attribution research. Several authors (Brickman et al., 1982; Michela & Wood, 1986; Zich and Temoshok,

1988) have discussed the importance of separating the concepts of behavioral self-responsibility for cause, self-blame (attributing cause to self, but perhaps with an added self-punitive element), responsibility for outcome, and self-involvement in affecting improvement (e.g., alteration of health habits, such as reducing stress; quitting smoking; and adopting health-promoting behaviors, such as exercise).

In addition to differentiating among these concepts of attribution, several researchers have stressed that it is important to take into account differences among patient populations. Based on our experience with malignant melanoma (e.g., Temoshok et al., 1985), we suggest that (a) the anticipated morbidity and mortality of the disease or condition and (b) the certainty of such an outcome can be strong forces in determining the type of attributions made, as well as the impact of such attributions on psychological or emotional adjustment. Given that attributions and their effects may vary from one health condition to another, it is important to study attributions within the context of particular health problems.

STUDY OF ATTRIBUTION IN AIDS AND ARC

Aims and Hypotheses

One of our goals was to examine the relationships among attributions, levels of distress, and health-behavior change in PWA and PWARC. Specifically, we were concerned with the following three questions:

1. Do those people who attribute responsibility and/or blame to themselves for contracting AIDS or ARC incur more (or less) distress and/or engage in more (or less) health-behavior change than those who attribute causation to external factors? We hypothesized that holding oneself responsible for cause, as well as self-blame, would be significantly associataed with greater distress and fewer positive health-behavior changes.

2. Do those who attribute responsibility for possible improvement to themselves incur more (or less) distress and/or engage in more positive health-behavior change than those who attribute possible improvement to external factors? We hypothesized that attributions of responsibility for improvement would be associated with less distress and more positive health-behavior change.

3. Are the relationships between attribution, distress, and health-behavior change different for persons with AIDS and those with ARC? We hypothesized that there would be significant differences between the two groups, based on the differing prognosis for each condition.

Methods

Our subjects were 103 research participants (50 PWA and 53 PWARC) recruited sequentially between April 1984 and September 1985 from the San Francisco General Hospital AIDS outpatient clinic and Custom Health Care, a large private medical clinic in San Francisco. The criteria for study eligibility included: (a) being a gay or bisexual man, and (b) a recent diagnosis of AIDS or ARC. PWA and PWARC participants were similar in age and education. Not suprisingly, PWA reported greater unemployment than PWARC.

In the context of a two-hour audiotaped psychosocial interview, attribution and life-change data were collected. Measures of psychosocial distress were included in a self-report package completed within two weeks after the interview. Self-report distress scales were factor analyzed using a principal components analysis from which a general dysphoria variable was retained and used in correlations with attribution and health-behavior change variables. A more detailed description of the methods used in this study can be found in Moulton, Sweet, Temoshok, and Mandel (1987).

Results

The pattern of results differed between PWA and PWARC, as we had initially hypothesized. Percent attributed to self-causation for contracting AIDS was significantly positively correlated with distress among PWA ($r = .37, p \le .05$). However, no such relationship was found among ARC subjects. We also found that percent attributed to self-responsibility for possible improvement was significantly negatively correlated with distress among the ARC group ($r = -.30, p \le .05$), although not in the AIDS group.

In terms of health-behavior change, percent attributed to self-responsibility for possible improvement was significantly positively correlated with increased health-behavior change among PWA ($r = .34, p \le .05$), while negatively correlated with hopelessness ($r = -.25, p \le .01$) and positively correlated with the vigor-activity subscale ($r = .24, p \le .01$) of the Profile of Mood States (POMS; Shacham, 1983) among PWARC.

Finally, we looked at those who blamed themselves versus those who did not. Self-blamers were not significantly different in distress or health-behavior change.

We speculated that the differential findings found between the AIDS and ARC groups may be related to the real and perceived prognostic differences between the two groups. At the time of this study (1984-1985), AIDS was considered to be a progressively deteriorating condition ending in death. ARC was thought to be a less severe and possibly changeable condition with a better prognosis. In our study, most ARC subjects were, in fact, not severely disabled. The positive correlation in the AIDS group between percent attributed to self-causation and distress was expected, given the perceived gravity of the disease relative to ARC. Assuming self-responsibility for the cause of a condition that is seemingly unchangeable, as well as severe and pervasive, is likely to be more distressing than attributing cause to external factors such as chance or someone else. In contrast, we would not expect the same relationship between distress and self-cause attributions in the ARC group, because although ARC symptoms may even be severe and pervasive, ARC was not, particularly at that time, thought to be a fatal condition.

A similar line of reasoning may be applied to explain the negative correlation in the ARC group between percent attributed to self-responsibility for improvement in disease status and levels of distress. We would expect that for a condition in which a negative outcome is less certain and disability may not be as severe, as we find in ARC, the belief that one can, to some extent, affect one's health would lead to a perceived sense of control associated with decreased distress.

Within the AIDS group, percent attributed to self-responsibility for improvement was correlated with health-behavior change. Unfortunately, health-behavior change was not associated with reduction in distress among PWA. Health-behavior changes may have been initiated among PWA out of a sense of hope of a positive effect but may have resulted in a deteriorating situation.

Although engaging in health-behavior change may not reduce distress significantly in the AIDS group, such behavior change appears to be an important coping mechanism among PWARC, despite the fact that there is, as yet, no evidence that any change in behavior is related to actual change in survival or longevity. The negative correlation between hopelessness and health-behavior change and the positive correlation between the vigor-activity dimension of the POMS and health-behavior change suggests that modifying health-behaviors is associated with reductions in distress and an increased sense of well-being among PWARC.

In our study, we differentiated the concepts of self-attribution for cause (holding oneself responsible for cause) and self-blame (self-attribution with, perhaps, a more punitive element). We were surprised that self-blamers were not more distressed than non-self-blamers in either the AIDS and ARC groups. Apparently, the distress associated with attributions of responsibility for cause of disease in the AIDS (or ARC) group was not the result of the punitive component associated with self-blame. It is also possible that many subjects may have been inclined to deny self-blame in order to protect self-esteem. Such reporting bias could distort any underlying relationship between self-blame and distress.

It is important to note that for the vast majority of our subjects, the cause of AIDS was not definitively known at the time they contracted the disease. Therefore, it would not be expected that distress would arise from blaming themselves for developing AIDS (or ARC), since they only learned of the disease etiology *after* they had contracted the Human Immunodeficiency Virus (HIV). However, a study conducted with persons contracting HIV since it has been identified as the cause of AIDS could yield quite different results since it is clear that the two major means of contracting HIV are related to personal behavior: unsafe sexual practices with persons infected with the virus and intravenous drug use with contaminated needles.

CLINICAL IMPLICATIONS

While the manner in which individuals contract AIDS or ARC is of little relevance to their current health care, attributions of personal responsibility for contracting the disease are a cause of distress among PWA. This distress, associated with holding oneself responsible for cause, is likely to increase beyond levels found in the current study because nearly all of those contracting HIV today are aware that exposure to the virus occurs largely through high-risk behaviors. Thus, distress associated with self-attribution for the cause of AIDS is likely to be even more salient a problem for the HIV-infected individual, PWA, and PWARC diagnosed later in the epidemic.

There are several dangers and costs associated with allowing such unproductive (though understandable) perceptions about contracting AIDS and ARC to continue unabated in PWA and PWARC. The model of learned helplessness in the development of clinical depression can be used to understand how attributing the cause of AIDS to oneself can lead to distress. According to theory (e.g., Peterson & Seligman, 1984; Seligman, Abramson, Semmel, & von Baeyer, 1979), individuals who construe the causes of bad events as *internal, stable*, and *global* are more susceptible to depression. Having AIDS or ARC is the type of powerful situation that can foster stable and global helplessness-inducing attributions (e.g., "It's going to last forever, and it is going to undermine everything I do."). If individuals also construe the cause of AIDS as "internal" (i.e., "It's my fault."), then they have the three basic ingredients for developing depression. While people with ARC may not be as susceptible to such cognitions because ARC has not been considered to be as stable and global, this may change, as an increasingly large percentage of PWARC progress each year to develop clinical manifestations of AIDS.

Clinical depression is not the only risk from causal attributions of self-responsibility and the belief that one is helpless to affect health outcomes. Suicidal ideation resulting from distress and/or depression is a possibility with which the clinician must contend. Goldblum (1987) discussed the risks of suicide at different time points in the progression of HIV disease. The initial point of vulnerability may occur at the time of diagnosis or shortly thereafter. Distress associated with attributions of self-causation and beliefs that one has little personal control over one's health could well undermine any perceived hope for improvement in one's condition, limit the use of available social support, or lead to interpretation of the diagnosis as an immediate death sentence. After a second bout of Pneumocystis Carinii pneumonia (PCP), a further advance of Kaposi's sarcoma (KS) lesions, or the presence of a new opportunistic infection, the belief that one's health-behavior changes are of any consequence can be shaken. Finally, thoughts of defeat and suffering may predominate as individuals approach death. Pain, loss of control, and helplessness may undermine any sense of the efficacy of interventions undertaken or any sense that personal involvement may affect health outcome. At this time, hopelessness may again surface and increase the risk of suicide. To lessen feelings of helplessness and loss of control, PWA and PWARC should be encouraged to participate in decision making about their health care (at all points along the continuum of HIV illness) and to engage in health-promoting behaviors.

One method of reducing distress in those with AIDS and ARC suggested by the current study is to support the belief that improvement in health may be attained by engaging in health behaviors such as moderate exercise, relaxation, improved diet, and other health-promoting activities. While these activities have not yet been shown to have a positive physical benefit, our study shows that in the ARC group, these activities have positive mental health benefits. Additional support for our contention that active involvement in one's health is associated with better psychological adjustment is found in the work of Namir, Wolcott, Fawzy, and Alumbaugh (1987; see Chapter 9, this volume). In this work on coping among AIDS patients, active behavioral methods of coping were related to lower total mood disturbance and higher self-esteem. Such coping methods included activities such as increasing vitamin intake and improving diet, developing oneself more as a person, trying to find out more about one's illness, and going to a friend or professional for advice on how to change things in the situation.

Other activities which might promote feelings of involvement and personal control are:

(1) involvement in political and social activities related to rights and services for those with AIDS and ARC;
(2) participation in AIDS forums and research, sharing personal experiences and knowledge;
(3) promotion of health and sexual practices that might reduce the risk of others contracting AIDS; and
(4) involvement with physicians and other health-care specialists in personal health-care decision making.

In summary, we wish to reiterate that the psychological distress associated with having AIDS and ARC has implications as important as the obvious physical distress caused by this disease. People with AIDS and ARC should be encouraged to be involved in health-care decision making and feel empowered to affect their lives on many levels. However, responsibility for and involvement in health-promoting behavior and health-care decisions should not be confused with responsibility for cause of disease.

REFERENCES

Abrams, D. I., & Finesinger, J. E. (1953). Guilt reactions in patients with cancer. *Cancer, 6,* 474-482.

Angell, M. (1985). Disease as a reflection of the psyche. *New England Journal of Medicine, 312,* 1570-1572.

Bard, M., & Dyk, R. B. (1956). The psychodynamic significance of beliefs regarding the cause of serious illness. *The Psychoanalytic Review, 43,* 146-162.

Brickman, P., Rabinowitz, V. C., Karuza, J., Coates, D., Cohn, E., & Kidder, L. (1982). Model of helping and coping. *American Psychologist, 37,* 368-384.

Cassileth, B. R., Lusk, E. J., Miller, D. S., Brown, L. L., & Miller, C. (1985). Psychosocial correlates of survival in advanced maligant disease. *New England Journal of Medicine, 312,* 1551-1555.

Fletcher, J. (1984). Homosexuality: Kick and kickback. *Southern Medical Journal, 77,* 149-150.

Forstein, M. (1984). The psychological impact of the acquired immunodeficiency syndrome. *Seminars in Oncology, 11,* 77-82.

Goldblum, P. (1987). Suicide: Clinical aspects. In M. Helquist (Ed.), *Working with AIDS: A resource guide for mental health professionals* (pp. 156-161). San Francisco: University of California, San Francisco AIDS Health Project.

Janoff-Bulman, R. J., & Wortman, C. B. (1977). Attributions of blame and coping in the "real world": Severe accident victims react to their lot. *Journal of Personality and Social Psychology, 35* 351-363.

Mastrovito, R. (1974). Cancer: Awareness and denial. *Clinical Bulletin, 4,* 142-146.

Michela, J. L., & Wood, J. V. (1986). Casual attributions in health and illness. In P. C. Kendell (Ed.), *Advances in cognitive-behavioral research and therapy* (Vol. 5, pp. 179-235). New York: Academic Press.

Moulton, J. M., Sweet, D. M., Temoshok, L., & Mandel, J. S. (1987). Attributions of blame and responsibility in relation to distress and health behavior change in people with AIDS and AIDS-related complex. *Journal of Applied Social Psychology, 17,* 493-506.

Namir, S., Wolcott, D. L., Fawzy, F. I., & Alumbaugh, M. J. (1987). Coping with AIDS: Psychological and health implications. *Journal of Applied Social Psychology, 17,* 309-328.

Peterson, C., & Seligman, M. E. P. (1984). Causal explanations as a risk factor for depression: Theory and evidence. *Psychological Review, 91,* 347-374.

Seligman, M. E. P., Abramson, L. Y., Semmel, A., & von Baeyer, C. (1979). Depression attributional style. *Journal of Abnormal Psychology, 88,* 242-247.

Shacham, S. (1983). A shortened version of the Profile of Mood States. *Journal of Personality Assessment, 47,* 305-306.

Taylor, S. E. (1984). Adjustment to threatening events: A theory of cognitive adaption. *American Psychologist, 38,* 1161-1173.

Taylor, S. E., Lichtman, R. R., & Wood, J. V. (1984). Attributions, beliefs about control, and adjustment to breast cancer. *Journal of Personality and Social Psychology, 46,* 489-502.

Temoshok, L., Heller, B. W., Sagebiel, R. W., Blois, M. S., Sweet, D. M., DiClemente, R. J., & Gold, M. L. (1985). The relationship of psychosocial factors to prognostic indicators in cutaneous malignant melanoma. *Journal of Psychosomatic Research, 29,* 139-153.

Weisman, A. D. (1976). Coping with an untimely death. In R. J. Moss (Ed.), *Human adaptation* (pp. 261-274). Lexington, MA: Heath.

Zich, J., & Temoshok, L. (1988). *Blaming the victim: A closer look at the biopsychosocial model of disease.* Manuscript in preparation.

Perceptions of Social Support, Distress, and Hopelessness in Men with AIDS and ARC: Clinical Implications

12

Jane Zich
Lydia Temoshok
Department of Psychiatry/Langley Porter Psychiatric Institute;
School of Medicine
University of California, San Francisco

Acquired immunodeficiency syndrome (AIDS) is probably the most frightening public-health problem in this century. In addition to the overwhelming physical debilitation caused by the disease, AIDS has a profound psychosocial impact. The problem of social isolation and the responses of the social system to persons with AIDS and related conditions have been discussed by numerous authors (Christ, Wiener, & Moynihan, 1986; Coates, Temoshok, & Mandel, 1984; Dilley, Ochitill, Perl, & Volberding, 1985; Forstein, 1984; Green & Miller, 1986; Miller, 1986; Morin & Batchelor, 1984; Siegel, 1986); the more general problem of living with a stigmatizing disease or disability is presented in detail by Goffman (1963).

Empirical studies of the relationship between social support and adjustment to AIDS, however, are limited. In their study of 21 homosexual or bisexual male outpatients with AIDS or ARC, Donlou, Wolcott, Gottlieb, and Landsverk (1985) used a "Resources and Social Supports Questionnaire." They reported that the total-social-support scale was not significantly correlated with measures of mood disturbance nor with a measure of self-esteem. In a study of psychosocial predicators of reported behavior change in homosexual men at risk for AIDS (Emmons et al., 1986), supportive social norms were significantly related to attempts to reduce the number of one's sexual partners. No significant relationship was found, however, between a measure of gay social network affiliation and any behavioral outcome.

Nonetheless, a large literature suggests that social support may be a critical variable to include in any psychosocial study of AIDS-spectrum disorders. For over a decade, social support has been posited to be a significant factor in health and illness from both an empirical (Berkman & Syme, 1979; Bloom & Spiegel, 1984; Funch & Marshall, 1983; Hibbard, 1985; House, Robbins, & Metzner, 1982; Medalie & Goldbourt, 1976) and a theoretical perspective (Berkman, 1984; Cohen & McKay, 1984; Gottlieb, 1983; Hammer, 1983; Pearlin, Lieberman, Menaghan, & Mullan, 1981; Wallston, Alagna, DeVellis, & DeVellis, 1983; Wortman, 1984).

Breast cancer has been the health problem most frequently examined in relation to social support (see reviews by Meyerowitz, 1980; Watson, 1983; Wortman, 1984), but social support has also been examined in relation to numerous other medical disorders (e.g., Dimond, 1979; Evans & Northwood, 1983; Jensen, 1983; Medalie & Goldbourt, 1976; Shearn & Fireman, 1985; see review by DiMatteo & Roy, 1985).

Enthusiasm among social scientists for social support as either a causal agent or powerful buffering mechanism in disease morbidity and mortality has been tempered in recent years by a number of critical reviews (Kessler, Price, & Wortman, 1985; Shinn, Lehmann, & Wong, 1984; Shumaker & Brownell, 1984; Singer & Lord, 1984; Starker, 1986; Wallston et al., 1983; Wortman, 1984). Even so, reviewers generally agree that social support has both theoretical and practical importance as a health-related resource which may prove more modifiable than other resources (Cassel, 1976).

In an effort to foster more sophisticated and complete social-support data bases, several reviewers have proposed guidelines for future research (Cohen & McKay, 1984; Shumaker & Brownell, 1984; Wallston et al., 1983; Wortman, 1984). Among the dimensions cited for inclusion in indices of social support are: perceived availability of support (Berkman, 1984; Cohen & McKay, 1984; Wortman, 1984); perceived desirability of support (Eckenrode, 1983; Funch & Marshall, 1984; Shinn et al., 1984; Starker, 1986); frequency of use (Wortman, 1984); and perceived helpfulness, harmfulness, or satisfaction with the support (Sandler & Barrera, 1984; Vachon et al., 1982; Watson, 1983; Wortman, 1984). The importance of assessing different types of social support has been emphasized by numerous reviewers (Sandler & Barrera, 1984; Wallston et al., 1983; Wortman, 1984).

Consistent with these guidelines, we employed a social support questionnaire (based on the content analytic work of Gottlieb, 1978, and then translated into an abbreviated self-report questionnaire by the first author) for use in a longitudinal study of men with AIDS and AIDS-related complex (ARC). This paper presents findings from the initial administration of the questionnaire, given to individuals shortly after they were indentified by their physicians as having either AIDS or ARC. Questionnaire responses are examined in relation to indices of psychological distress, hardiness, and number of reported physical symptoms. It was hypothesized that social support would be positively associated with measures of hardiness and negatively related to self-report measures of physical and psychological distress.

METHODS

Recruitment

Sequential samples of eligible health-care consumers from San Francisco General Hospital's (SFGH) Acquired Immune Deficiency Outpatient Clinic and from Custom Health Care were invited to participate in the study by their health care providers. Both persons with AIDS and ARC were recruited through SFGH. Only persons with ARC were recruited through Custom Health Care, a large private medical clinic in San Francisco. Use of two recruitment centers was necessary in order to assure an adequate sample of ARC participants.

Criteria for eligibility into the study included: (1) the participant must be a gay or bisexual man (operationally defined by acknowledging sexual intercourse with one more more men during the year preceding onset of illness or symptoms); and (2) the participant must have a recent diagnosis of AIDS or ARC.

Diagnosis of AIDS was based on the Centers for Disease Control's definition of AIDS at the time the study began (early 1984). No added exclusionary criteria were used. Hence, the sample included men with Kaposi's sarcoma (KS) only, with *Pneumocystis carinii* pneumonia (PCP) only, with both KS and PCP (KS/PCP), and with KS/PCP plus other opportunistic infections.

Because the diagnosis of AIDS is a severe stressor and often requires extensive medical treatment and follow-ups, patients were not approached during the initial two weeks after diagnosis. However, in order to gather data related to the initial adjustment phase and to diminish, as much as possible, the variability in psychological reaction attributable to time, all subjects were interviewed within eight weeks post-diagnosis. Thus, the initial interviews occurred two to eight weeks after diagnosis.

Since no formal diagnostic criteria for an ARC diagnosis existed at the time the study began, the diagnosis was operationally defined in consultation with physicians at the SFGH AIDS clinic. An ARC diagnosis required at least two of the following indices of disturbed immune functioning: herpes zoster; white blood cell count below 4.0; globulin levels above 3.3; anergy to skin tests; decreased platelet count (below 100,000); helper/suppressor T-cell ratio less than 1.0; persistent, unexplained diarrhea; oral (not esophageal) thrush; active CMV infection; unexplained lymphadenopathy in at least two sites (excluding inguinal) of three month duration; unexplained fevers or night sweats; unexplained cough for greater than 30 days; unexplained anemia; and severe recurrent herpes simplex.

As the onset of ARC symptoms is often insidious and not usually marked by the sudden presence of opportunistic infection, and because no formal criteria for an ARC diagnosis existed at the time of the study, the date of physician's diagnosis of ARC has an ambiguous meaning. The diagnosis in the case of persons with ARC may have been triggered as much by the study inclusion criteria distributed to the physicians as by a change in the participants' symptoms or medical status. Thus, it is unclear at what point in the adjustment process persons with ARC entered the study.

Eligible persons with AIDS and ARC were told about the study by their physicians or nurse practitioners. Individuals interested in participating were then introduced to, or subsequently contacted by, a representative of the study, at which point the project was described in detail. Issues of confidentiality were discussed at length.

Participants

Fifty persons with AIDS and 53 persons with ARC participated in the study. All AIDS participants were recruited through SFGH. Thirty-five, or 66%, of the ARC participants were recruited through SFGH; the remainder were recruited through Custom Health Care.

AIDS and ARC participants were similar in age and education. For the AIDS group, the average age was 35, ranging from 24 to 56 years. Forty-six percent had completed some college. Nearly 40% had graduated from college or undertaken postgraduate training. For the ARC group, the mean age was 37, with a range from 23 to 62 years. Forty-six percent had completed some college. Forty-nine percent had graduated from college or undertaken postgraduate training.

In contrast to these similarities, AIDS and ARC groups differed in employment status. Forty-seven percent of ARC participants were employed full time, while 25% were unemployed. As might be expected due to medical status, more AIDS participants (67%) were unemployed. Twenty-two percent were working either full time or part time. Average income in the previous year, prior to taxes, was $12,000-$15,000 for both groups.

Measures

Measures were administered through two methods. Some of the measures were incorporated into a structured interview. Other measures were presented as part of a self-report questionnaire packet. In the present paper, only the reported physical symptoms data were obtained through interview. All other data were derived from the self-report questionnaires.

Structured Interview.

A two-hour audiotaped interview was scheduled and conducted by one of three male psychologists (one practicing clinical psychologist and two advanced graduate students in clinical psychology), who then served as the participant's interviewer throughout the study. The structured interview addressed reactions to diagnosis, current symptoms, major life events, attributions for cause and improvement in medical condition, recent behavior change, emotional adjustments, coping strategies, and other dimensions which will be examined in subsequent reports.

Self-report Questionnaire Packet.

A self-report packet was given to all participants following the interview, with instructions to complete the packet within one week and return it by mail in the provided stamped, addressed envelope. All materials were identified by subject identification number only. This constituted the first wave of data collection. Only the measures pertinent to the current topic are included in the following description, analysis, and discussion.

(1) A social support questionnaire was developed by the first author, based on the content analytic work of Gottlieb (1978). Gottlieb's qualitative analyses yielded four major categories of informal helping:

1. Emotionally sustaining behaviors (e.g., "someone to talk to")
2. Problem-solving behaviors (e.g., "someone who offers suggestions")
3. Indirect personal influence (e.g., "someone who conveys a willingness to help")
4. Environmental action (e.g., "someone who intervenes in the environment to reduce stress")

Three examples from each of the first two categories and one example from each remaining category were included in the social support questionnaire. Respondents were asked to indicate, on a five-point scale, how desirable each type of help was to them, how available it was, how often they used it, and how useful it was if used. For both AIDS and ARC participants, it was expected that degree of social support would be positively related to psychological hardiness and negatively correlated with indices of distress. No specific hypotheses were made regarding relationships among specific categories of social support.

Items were selected a priori to compose the following scales, which are listed along with their separate standardized coefficient alpha reliabilities (Cronbach, 1951; Nunnally, 1978):

Eight-item scales regarding help
1. Total "How desirable?" (.89)
2. Total "How available?" (.88)

3. Total "How often used?" (.85)

4. Total "How useful?" (.84)

Three-item scales regarding help (items from these scales are a subset of the scales above)

1. Emotionally sustaining—"How desirable?" (.88)

2. Emotionally sustaining—"How available?" (.86)

3. Emotionally sustaining—"How often used?" (.79)

4. Emotionally sustaining—"How useful?" (.74)

5. Problem-solving—"How desirable?" (.72)

6. Problem-solving—"How available?" (.64)

7. Problem-solving—"How often used?" (.65)

8. Problem-solving—"How useful?" (.73)

(2) McNair's Profile of Mood States (POMS) was included to determine current mood states. The POMS is an adjective rating scale, with documented reliability and validity, which measures the following dimensions of mood: tension/anxiety; depression/dejection; anger/hostility; vigor/activity (reverse scored); fatigue/inertia; and confusion/bewilderment (McNair, Lorr, & Doppleman, 1971).

The POMS Short Form (Shacam, 1983) was used in this study. The POMS was predicted to be associated with lower levels of perceived social support for both AIDS and ARC participants.

(3) Kobasa's "Hardiness' measure [an abbreviated form (Kobasa, 1983, personal communication to the second author)] served as a measure of psychological strength, coping resources, and adaptive capacities. It was included to provide a more comprehensive assessment of individual adjustment. Conceptually, personality-based "hardiness" is a composite of commitment, control, and challenge (Kobasa, Maddi, & Courington, 1980). The commitment subscale measures involvement with life, including involvement and investment in the interpersonal sphere. The control subscale taps feelings of effectiveness versus helplessness. The challenge subscale addresses a person's tendency to perceive stress as challenging rather than threatening. From a construct validity perspective, the commitment subscale was expected to be most strongly correlated with social support for both AIDS and ARC participants.

(4) An abbreviated 20-item version (Bendig, 1956) of the Taylor Manifest Anxiety Scale (MAS; Taylor, 1953) was used to estimate how much a person is consciously distressed by current stressors. Higher scores on this measure were predicted to correlate negatively with degree of perceived social support for both AIDS and ARC participants.

(5) The Beck Hopelessness Scale was used to measure level and degree of hopelessness experienced by participants and to detect respondent's negative expectancies. The underlying assumption of the scale is that hopelessness can be readily operationalized as a system of cognitive schema, whose common denominator is negative expectation about the future (Beck, Weisman, Lester, & Trexler, 1974). The Hopelessness Scale has been shown to be strongly positively correlated with measures of suicidal intent (Beck, Kovacs, & Weissman, 1975; Dyer & Kreitman, 1984; Goldney, 1981; Nekanda-Trepka, Bishop, & Blackburn, 1983; Wetzel, 1976). It was predicted that hopelessness would be negatively correlated with perceived degree of social support for both AIDS and ARC participants.

RESULTS

Social Support and Distress

As a first step in the data analysis, we examined the relationship between social support ratings and indices of psychological distress. Because the patterns of ratings across Desirability, Availability, Frequency of Use, and Usefulness were highly similar for all eight social support items (see Table 12.1), ratings for each of the social support dimensions were summed across items, yielding the following variables: Total Desirability rating, Total Availability rating, Total Use rating, and Total Usefulness rating. These four total ratings were then correlated with the psychological scales and with the total number of physical symptoms reported by each participant. Analyses were conducted separately for the AIDS group and the ARC group (see Table 12.2).

While none of the total social support ratings correlated significantly with the number of physical symptoms reported by people with ARC, the Total Availability rating correlated strongly ($r = -.44$, $p < .005$) with reported physical symptoms for persons with AIDS. As this is a negative correlation, the finding indicates that the greater the number of physical symptoms a person with AIDS reports, the less available he perceives help to be. This does not appear to reflect a greater demand for social support on the part of the person with AIDS, since Desirability and Used ratings are not significantly correlated with number of reported physical symptoms.

One possible explanation for the finding is that both number of physical symptoms reported and rating of available help reflect a negative reporting bias in distressed individuals with AIDS. If so, number of physical symptoms reported and indices of psychological distress should be positively correlated, but only for the AIDS group. As shown in Table 12.2, this was, in fact, the case. However, the pattern of correlations between physical symptoms and psychological distress differed from the pattern found for social support ratings and psychological distress. Specifically, physical symptoms were

TABLE 12.1
Means and Standard Deviations for Each Type of Help

Category of Help		How Desirable		How Available		How Often Used		How Useful	
		AIDS	ARC	AIDS	ARC	AIDS	ARC	AIDS	ARC
Someone to talk to	X̄	4.72	4.40	3.00	2.77	(2.66 * 2.27)		4.70	4.56
	SD	0.50	1.07	0.99	0.94	0.90	0.84	0.61	0.67
Someone who understands your problems or feelings	X̄	4.64	4.33	2.78	2.52	2.28	2.04	4.54	4.48
	SD	0.63	1.06	1.06	1.13	0.88	0.93	0.71	0.74
Someone who expresses confidence in you	X̄	4.38	4.35	2.76	2.42	2.18	1.96	4.39	4.39
	SD	0.67	1.03	1.02	1.07	0.96	0.95	0.76	0.81
Someone who gives you suggestions or advice about how to solve a problem	X̄	4.06	3.92	2.38	2.51	1.86	1.96	4.10	4.16
	SD	0.79	1.08	1.07	1.03	0.95	0.77	0.89	0.64
Someone who explains or shows you how they dealt with problems similar to your own	X̄	4.22	3.98	2.00	2.04	1.62	1.76	4.19	4.08
	SD	0.82	1.02	0.97	0.93	1.08	0.87	0.88	0.85
Someone to whom you can turn when you need to borrow something or need help with an errand	X̄	4.33	4.36	2.65	2.34	1.69	1.56	4.40	4.42
	SD	0.69	0.96	1.16	1.10	0.88	0.76	0.92	0.70
Someone who is there for you	X̄	4.79	4.77	3.04	2.60	(2.43 * 1.87)		4.77	4.58
	SD	0.41	0.72	1.18	1.25	0.99	1.14	0.48	0.68
Someone who will do something to change your situation so you'll be under less stress	X̄	4.08	3.88	(2.34 * 1.51)		1.45	1.04	4.23	3.84
	SD	1.03	1.30	1.32	1.14	1.16	0.92	0.87	1.18
Total	X̄	35.42	34.17	20.98	19.04	16.31	14.58	35.47	34.44
	SD	3.65	6.45	6.65	6.08	5.67	4.92	4.29	4.14

Note: Scales are scored 1–5, from 1 (extremely undesirable; never available; never used; very harmful) to 5 (extremely desirable; always available; constantly used; very helpful). (*) indicates a significant difference between AIDS and ARC means at $p < .05$ level.

TABLE 12.2
Correlations of Social Support Summed Ratings with Self-Report Scales of Distress,
Mood, "Hardiness," and Number of AIDS-related Symptoms

	Ratings of Help									
	How Desirable		How Available		How Often Used		How Useful		Number of Symptoms	
Scales of Help	AIDS	ARC	AIDS	ARC	AIDS	ARC	AIDS	ARC	AIDS	ARC
Taylor Manifest Anxiety Scale	-.01	.17	-.24	-.15	-.03	-.12	-.00	-.02	.01	.20
Beck Hopeless-ness Scale	-.26[a]	-.05	-.47[d]	-.37[b]	-.45[c]	-.41[b]	-.38[b]	-.25	.04	.00
POMS Confusion	.11	-.20	-.22	-.26	-.03	-.04	-.17	-.09	.18	.05
POMS Depression-Dejection	-.06	-.08	-.43[c]	-.43[c]	-.34[b]	-.40[b]	-.25	-.23	.31[b]	.01
POMS Fatigue-Inertia	.04	-.02	-.14	-.15	.05	.03	-.07	-.04	.01	.16
POMS Tension-Anxiety	-.06	-.13	-.25	-.32[b]	-.22	-.14	-.24	-.12	.39[c]	.19
POMS Vigor-Activity	.18	.03	.30[b]	.23	-.01	.06	.06	.10	-.11	-.12
POMS Anger-Hostility	-.01	-.10	-.24	-.44[d]	-.08	-.31[b]	-.40[b]	-.03	.23	.20
"Hardiness"	-.02	.19	.46[d]	.58[d]	-.23	.43[c]	.21	.31	.09	-.03
Number of Symptoms	-.00	.06	-.44[d]	-.13	-.26	-.08	.01	-.17		
Hard Symptoms	.01	.19	-.32[b]	-.09	-.19	-.05	.08	-.07		
Soft Symptoms	-.03	.10	-.45[d]	.12	-.30[b]	.17	-.04	-.01		

[a] $p < .10$
[b] $p < .05$
[c] $p < .01$
[d] $p < .005$

correlated with depression and tension measures for AIDS only; whereas, social support (Availability and Used) ratings were strongly correlated with depression for both AIDS and ARC groups. Additionally, while hopelessness was strongly correlated with ratings of social support for both AIDS and ARC groups, hopelessness was not correlated with physical symptoms for either group. Hence, the correlations of social support with psychological distress measures and with reported physical symptomatology, although related, appear to involve more than redundant information.

As Table 12.2 shows, for both AIDS and ARC participants, Availability and Used ratings were strongly negatively correlated with several of the psychological indices of distress, particularly depression and hopelessness. For persons with ARC, ratings were also strongly negatively correlated with anger. In contrast, Desirability and Useful ratings were associated with psychological indices no more frequently than would be expected by chance. This finding may, in part, be due to a structural difference between the rating scales. While the rating scale for Availability and Used ranged from neutral (or never) to strongly positive (or very frequently), the Desirability and Useful scales were bipolar, ranging from an extremely negative to an extremely positive pole. It may be that our respondents tended to endorse the positive end of rating scales. Consequently, variance in ratings and the likelihood of finding significant correlations were substantially reduced when the rating scales were bipolar. This possibility is supported by the tendency toward higher means and lower standard deviations for the Desirability and Useful ratings, as compared to the Availability and Used ratings (see Table 12.1).

Emotionally Sustaining Versus Problem-solving Help

In the second step of the data analyses, we examined the hypothesis that some types of help may be preferable to others. Specifically, we examined the ratings for emotionally sustaining forms of help ("someone to talk to"; "someone who understands your problems or feelings"; "someone who expresses confidence in you") versus ratings for problem-solving help ("someone who gives you suggestions or advice about how to solve a problem"; "someone who explains or shows you how they dealt with problems similar to your own"; "someone to whom you can turn when you need to borrow something"). Ratings from the three emotionally sustaining (ES) items were summed to yield the following variables: ES Desirable, ES available, ES Used, and ES Useful. Similarly, ratings from the three problem-solving (PS) items were summed to yield four variables: PS Desirable, PS Available, PS Used, and PS Useful.

Since findings were the same for ARC and AIDS groups separately as well as combined, only paired difference tests for the combined group are reported. As shown in Table 12.3, emotionally sustaining help was viewed as more

TABLE 12.3
Tests of Differences Between Emotionally Sustaining (ES) and Problem-solving (PS)
Help Ratings for AIDS and ARC Groups Combined

		Mean	Standard Deviation	t-Test	df	p
How Desirable	PS	12.18	2.18	-6.38	97	.0001
	ES	13.56	2.22			
How Available	PS	6.95	2.40	-6.19	95	.0001
	ES	8.19	2.78			
How Often Used	PS	4.21	2.05	-7.80	95	.0001
	ES	6.74	2.32			
How Useful	PS	12.67	1.99	-5.78	93	.0001
	ES	13.59	1.72			

desirable ($t = -6.38$, $df = 97$, $p < .0001$), more available ($t = -6.19$, $df = 95$, $p < .0001$), more often used ($t = -7.80$, $df = 95$, $df = .0001$), and more useful when used ($t = -5.78$, $df = 93$, $p < .0001$) than was problem-solving help.

Relationship Between Social Support and Hardiness

Finally, social support was examined in relationship to Kobasa's hardiness indices. As shown in Table 12.4, 14 out 32 correlations between social support

TABLE 12.4
Correlations Between Social Support Ratings and Kobasa Measures of "Hardiness'

Kobasa Measure:	Ratings of Help							
	How Desirable		How Available		How Often Used		How Useful	
	ES	PS	ES	PS	ES	PS	ES	PS
Control	.09	.08	.53***	.30***	.40***	.07	.24*	.04
Commitment	.28**	.25*	.59***	.32***	.52***	.19	.30***	.11
Challenge	-.03	.03	.02	-.11	-.08	-.07	-.05	.08
[1]Hardiness	.17	.17	.59***	.30**	.46***	.13	.29*	.12

[1]Control, Commitment, and Challenge are taken as subscales of the total Hardiness
Scale.
*$p < .05$
**$p < .01$
***$p < .005$

ratings and dimensions of hardiness are significant and positive. It appears that ratings of emotionally sustaining support are more consistently significantly associated with the Kobasa scales than are indices of problem-solving help. Specifically, there are no significant correlations between hardiness measures and problem-solving use or usefulness. Also striking about the pattern of results is the consistent lack of significant correlations between the challenge subscale and all ratings of social support.

The two subscales of the Kobasa hardiness measure that are associated most strongly with social support ratings are commitment and control. As previously noted, the commitment subscale taps degree of involvement with others and commitment to the interpersonal as well as the work-related world. As predicted from a construct validity perspective, persons who score higher on the commitment subscale perceive social support as more desirable, available, and useful. They also indicate a higher frequency of use for this resource. The overlap between the Kobasa commitment subscale and the social support questionnaire appears to be considerable. In a regression analysis predicting to overall level of dysphoria (Temoshok, Sweet, Moulton, & Zich, 1987), Kobasa hardiness measures accounted for the most variance, and social support ratings did not add significantly to this prediction.

The hardiness control subscale, theoretically, taps feelings of effectiveness versus helplessness. The positive correlation with indices of social support may indicate that persons who feel less in control of their lives also feel helpless interpersonally. Their lower ratings of social support availability, frequency of use, and usefulness when used may indicate either actual or perceived helplessness in mobilizing desired social support. Since the control subscale is not significantly correlated with perceived desirability of social support, the control factor does not seem to indicate how desirable people find social support to be, but rather how effective people feel they have been in securing the desired support.

DISCUSSION

Physical Symptoms and Perceived Availability of Social Support

Among persons with AIDS, the greater the number of physical symptoms a person reports, the less likely he is to perceive social support as available. Perhaps relevant to this finding is a study by Holahan and Moos (1982). In a large-scale investigation of social support and adjustment, Holahan and Moos found decreased levels of social support to be associated with increased levels of psychosomatic complaints. Their results highlight the possibility that number of self-reported physical problems may be more reflective of psychological distress than of medical status.

The fact that number of physical symptoms, in our study, was positively correlated with depression and tension/anxiety for persons with AIDS (the group in which a significant, negative correlation between physical symptoms and social support was found) is consistent with this interpretation. However, it does not seem to be the case that our physical symptoms measure simply tapped the vegetative signs of depression. Although some of the AIDS-related symptoms in our checklist may be considered depressive equivalents (e.g., fatigue, loss of sleep, weight loss), others are "hard" symptoms, such as herpes, anemia, and fungal infections. The "hard" as well as the "soft" symptoms were significantly negatively correlated with perceived availability of social support.

This pattern of results does not rule out an underlying reporting bias, but it does suggest that our findings reflect more than a mere correlation of self-reported depression with self-reported vegetative symptoms of depression. We are left wondering about this finding that persons with AIDS who report the most physical distress are also those who are most psychologically distressed, yet perceive the least social support to be available to them. The relative lack of perceived social support is not attributable to a disinterest in social support, because ratings of social support desirability were not correlated with physical distress. This finding that it is not the desirability of social support, but rather its perceived availability that varies with number of physical symptoms, is consistent with reports in the cancer literature. Among cancer patients, those with worse prognoses are less likely to receive social support than are their healthier counterparts (Dunkel-Schetter & Wortman, 1982; Kessler et al., 1985; Peters-Golden, 1982).

Such a relationship may be due to several factors. For example, as a result of changes in expectations, roles, interests, or capabilities, a person's customary social support system may be radically altered by serious illness, and this alteration may often involve a reduction in contact with friends and acquaintances. Increasingly, then, the seriously ill may need to rely on professional helpers for social support, and these professionals may, in turn, experience burnout if they work for extended periods of time with the severely ill (Schmale, 1984; Shumaker & Brownell, 1984).

The issue of burnout is frequently raised, anecdotally, by health-care providers in both the U.S. and abroad who speak of the difficulties resulting from seeing so many people (who are often the provider's age or younger) deteriorate and die from AIDS (McKusick et al., 1986; Miller, 1988). Sometimes these care providers may themselves be at high risk for contracting the disease or may have close friends who have died or are dying from AIDS. Under any of these conditions, balancing emotional involvement in an individual patient's care with a self-protective distancing may be a continually taxing struggle, despite periods of pronounced satisfaction with the meaningfulness of one's work.

Decreased social support may also be the result of a stigmatizing disease (Goffman, 1963). Persons with more medical symptoms may be less able to keep their condition hidden, or the salience of their symptoms may lead to more frequent rejections. If this is coupled with a self-protective withdrawal from social situations, opportunities to experience or even perceive social support availability will be radically curtailed.

A third possible explanation of why those who appear to be most ill perceive social support to be least available is that persons who are most ill do not feel capable of reciprocating the help (Gottlieb, 1983; Wortman, 1984). They may feel unentitled to help, or unable to meet the social requirements of accepting help, which may contribute to the perception that help is out of reach. This may be particularly true for individuals who had prided themselves on their self-reliance or their helpfulness toward others prior to contracting AIDS. For such individuals, the interpersonal and intrapsychic upheavals may be as pronounced as the physical effects of AIDS.

Attempts to supply support are apt to be ineffectual at best and intrusive at worst if an individual is unable or unwilling to accept help because of deeply held values. It is for this reason that any social support intervention must be undertaken in a collaborative spirit with respect for the values, beliefs, personal style, and pacing preferences of the person for whom they are intended. Otherwise, well-intentioned "interventions" will amount to little more than coercion at the very time when freedom of choice may be of utmost importance to the individual.

Perceptions of Social Support, Hopelessness, and Depression

For persons with AIDS and those with ARC, the more available social support was perceived to be, the less hopelessness and depression was reported. For persons with ARC, decreased availability of social support was associated with anger, as well as hopelessness and depression. These results are consistent with Antonovsky's (1979) conclusion that those with high life change and low social support are more likely to have the highest levels of distress. It is also consistent with Aneshensel and Stone's (1982) finding that lack of social support contributes to the creation of depressive symptoms. It may be, however, that depressed persons, particularly those who feel hopeless, do not perceive supports that are, in fact, available; or that their social support system has deteriorated as a result of depressive behaviors.

Increased distress does not necessarily mean poorer adaptation. Some degree of anxiety, anger, and depression may be normal and even adaptive (Kessler et al., 1985; Meyerowitz, 1980). Meyerowitz (1980) suggests that it is only when the person's emotional discomfort does not decrease over time that it is considered a cause for concern.

Additionally, the established relationship between hopelessness and suicidal intent (Beck, Kovacs, & Weissman, 1975; Dyer & Kreitman, 1984; Goldney, 1981; Nekanda-Trepka, Bishop, & Blackburn, 1983; Wetzel, 1976), and our data linking lower levels of perceived social support with hopelessness as well as depression, suggest that despondent persons with AIDS and ARC should be queried about the adequacy of their social support. Conversely, persons reporting low social support should be given ample opportunities to discuss feelings of hopelessness, suicidal ideation, and factors contributing to it.

It is in the area of suicide intervention, that the previously mentioned issue of coerciveness in well-intentioned interventions reaches its most disquieting extremes, as documented by sobering reflections from clinicians and philosophers alike (Battin, 1983; Clements, Sider, & Perlmutter, 1983; Goldblum, 1986; Goldblum & Moulton, 1986; Hill, 1983; Maris, 1983, 1986; Mayo, 1983, 1984; Motto, 1972, 1983; Pohmeier, 1985; Regan, 1983; Sartorius, 1983; Scholten, 1986). It is not our intention to propose a solution for either the euthanasia or "assisted suicide" controversy. We want, however, to highlight the very real possibility that, for some persons with AIDS who express a wish to die, the desire to end life might be sufficiently due to potentially modifiable circumstances, such as the extent and quality of the person's social-support system, that intervening in these realms could literally make the difference between life and death—not by restraining a person from carrying out a decision, but by increasing awareness of alternatives that lead to a different choice. Enhancing the person's perceived quality of life may, in addition to making life seem worthwhile, allow for a death with greater dignity and sense of completion.

It would be negligent for clinicians to assume that because AIDS is a devastating illness with no known cure, all suicidal statements by persons with AIDS are unambivalent, well reasoned, and based on unalterable factors. Despite pronounced physical debilitation and emotional suffering, persons with AIDS who state an intention to die may still be asking for help. Therefore, it is imperative for clinicians to guard against premature assumptions about the motivation behind suicidal ideation in a person with AIDS (and related syndromes) and to explore, instead, the full range of factors which may be contributing to the person's suicidal wishes.

The first task of the clinician, then, remains, as it always has been, to understand the person's suicide wish—never to presume comprehension of it. Distinguishing between factors which appear to be modifiable and those unlikely to change may lead to more informed and responsible choices for both the clinician and the person considering suicide. Neither guidelines nor laws can save us from our consciences. Clinicians, as well as patients and their families and friends, must struggle individually with the question of what is ethical, responsible, and humane.

Emotionally Sustaining Versus Problem-Solving Types of Help

All types of help were rated as desirable by both persons with AIDS and with ARC. Furthermore, the impact of social support was perceived to be considerable. When study participants were asked what helped most in coping with any difficult times they may have experienced since their diagnosis, social support was found to be most helpful at all points in the coping process (Moulton, 1985). The support of lovers, friends, and families was perceived as crucial in regaining and maintaining equilibrium.

In particular, our findings indicate that emotionally sustaining types of help are seen as more desirable, more available, more frequently used, and more useful when used than are problem-solving types of help. Perhaps emotionally sustaining types of help are simply more valued and more valuable than problem-solving types of help. Alternately, it may be that, whereas emotionally sustaining help can come from a broad range of social support agents, problem-solving support requires an expert, if it is to be perceived as truly helpful. The "expert" might be a person with expertise in medicine (Meyerowitz, 1980) or with expertise in coping with the illness because he himself has it (cf. Wortman, 1984, on the value of "a similar other" as a helper). For example, numerous persons with AIDS have commented on the importance of talking with someone else who has AIDS, particularly someone who is coping well with it. If, however, a "non-expert" attempts to offer such problem-solving help, it may be experienced as annoying, unhelpful, or simply patronizing. On the average, then, problem-solving help might be rated lower by participants because they had experienced both helpful and annoying forms of it.

The Relationship Between Hardiness and Social Support

As expected, from a theoretical perspective, social-support measures were most consistently correlated (positively and significantly) with the commitment subscale of Kobasa's hardiness index. Part of Kobasa's (1979) definition of commitment is that "committed persons feel an involvement with others. ... Committed persons have both a reason to and an ability to turn to others for assistance in times demanding readjustment" (p. 4).

In a subsequent paper, Kobasa, Maddi, Puccetti, and Zola (1985) reported an obtained correlation between hardiness and social support which "suggests that some meanings of the latter may overlap with the former... when hardiness is controlled statistically... perhaps all that is left are the more passive implications of social support" (p. 532).

In our study, we found that while hardiness measures in general were positively correlated with measures of social support, the correlations were more frequent and pronounced for emotionally sustaining types of help, as compared to problem-solving types of help. This suggests that hardiness has more in common with the expressive rather than with the instrumental aspects of social support. The overlap appears to be considerable.

In a study of the effectiveness of hardiness, exercise, and social support as resources against illness, Kobasa et al. (1985) found that while hardiness accounted for most of the variance in the obtained correlation with health outcome, it was also true that having all three resources was superior to having two resources, which was superior, in turn, to having only one resource.

Perhaps, as Pearlin et al. (1981) suggested, when stress occurs, coping style or personality variables (such as hardiness) may be the first line of defense and account for most of the adjustment variance. If this first line of defense fails, however, then social support may prove critical. Other researchers have suggested that support may be less important for persons with a self-reliant style of coping (Funch & Marshall, 1984). Such a style, however, may be difficult to maintain when one is seriously ill. As the demands of a debilitating medical condition increase, social supports may become more powerful predictors of outcome. This possibility is consistent with the preliminary analysis of our follow-up data (Temoshok et al., 1987).

Caveats

Several cautions are warranted in interpreting these results. First, findings presented in this paper are based solely on the initial wave of psychosocial data collection. Consequently, they are cross-sectional in nature and, thus, cannot address issues of causality. Second, data were collected at a particular point in the disease adaptation process (i.e., during the initial period of adjustment to diagnosis). A markedly different pattern of relationships might be present at a later stage in the adjustment process. Third, participants were residing in San Francisco, a city which is often held up as a model in terms of its medical care and grass-roots social, political, and educational resources for persons with AIDS—particularly gay men with AIDS. As such, the amount of perceived support in San Francisco for a gay man with AIDS is apt to be substantially more varied and accessible than would be true in most other cities in the United States.

Fourth, unlike many other diseases, AIDS is a relatively recent phenomenon with immense public-health impact. Since 1981, there has been an explosion of new medical information, new treatments, and new AIDS support agencies appearing on the scene in rapid succession. Public hysteria waxes and wanes, as does funding for AIDS research and services. Policies with profound implications for the physical, financial, and psychological well-being of persons with AIDS and ARC are proposed with lightning rapidity. These issues create much uncertainty as to whether, for example, antibody testing will remain anonymous, or whether health-insurance coverage will be available for men at risk for AIDS. Resources that provide a range of social-support functions may alternately be bolstered or undermined by shifts in public policy and attitudes. Each new wave of media attention can create a new "crisis of adaptation" for the person with AIDS or ARC. And each newly adopted policy in health care and insurance benefits can have profound effects, not only on the quality of life, but also on the availability of social supports for the individual with AIDS or ARC who relies on the emotionally sustaining aspects of medical care, as well as on its medical regimens and technology.

Because society is also adapting to AIDS, it is imperative to recognize that the context in which a given individual is reacting to a diagnosis of AIDS or ARC is in the state of flux. Thus, findings about the pattern of social-support perceptions in relation to physical symptoms, hardiness, and psychological distress may prove markedly different in 1989 or 1990 than has been true for 1984 and 1985.

Several other methodological limitations of the study should be noted. While our measure of social support adhered to many of the guidelines recommended by previous researchers in this area, other dimensions recommended for inclusion were not examined, yet may prove critical. Such dimensions could include: network size and structure, characteristics of support providers, objective indices of social-support episodes, distinctions between formal and informal support, assessment of reciprocity, and delination of specific adjustment tasks and related social-support needs (Cohen & McKay, 1984; Shumaker & Brownell, 1984; Wallston et al. 1983; Wortman, 1984).

As there are no criteria for "adequate social support" for persons with AIDS and ARC, we were particularly interested in the *perceived* adequacy in terms of its availability, desirability, frequency of use, and usefulness when used. The problem with self-report measures based on a person's perception is that measures may not be independent. Several reviewers have addressed the advantages and disadvantages of employing self-report measures of social support (Shumaker & Brownell, 1984; Starker, 1986; Wortman, 1984).

Finally, because the ARC sample was drawn from two facilities, whereas the AIDS sample was drawn only from one of these facilities, any differences between AIDS and ARC groups must be viewed cautiously, since differences may reflect differences in the population from which the samples were drawn, rather than differences due to the adjustment reactions to AIDS versus ARC. Analyses suggested, however, that the AIDS and ARC samples were similar on a range of demographic and psychological indices. Also, as previously noted, date of diagnosis and onset of related symptoms appeared to be more clear-cut for persons with AIDS than for persons with ARC. Although we attempted to match AIDS and ARC samples on time since diagnosis, it cannot be assumed that the AIDS group and the ARC group were at a comparable stage in adjustment to diagnosis. Differences between AIDS and ARC groups might have resulted from this discrepancy in adjustment stage.

CONCLUSIONS

As Watson (1983) noted, "The assumption that any support is beneficial, no matter what form it takes, is dangerous...there is the risk that, for a few people, intervention may cause unnecessary distress in the process of trying to change their psychological responses" (p. 843).

Keeping this caution in mind, findings from our study suggest it may be valuable to assess further the possibility that enhancing social support could have a clinically significant effect on quality of life for many persons with AIDS and ARC. In particular, we would like to alert health-care workers to three findings: (1) Persons with AIDS who experienced or reported multiple physical symptoms were apt to perceive social support as relatively unavailable to them; (2) although problem-solving types of help were valued by persons with AIDS and ARC, emotionally sustaining types of help were generally rated as more desirable and more useful; and (3) hopelessness, an index of suicidality, was strongly correlated with the perceived availability of support and was not correlated with reported physical symptoms. This last finding suggests that when a person with AIDS expresses an interest in committing suicide, it should not be assumed that his or her intention to die is based predominantly on an untreatable, and probably worsening, physical condition. The possibility that social support, and other modifiable psychosocial resources, may significantly affect both quality of life and desire to live must be recognized. When social support does seem to be a significant factor in the person's quality of life, providing the person with the option of an individualized assessment of specific social-support needs and preferences, followed by a collaboratively designed intervention is recommended. On the whole, these findings suggest that when caring for a person with AIDS or ARC, "just listening" may be a particularly valuable and valued use of a clinician's time.

Both clinicians and researchers need to recognize that primary support networks may be depleted by the seriously ill (Hammer, 1983). When this happens, the extended network takes on added importance. This is likely to be the case for many persons with AIDS. As the person's core network is depleted, community agencies and health-care providers, as well as interviewers for research projects, can become increasingly important sources of social support. Even if family and friends do stay actively involved, community-based programs for persons with AIDS and ARC remain essential. As Pilisuk and Minkler (1985) noted:

> The effectiveness of families and other micro-level support systems is seen as heavily dependent upon the adequacy of programs and policies on the local, state and national levels which provide help with income maintenance, hous-

ing, transportation and other basic necessities. The cutting back of these more basic programs and services will be seen to disrupt the delicate web of natural relationships. (p. 106)

Our initial findings demonstrate that perceptions of social support are significantly related to distress levels in persons with AIDS and ARC. Analysis of the study's follow-up data may help to illuminate the sequential processes involved in these relationships, including their impact on health, and suggest ways to optimize social support, particularly for those markedly distressed persons who perceive such help to be highly desirable, but relatively unavailable. In the meantime, it is recommended that clinicians and researchers recognize that social supports are perceived as highly desirable by both persons with ARC and AIDS and that such resources may have significant impact on both health and the quality of life available to persons suffering from these conditions.

ACKNOWLEDGMENTS

This research was supported by NIMH grant # 39344 (Lydia Temoshok, Ph.D., Principal Investigator). Dr. Zich's involvement in the research was supported by National Research Service Award #1F32 MH09046 and by Clinical Investigator Award #1 K08 MH00608, both from the National Institute of Mental Health.

Special thanks are extended to Joseph Brewer, M.A., for his comments regarding the selection of specific items for the Social Support Questionnaire. Additionally, the authors wish to acknowledge our colleagues in UCSF-BAP involved in various aspects of the ongoing NIMH-supported longitudinal investigation of persons with AIDS and ARC. These UCSF-BAP co-investigators are: Joseph Brewer, M.A.; Evan Elkin, B.A.; Suzanne Engleman, Ph.D.; Robert Fagan, B.A.; Robert Gorter, M.D.; Thomas Irish, Ph.D., Christopher Mead, Ph.D.; Jeffrey Mandel, Ph.D., M.P.H.; Jeffrey Moulton, Ph.D.; George Solomon, M.D.; David M. Sweet, M.A.; and William Woods, Ph.D. Consultants to the group have been: Claus Bahnson, Ph.D.; Thomas J. Coates, Ph.D.; and Edward Morales, Ph.D. We are grateful to Paul Volberding, M.D., and Donald Abrams, M.D., of Ward 86 at San Francisco General Hospital and to Richard Hamilton, M.D., of Custom Health Care for their continuing valuable support of our research. We wish to thank David Sweet, who conducted the data analyses. Additionally, we appreciate the care and time given by Vernnez Rockett, Faustina Shia, and Michelle Won in preparing this manuscript. Finally, we wish to express our appreciation to the participants in our research for sharing their time and their personal experience, as well as to the persons with AIDS and ARC who served as consultants to this project.

This chapter is based, in part, on an article published in the *Journal of Applied Social Psychology*: Zich, J., & Temoshok, T. (1987). Perceptions of social support in men with AIDS and ARC: Relationships with distress and hardiness. *JASP, 17*, 193-215.

Requests for reprints should be sent to Dr. Jane Zich, Division of General Internal Medicine—Behavioral Medicine Unit, Room 433, Ambulatory Care Center, 400 Parnassus Avenue, San Francisco, CA 94143.

REFERENCES

Aneshensel, C. S., & Stone, J. D. (1982). Stress and depression: A test of the buffering model of social support. *Archives of General Psychiatry, 39*, 1392-1396.

Antonovsky, A. (1979). *Health, stress, and coping.* San Francisco: Jossey-Bass.

Battin, M. (1983). Suicide and moral theory. *Suicide and Life-Threatening Behavior, 13*, 231-239.

Beck, A. T., Kovacs, M., & Weissman, A. (1975). Hopelessness and suicidal behavior: An overview. *Journal of the American Medical Association, 234*, 1146-1149.

Beck, A. T., Weisman, A., Lester, D., & Trexler, L. (1974). The measurement of pessimism: The hopelessness scale. *Journal of Consulting and Clinical Psychology, 42*, 861-865.

Bendig, A. W. (1956). The development of a short form of the Manifest Anxiety Scale. *Journal of Consulting Psychology, 5*, 384.

Berkman, L. F. (1984). Assessing the physical health effects of social networks and social support. *Annual Review of Public Health, 5*, 413-432.

Berkman, L. F., & Syme, L. (1979). Social networks, host resistance, and mortality: A nine-year follow-up study of Alameda County residents. *American Journal of Epidemiology, 109*, 186-204.

Bloom, J. R., & Spiegel, D. (1984). The relationship of two dimensions of social support to the psychological well-being and social functioning of women with advanced breast cancer. *Social Science and Medicine, 19*, 831-837.

Cassel, J. (1976). The contribution of the social environment to host resistance. *American Journal of Epidemiology, 104*, 107-123.

Christ, G. H., Wiener, L., & Moynihan, R. T. (1986). Psychosocial issues in AIDS. *Psychiatric Annals, 16*, 173-179.

Clements, C., Sider, R., & Perlmutter, R. (1983). Suicide: Bad act or good intervention. *Suicide and Life-Threatening Behavior, 13*, 28-41.

Coates, T. J., Temoshok, L., & Mandel, J. (1984). Psychosocial research is essential to understanding and treating AIDS. *American Psychologist, 39*, 1309-1314.

Cohen, S., & McKay, G. (1984). Social support, stress, and the buffering hypothesis: A theoretical analysis. In A. Baum, S. E. Taylor, & J. E. Singer (Eds.), *Handbook of psychology and health: Volume IV* (pp. 253-267). Hillsdale, NJ: Lawrence Erlbaum Associates.

Cronbach, L. J. (1951). Coefficient alpha and the internal structure of tests. *Psychometrika, 16*, 297-334.

Dilley, J. W., Ochitill, H. N., Perl, M., & Volberding, P. A. (1985). Findings in psychiatric consultations with patients with acquired immune deficiency syndrome. *American Journal of Psychiatry, 142*, 82-85.

DiMatteo, M. R., & Hays, R. (1985). Social support and serious illness. In B. H. Gottlieb (Ed.), *Social networks and social support*, (pp. 117-148). Beverly Hills, CA: Sage Publications.

Dimond, M. (1979). Social support and adaptation to chronic illness: The case of maintenance hemodialysis. *Research in Nursing and Health, 2*, 101-108.

Donlou, J. N., Wolcott, D. L., Gottlieb, M. S., & Landsverk, J. (1985). Psychosocial aspects of AIDS and AIDS-related complex: A pilot study. *Journal of Psychosocial Oncology, 3*, 39-55.

Dunkel-Schetter, C., & Wortman, C. (1982). The interpersonal dynamics of cancer: Problems in social relationships and their impact on the patient. In H. S. Friedman & M. R. DiMatteo (Eds.), *Interpersonal issues in health care*. New York: Academic Press.

Dyer, J. A., & Kreitman, N. (1984). Hopelessness, depression and suicidal intent in parasuicide. *British Journal of Psychiatry, 144*, 127-133.

Eckenroide, J. (1983). The mobilization of social supports: Some individual constraints. *American Journal of Community Psychology, 11*, 509-528.

Emmons, C. A., Joseph, J. G., Kessler, R. C., Wortman, C. B., Montgomery, S. B., & Ostrow, D. G. (1986). Psychosocial predictors of reported behavior change in homosexual men at risk for AIDS. *Health Education Quarterly, 4*, 331-345.

Evans, R. L., & Northwood, L. K. (1983). Social support needs in adjustment to stroke. *Archives of Physical Medicine and Rehabilitation, 64*, 61-64.

Forstein, M. (1984). The psychosocial impact of the acquired immune deficiency syndrome. *Seminars in Oncology, 11*, 77-82.

Funch, D. P., & Marshall, J. (1983). The role of stress, social support and age in survival from breast cancer. *Journal of Psychosomatic Research, 27*, 77-83.

Funch, D. P., & Marshall, J. R. (1984). Self-reliance as a modifier of the effects of life stress and social support. *Journal of Psychosomatic Research, 28*, 9-15.

Goffman, E. (1963). *Stigma: Notes on the management of spoiled identity*. New York: Simon & Schuster.

Goldblum, P. (1986). Diagnosis/treatment—suicide: Clinical Aspects. *Focus: A Review of AIDS Research, 2*, 2-3.

Goldblum, P., & Moulton, J. (1986). AIDS-related suicide: A dilemma for health care providers. *Focus: A Review of AIDS Research, 2*, 1-2.

Goldney, R. D. (1981). Attempted suicide in young women: Correlates of lethality. *British Journal of Psychiatry, 139*, 282-290.

Gottlieb, B. H. (1978). The development and application of a classification scheme of informal helping behaviors. *Canadian Journal of Behavior Sciences, 10*, 105-115.

Gottlieb, B. H. (1983). Social support as a focus for integrative research in psychology. *American Psychologist, 38*, 278-287.

Green, J., & Miller, D. (1986). Hospital counseling: Structure and training. In J. Green & D. Miller (Eds.), *The management of AIDS patients* (pp. 187-194). London: MacMillan Press.

Hammer, M. (1983). "Core" and "extended" social networks in relation to health and illness. *Social Science and Medicine, 17*, 405-411.

Hibbard, J. H. (1985). Social ties and health status: An examination of moderating factors. *Health Education Quarterly, 12*, 23-34.

Hill, T. (1983). Self-regarding suicide: A modified Kantian view. *Suicide and Life-Threatening Behavior, 13*, 254-275.

Holahan, C. J., & Moos, R. H. (1982). Social support and adjustment: Predictive benefits of social climate indices. *American Journal of Community Psychology, 10*, 403-415.

House, J. S., Robbins, C., & Metzner, H. L. (1982). The association of social relationships and activities with mortality: Prospective evidence from the Tecumseh community health study. *American Journal of Epidemiology, 116*, 123-140.

Jensen, P. S. (1983). Risk, protective factors, and supportive interventions in chronic airway obstruction. *Archives of General Psychiatry, 40*, 1203-1207.

Kessler, R. C., Price, R. H., & Wortman, C. B. (1985). Social factors in psychopathology: Stress, social support, and coping processes. *Annual Review of Psychology, 36*, 531-572.

Kobasa, S. C. (1979). Stressful life events, personality, and health: An inquiry into hardiness. *Journal of Personality and Social Psychology, 37*, 1-11.

Kobasa, S. C., Maddi, S. R., & Courington, C. (1981). Personality and constitution as mediators in the stress-illness relationship. *Journal of Health and Social Behavior, 22*, 368-378.

Kobasa, S. C., Maddi, S. R., Puccetti, M. D., & Zola, M. A. (1985). Effectiveness of hardiness, exercise, and social support as resources against illness. *Journal of Psychosomatic Research, 29*, 525-533.

Maris, R. (1983). Suicide: Rights and responsibility. *Suicide and Life-Threatening Behavior, 13,* 223-230.

Maris, R. (1986). Basic issues in suicide prevention: Resolutions of liberty and love (The Dublin Lecture). *Suicide and Life-Threatening Behavior, 16,* 326-334.

Mayo, D. (1983). Contemporary philosophical literature on suicide. *Suicide and Life-Threatening Behavior, 13,* 313-345.

Mayo, D. (1984). Confidentiality in crisis counseling: A philosophical perspective. *Suicide and Life-Threatening Behavior, 14,* 96-112.

McKusick, L., Horstman, W., Abrams, D., & Coates, T. (1986). The impact of AIDS on primary practice physicians. Paper presented at IInd International Conference on AIDS, Washington, DC.

McNair, D., Lorr, M., & Doppleman, L. F. (1971). *Edits manual: Profile on Mood States.* San Diego: Educational and Industrial Testing Service.

Medalie, J. H., & Goldbourt, U. (1976). Angina pectoris among 10,000 men. II. Psychosocial and other risk factors as evidenced by a multivariate analysis of a five-year incidence study. *The American Journal of Medicine, 60,* 910-921.

Meyerowitz, B. E. (1980). Psychosocial correlates of breast cancer and its treatments. *Psychological Bulletin, 87,* 108-131.

Miller, D. (1986). Psychology, AIDS, ARC, and PGL. In J. Green & D. Miller (Eds.), *The management of AIDS patients* (pp. 131-150). London: MacMillan Press.

Miller, D. (1988). HIV and social psychiatry. *British Medical Bulletin, 44,* 130-148.

Morin, S. F., & Batchelor, W. F. (1984). Responding to the psychological crisis of AIDS. *Public Health Reports, 99,* 4-9.

Motto, J. (1972). The right to suicide: A psychiatrist's view. *Suicide and Life-Threatening Behavior, 13,* 183-188.

Motto, J. (1983). Clinical implications of moral theory regarding suicide. *Suicide and Life-Threatening Behavior, 13,* 304-312.

Moulton, J. M. (1985). *Adjustment to a diagnosis of AIDS and related conditions: A cognitive and behavioral approach.* Unpublished doctoral dissertation. California School for Professional Psychology, Berkeley, CA.

Nekanda-Trepka, C. J., Bishop, S., & Blackburn, I. M. (1983). Hopelessness and depression. *British Journal of Clinical Psychology, 22,* 49-60.

Nunnally, J. C. (1978). *Psychometric theory* (2nd ed.). New York: McGraw-Hill.

Pearlin, L. I., Lieberman, M. A., Menaghan, E. G., & Mullan, J. T. (1981). The stress process. *Journal of Health and Social Behavior, 22,* 337-356.

Peters-Golden, H. (1982). Breast cancer: Varied perceptions of social support in the illness experience. *Social Science and Medicine, 16,* 483-491.

Pilisuk, M., & Minkler, M. (1985). Supportive ties: A political economy perspective. *Health Education Quarterly, 12,* 93-106.

Pohlmeier, H. (1985). Suicide and euthanasia—special types of partner relationships. *Suicide and Life-Threatening Behavior, 15,* 117-123.

Regan, D. (1983). Suicide and the failure of modern moral theory. *Suicide and Life-Threatening Behavior, 13,* 276-292.

Sandler, I. N., & Barrera, M., Jr. (1984). Toward a multimethod approach to assessing the effects of social support. *American Journal of Community Psychology, 12,* 37-52.

Sartorius, R. (1983). Coercive suicide prevention: A libertarian perspective. *Suicide and Life-Threatening Behavior, 13,* 293-303.

Schmale, A. H. (1984). Response to "social support and the cancer patient." *Cancer,* May 15 (Supplement), 2360-2362.

Scholten, H. (1986). Court decision: Justification of active euthanasia. *Medicine and Law, 5,* 169-172.

Shacam, S. (1983). A shortened version of the Profile of Mood States. *Journal of Personality Assessment, 47,* 305-306.

Shearn, M. A., & Fireman, B. H. (1985). Stress management and mutual support groups in rheumatoid arthritis. *The American Journal of Medicine, 78,* 771-775.

Shinn, M., Lehmann, S., & Wong, N. W. (1984). Social interaction and social support. *Journal of Social Issues, 40,* 55-76.

Shumaker, S., & Brownell, A. (1984). Toward a theory of social support: Closing conceptual gaps. *Journal of Social Issues, 40,* 11-36.

Siegel, K. (1986). AIDS: The social dimension. *Psychiatric Annals, 16,* 168-172.

Singer, J. E., & Lord, D. (1984). The role of social support in coping with chronic or life-threatening illness. In A. Baum, S. E. Taylor, & J. E. Singer (Eds.), *Handbook of psychology and health: Volume IV* (pp. 269-277). Hillsdale, NJ: Lawrence Erlbaum Associates.

Starker, J. (1986). Methodological and conceptual issues in research on social support. *Hospital and Community Psychiatry, 37,* 485-490.

Taylor, J. A. (1953). A personality scale of manifest anxiety. *Journal of Abnormal and Social Psychology, 48,* 285-290.

Temoshok, L, Sweet, D., Moulton, J., & Zich, J. (1987). *A longitudinal study of distress and coping in men with AIDS and AIDS-related complex.* Poster presented at the IIIrd International Conference on Acquired Immunodeficiency Syndrome, Washington, DC.

Vachon, M. L., Rogers, J., Lyall, W. A., Lance, W. J., Sheldon, A. R., & Freeman, S. J. (1982). Predictors and correlates of adaptation to conjugal bereavement. *American Journal of Psychiatry, 139,* 998-1002.

Wallston, B. S., Alagna, S. W., DeVellis, B. M., & DeVellis, R. F. (1983). Social support and physical health. *Health Psychology, 2,* 367-391.

Watson, M. (1983). Psychosocial intervention with cancer patients: A review. *Psychological Medicine, 13,* 839-846.

Wetzel, R. D. (1976). Hopelessness, depression, and suicide intent. *Archives of General Psychiatry, 33,* 1069-1073.

Wortman, C. (1984). Social support and the cancer patient: Conceptual and methodologic issues. *Cancer,* May 15 (Supplement), 2339-2360.

Social Support Questionnaire

Below is a list of eight types of help/support. After the name for each category of help/support is an example of what is meant by the category. Your own examples may be somewhat different from the one provided, so long as they seem to you to be examples of the category you are being asked to rate.

For each category of help/support, please indicate how (1) DESIRABLE you believe this type of help/support would be *for you at this time in your life*, (2) how AVAILABLE this type of help/support would be if you wanted it, (3) how often you have EXPERIENCED this type of help/support *during the past month*, and (4) how USEFUL this type of help/support has been when you did receive it.

INDICATE YOUR RATING BY CIRCLING THE NUMBER ON THE SCALE WHICH BEST DESCRIBES *YOUR EXPERIENCE DURING THE PAST MONTH.*

225

Category of Help/Support and Example	How desirable to you?					How available is it?					How often actually used?					How useful to you?				
	extremely undesirable	somewhat undesirable	neutral	somewhat desirable	extremely desirable	always	often	sometimes	rarely	never	constantly	often	sometimes	rarely	never	very harmful	somewhat harmful	no impact/didn't occur	somewhat helpful	very helpful
1. Someone to talk to. ("He/she'll talk things over with me.")	1	2	3	4	5	1	2	3	4	5	1	2	3	4	5	1	2	3	4	5
2. Someone who understands your problems or feelings. ("He/she knows what I'm going through.")	1	2	3	4	5	1	2	3	4	5	1	2	3	4	5	1	2	3	4	5
3. Someone who expressed confidence in you. ("He/she seems to have faith in me.")	1	2	3	4	5	1	2	3	4	5	1	2	3	4	5	1	2	3	4	5

4. Someone who gives you suggestions or advice about how to solve a problem. ("He/she advised me to try something different.")

    1 2 3 4 5   1 2 3 4 5   1 2 3 4 5

5. Someone who explains or shows you how they dealt with problems similar to your own. ("Just seeing how he/she handles situations helps me know what to do.")

    1 2 3 4 5   1 2 3 4 5   1 2 3 4 5

6. Someone to whom you can turn when you need to borrow something like a household object or money or need help with an errand. ("He/she came over and helped me move so I wouldn't have to do it by myself.")

    1 2 3 4 5   1 2 3 4 5   1 2 3 4 5

7. Someone who is there for you. ("I can always count on him/her.")

    1 2 3 4 5   1 2 3 4 5   1 2 3 4 5

8. Someone who will do something to change your situation so you'll be under less stress. ("He/she helped by talking to the landlord and convincing him to wait for the money for a while.")

    1 2 3 4 5   1 2 3 4 5   1 2 3 4 5

227

Neuropsychological Impairment in AIDS

13

Susan Tross, Ph.D.
Clinical Assistant Psychologist, Psychiatry Service,
Memorial Sloan Kettering Cancer Center;
Assistant Professor of Psychology in Psychiatry
Cornell University Medical College
University of California, San Francisco

SCOPE OR PROBLEM

Neurological impairment is now recognized as a serious and common complication of HIV brain infection in the setting of frank AIDS (Navia, Jordan, & Price, 1986). By the final phase of illness, approximately two thirds of all people with AIDS (PWAs) manifest a pattern of diffuse impairment, known as the AIDS dementia complex (ADC). An additional quarter manifest more limited symptoms (Price et al., 1988). Furthermore, at autopsy, neuropathological evidence of CNS disease has been detected in 78% of the brains studied (Nielsen, Petito, Urmacher and Posner, 1984).

CLINICAL DESCRIPTION OF ADC

As the most common neurological complication of AIDS, ADC has also been the best characterized—on clinical, neuropsychological, and neuropathological terms. Early clinical reports described the presence of global organic brain syndromes, marked by highly variable cognitive, motor, and behavioral symptoms (Bredesen & Messing, 1983; Britton, Marquardt, Koppel, Garvey and Miller, 1982; Horowitz Benson, Gottlieb, Davos, & Bentson, 1982). Initially, these were characterized as subacute encephalitis (SE; Nielsen et al., 1984; Snider et al., 1983). However, the assumptions of subacuteness and encephalitis are less appropriate for a condition now generally recognized as chronically progressive and sometimes unassociated with encephalitic inflammation (Price et al. 1988).

229

The concept of ADC was developed in seminal work of Price and his multidisciplinary research team in the Department of Neurology, MSKCC, and in which the author was a collaborator (Navia, Jordan, & Price, 1986: Navia Cho, Petito & Price, 1986). The presence of global cognitive deterioration, along with motor and behavioral symptoms, in the absence of impaired consciousness was documented in the clinical histories of two thirds of a series of 70 autopsied AIDS patients. In the majority of patients, the progression to global impairment was rapid—occurring within two months of the onset of any cognitive symptoms.

In its early course, ADC is especially marked by cognitive symptoms, particularly mental slowing and deficits in recent memory and attention, which are manifested by the majority of patients. At the same time, approximately one half of these patients present with motor symptoms in the form of increased apathy and withdrawal. Neurological signs, detected by examination, are relatively limited to slowing and blunted affect (½ of patients), gait problems and ataxia (½), and hyperreflexia, especially in the lower extremities (1/3).

In its later course, ADC may resemble a full-blown, incapacitating geriatric-like dementia. Global cognitive impairment was identified in 45 out of 46 patients. Slowing, in both the verbal and motor nodes, was detected in 38 patients. At this stage, motor symptoms were common, including: ataxia (N = 32); hypertonia (N = 22); incontinence (N = 21); tremor (N = 20); frontal release signs (N = 17); and weakness, especially of the lower extremities (N = 15).

HIV ETIOLOGY OF ADC

The causal role of HIV brain infection in these neurological complications is well documented (Ho Rota & Schooley, 1985; Levy Shimabukuro, Hollander, Millsant, Kaminsky, 1985; Shaw et al., 1985). HIV has been detected in the brains and CSF of PWAs with neurological complications (Ho et al., 1985; Levy et al., 1985; Shaw et al., 1985) and in the CSF of people with earlier forms of HIV disease (Ho et al., 1985). Ho et al. (1985) isolated HIV from the CSF of people at intermediate stages of HIV disease, including AIDS-related complex and aseptic meningitis immediately following seroconversion, from the sural nerve of a person with peripheral neuropathy and from the spinal cord of a patient with vacuolar myelopathy.

Other authors (Chiodi Asjo, & Fenyo, 1986: McArthur et al, 1988) have isolated HIV from the CSF of asymptomatic HIV seropositive individuals, especially, but not solely, if they had neuropsychiatric symptoms. Shaw et al. (1985) found even higher concentrations of HIV in the brain than in the lymph nodes, peripheral blood, or bone marrow.

NEURORADIOLOGIC CHARACTERIZATION OF ADC

Neuroradiologic methods have been variably useful in the detection of AIDS-related neurological complications. The most widely cited neurologic indicator of these complications is cortical atrophy, especially with ventricular dilation, observed on computed tomographic (CT) scan (Britton, 1984; Horowitz et al., 1982; Navia, Jordan, & Price, 1986; Snider et al, 1983). However, Navia, Jordan, and Price (1986) argue that CT scan may fail to detect actual abnormalities that MRI can identify.

NEUROPSYCHOLOGICAL CHARACTERIZATION OF ADC

In collaboration with Dr. Price and his colleagues, the current author has carried out a study out of neuropsychological deficits in AIDS patients (Tross et al., 1988). A comprehensive battery of neuropsychological tests was used, covering the major components of intellectual function. These included language ability, verbal and visual memory, attention, visuospatial, problem solving, and motor control.

Four groups of gay men were examined: an HIV seronegative group (N = 20); an HIV seropositive group (N = 16); newly diagnosed AIDS patients (N = 44); and AIDS patients referred for neurological consultation (N = 40). Only the two AIDS groups demonstrated significant impairment in motor speed and fine control, concentration, and visuospatial problem solving.

These deficits all share the common features of slowing on timed tasks and impairment in integrative thinking and novel mental processing and problem solving. At the same time, there was relative hold on overlearned tasks of verbal abstraction.

In the newly diagnosed AIDS group, the introduction of psychiatric interviews made it possible to examine the role of depression on neuropsychological impairment. There was no difference in the number of abnormal test results obtained by the five depressed patients and the nondepressed patients. Thus, it was reasonable to conclude that depression did not account for this impairment. There was also no evidence of impairment in the asymptomatic HIV seropositive group.

NEUROPATHOLOGICAL CHARACTERIZATION OF ADC

The presence of ADC has also been corroborated by neuropathological studies. In Navia et al.'s (1986) series of 70 AIDS brains, only 5 were neuropathologically normal; none of these had a history of ADC. While mild to moderate atrophy was evident in 28 out of 37 ADC brains, it was evident in only 2 out of 18 nondemented brains. In the total series, white and subcortical gray-matter involvement were most frequently detected. White-matter pathology was characterized by diffuse pallor (most frequently involved the basal ganglia and the thalamus). Multinucleated giant cells, derived from macrophages, were prominent in both gray- and white-matter pathology. Their presence was correlated with severity of dementia, positive history of major neurological signs, and insidious deteriorating clinical course.

Inflammation, consistent with viral infection, was common ($N = 52$), along with reactive astrocytosis. The investigators were able to define three clinical subgroups, at graduated levels of impairment, which were also characterized by distinct histopathological patterns.

SUBCORTICAL DEMENTIA

Taken together, these neurological, neuropsychological, and neuropathological findings argue for the presence of subcortical dementia, characterized by slowing on timed tasks and deficits in integrative thinking and novel mental processing and problem solving (Sidtis, Tross, Navia, Jordan, & Price, 1986). Subcortical dementia was first invoked by Albert, Feldman, and Willis (1974) to describe cognitive impairment in progressive supranuclear palsy and McHugh and Folstein (1975) to characterize Huntington's disease dementia. It has been described by Cummings and Benson (1984) as a clinical syndrome marked by

> forgetfulness, slowing of mental processes...impaired ability to manipulate acquired knowledge, and personality and affective changes, including apathy and depression...in which elementary linguistic, calculation, and learning processes are intact, but spontaneous use of stored information, ability to generate problem-solving strategies, and insight are impaired...and in which "pathologic" changes involve primarily, but not necessarily exclusively, the deep gray-matter structures, including the thalamus, basal ganglia, and related brain stem nuclei.

OTHER NEUROLOGICAL COMPLICATIONS

Other specific disorders of the central nervous system (CNS) may create neurological problems in patients with AIDS or HIV disease. These include CNS infections, cancers, vacuolar myelopathy, and peripheral neuropathies (Snider et al, 1983). The principal one is CNS toxoplasmosis, which presents as headache, focal dysfunction (i.e., hemiparesis, aphasia, central visual field deficit, etc.), and global mental status change (i.e., lethargy, confusion, disorientation).

Other CNS infections include: cryptococcal meningitis; progressive multifocal leukoencephalopathy, associated with papovavirus infection; herpes virus infection, especially herpes simplex; varicella zoster; and cytomegalovirus, which may cause retinopathy and blindness.

The major form of CNS cancer is primary CNS lymphoma. Vacuolar myelopathy, which may be manifested by progressive motor symptoms of spastic-ataxic paraparesis and eventually mutism, myoclonus, and incontinence, has been identified in 20 out of 89 brain and spinal-cord autopsy samples of PWAs (Petito et al, 1985). Peripheral neuropathies present as burning paresthesias and numbness. Due to their relative specificity, these disorders are easier to diagnose than ADC, and they must be ruled out before the diagnosis of ADC is made.

PROSPECT OF
NEUROPSYCHOLOGICAL IMPAIRMENT
IN ASYMPTOMATIC HIV INFECTION

Clearly, HIV brain infection is a necessary condition for the development of ADC. However, it is not clear whether it is a sufficient condition for the development of neuropsychological impairment in otherwise asymptomatic HIV seropositive individuals. At this time, there is conflicting evidence of both the presence (Grant et al, 1987; and absence (McArthur et al, 1988 Rubinow, Berrettini, Brouwers, & Lane, 1988; Tross et al., in press) of cognitive impairment in asymptomatic individuals. Further, these studies are methodologically limited by small sample sizes, multiple comparisons, and single-assessment designs, which diminish both their power and generalizability. However, there is also a substantive basis for the lack of conclusive results.

Price and his colleagues (Navia, Jordan, & Price, 1986) found that their ADC patient group could be differentiated from their nondemented patient group by their longer duration of AIDS diagnosis, their higher frequency of infection with micobacterium avium intracellular (MAI) and cytomegalovirus (CMV), and their lower frequency of diagnosis with Kaposi's sarcoma in the absence of a concomitant opportunistic infection. They suggested that these findings may be seen as evidence that the setting of significant immunodeficiency, as marked by the presence of opportunistic infection, is required for the development of ADC. They have recently concluded that "although this virus is 'neurotropic,' it is relatively nonpathogenic for the brain in the absence of immunosuppression" (p. 586, Price et al., 1988). Clearly, this is a compelling scientific and practical question in critical need of prospective, larger-scale research.

DIRECTIONS FOR FUTURE RESEARCH

The major role of the brain in HIV disease demands vigorous research initiatives to study its natural history. Little is known about possible functional and structural specificity of HIV brain infection, in which some capacities or structures may be spared while others are affected. Little is known about possible co-factors for clinical disease, which may promote early symptoms in some HIV seropositive individuals but not in others.

Future studies must also be designed to meet the special methodological challenges of this research. The differential diagnosis of evolving subcortical impairment from affective psychiatric symptoms, that may be primary or secondary to it, is especially problematic (Cummings & Benson, 1984). The mental slowing, integrative difficulty, concentration problems, impaired retrieval, and behavioral apathy that may be hallmarks of subcortical dysfunction may also be features of depression and/or anxiety. Multiple approaches to the assessment of affective symptoms are essential—these approaches must tap both subjective and clinical judgment.

Further, there is a particular need for such research among intravenous drug users (IVDUs). Although they are the second-largest risk group for AIDS, they have been virtually ignored in this literature. Only one published study (Silberstein et al., 1986) compared neuropsychological function in HIV seropositive and seronegative drug users. These authors reported poorer performance on selected tests of short-term memory, fine motor speed and control, and visuospatial problem solving in the seropositive group.

Major sociodemographic and medical differences between the gay male and IVDU risk groups make the generalizability of neuropsychological findings from the former to the latter highly problematic. IVDUs are generally poorer, less well-educated, and more likely to use English as a second language; they may also, obviously, either be male or female. The types and course of HIV disease may be different in them than in gay men. IVDUs are much less likely to have Kaposi's sarcoma and much more likely to acquire certain wasting infections, like tuberculosis; consequently, their course may be more rapid and their prognosis poorer.

This research will also have to take into account the special neuropsychological and psychiatric vulnerabilities of the IVDU. Even when they are in treatment, IVDUs are at higher risk for alcohol abuse and abuse of a variety of drugs, including their primary drug abuse, than the general population (Rounsaville Weissman, Kleber & Wilber, 1984). A series of studies have demonstrated that polysubstance abuse may cause neuropsychological deficits, even after abstinence has been achieved (Grant, 1976a; 1978; Parsons & Farr, 1981). IVDUs are also at higher risk for depression (Rounsaville et al., 1984).

IMPLICATIONS FOR CLINICAL INTERVENTION

Clinically, the prospect of neurological complications demands regular monitoring by the clinician and referral for neurological, neuropsychological, and psychiatric consultation, should they be detected. In order to serve the vast population that may require screening and surveillance, methods of assessment must be refined that are easy to administer, minimally demanding, and cost-effective, while meeting traditional prerequisites for sensitivity and specificity. This need is becoming especially critical as anti-viral therapies for HIV infection are being developed that may affect these complications.

It is also essential that the clinician approach the patient's problems in daily living with practicality, resourcefulness, and optimism. The patient's capacity for daily functioning may be enhanced by behavioral techniques and practical assistance used with other patients with cognitive impairment. These include maintenance of daily appointment logs and chore lists, taping of simple instructions to important household objects, and arrangements for a family member, friend, or volunteer buddy to check in with the patient on a daily basis (by visit or phone).

CONCLUSION

By the final phase of illness, HIV brain infection eventually causes diffuse cognitive impairment, known as AIDS Dementia Complex, in at least two thirds of all people with AIDS (Navia, Jordan, & Price, 1986). Such impairment is gradually being recognized earlier in the course of HIV disease in individuals with lymphadenopathy syndrome (Janssen et al., 1988). At this time, there is conflicting evidence of both its presence (Grant et al., 1987; McArthur et al., 1988; Silberstein et al., 1986) and absence (Rubinow et al., 1988; Tross et al., in press) in individuals with HIV infection, in the absence of other constitutional AIDS symptoms.

Price and his colleagues have explained the unstable association between HIV infection and neuropsychological impairment (Price et al., 1988). The question of whether otherwise asymptomatic HIV infection is a sufficient condition for the development of cognitive impairment remains a critical and unresolved issue in need of research. Studies are also needed to: (1) further describe the natural history of such impairment; (2) develop strategies for early assessment and differential diagnosis, particularly with respect to affective symptoms; and (3) characterize this impairment in the IVDU population.

REFERENCES

Albert, M. L., Feldman, R. G., & Willis, A. (1974). The "subcortical dementia" of progressive supranuclear palsy. *Journal of Neurological and Neurosurgical Psychiatry, 37,* 121–130.

Bredesen, D. G., & Messing, R. (1983). Neurological syndromes heralding the acquired immune deficiency syndrome. *Annals of Neurology, 14,* 141.

Britton, C. B., Marquardt, B., Koppel, G., Garvey, G., & Miller, J. R. (1982). Neurological complications of the gay immunosuppressed syndrome. Clinical and pathological features. *Annals of Neurology, 12,* 80.

Chiodi, F., Asjo, B., Fenyo, E. M. (1986). Isolation of human immunodeficiency virus from cerebrospinal fluid of antibody-positive virus carrier without neurological symptoms. *Lancet, 2,* 1276–1277.

Cummings, J. L., & Benson, D. F. (1984). Subcortical dementia: Review of an emerging concept. *Archives of Neurology, 41,* 874–879.

Grant, I., Atkinson, J. H., Hesselink, JR, Kennedy, C. J., Richman, D. D., Spector, S. A., & McCutcheon, J. A. (1987). Evidence for early central nervous system involvement in the acquired immunodeficiency syndrome (AIDS) and other human immunodeficiency virus (HIV) infections. *Annals of Internal Medicine, 107,* 828–836.

Ho, D., Rota, T. R., & Schooley, R. T. (1985). Isolation of HTLV-III from cerebrospinal fluid and neural tissues of patients with neurologic syndromes related to the acquired immune deficiency syndrome. *New England Journal of Medicine, 313,* 1493–1497.

Horowitz, S. L., Benson, DF, Gottlieb, MS, Davos, I., & Bentson, J. R (1982). Neurological complications of gay-related immunodeficiency disorder. *Annals of Neurology, 12,* 80.

Janssen, R., Saykin, A., Kaplan, J. E., Spira, T. J., Pinsk, P. S., Sprehn, G. C., Hoffman, J. C., Meyer, W. B., & Schonberger, L. B. (1988). Neurological complications of HIV infection in patients with lymphadenopathy syndrome. *Annals of Neurology, 23,* 49–55.

Levy, J. S., Shimabukiro, J., Hollender, H., Mills, J., & Kominsky, J. (1985). Isolation of AIDS-associated retroviruses from cerebrospinal fluid and brain of patients with neurological symptoms. *Lancet, II,* 586–588.

McArthur, J. C., Cohen, B. A., Farzedegan, H., Cornblath, D. R., Selnes, O. A., Ostrow, D., Johnson, R. T., Phair, T., & Polk, B. F. (1988). Cerebrospinal fluid abnormalities in homosexual men with and without neuropsychiatric findings. *Annals of Neurology, 23* (Supplement), S34–S37.

McHugh, P. R., & Folstein, M. F. (1975). Psychiatric syndromes of Huntington's chorea: A clinical and phenomenologic study. In D. F. Benson & D. Blumer (Eds.), *Psychiatric aspects of neurologic disease* (pp. 267–285). New York: Grune and Stratton.

Navia, B. A., Cho, E. S., Petito, C. K., & Price, R. W. (1986). The AIDS dementia complex: II. Neuropathology. *Annals of Neurology, 19,* 525–535.

Navia, B. A., Jordan, B. D., & Price, R. W. (1986). The AIDS dementia complex: I. Clinical features. *Annals of Neurology, 19,* 517–524.

Navia, B. A., et al. (1986). The AIDS dementia complex II. Neuropathology. *Annals of Neurology, 19,* 525–535.

Nielsen, S. L., Petito, C. K., Urmacher, C. D., & Posner, J. B. (1984). Subacute encephalitis in acquired immune deficiency syndrome: A post-mortem study. *American Journal of Clinical Pathology, 82,* 678–682.

Parsons, O. A., & Farr, S. P. (1981). The neuropsychology of alcohol and drug use. In S. Filskov & T. Boll (Eds.), *Handbook of clinical neuropsychology* (pp. 320–365). New York: Wiley.

Petito, C., Nana, B. A., Cho, E. S., Jordan, B. D., George, D. C., & Price, R. W. (1985). Myelopathy pathologically resembling subacute combined degeneration in patients with acquired immune deficiency syndrome. *New England Journal of Medicine, 312,* 874–879.

Price, R.W., Brew, B., Sidtis, J., Rosenblum, M., Scheck, A. C., & Cleary, P. (1988). The brain in AIDS: Central nervous system HIV-1 infection and AIDS dementia complex. *Science*, 239, 586-952.

Rounsaville, B. J., Weissman, M. M., Kleber, H. D., & Wilber, C. H. (1984). Psychiatric disorder in treated opiate addicts. In G. Serban (Ed.), *The social and medical aspects of drug abuse*. New York: Spectrum Publications.

Rubinow, D. R., Berrettini, C. H., Brouwers, P., & Lane, H. C. (1988). Neuropsychiatric consequences of AIDS. *Annals of Neurology*, 23 (Supplement), S24–S26.

Shaw, G., Harper, M. E., Hahn, B. H., Epstein, L. G., Gaidusek, D. C., Price, R. W., Navia, B. A., Petito, C. K., O'Hara, C. J., Groopman, J. E., Cho, E-S., Oleske, J. M., Wong-Staal, F., & Gallo, R. C. (1985). HTLV-III infection in brains of children and adults with AIDS encephalopathy. *Science*, 227, 177–182.

Sidtis, J., Tross, S., Navia, B. A., Jordan, B. D., & Price, R. W. (1986, June). *Neuropsychological characterization of the AIDS dementia complex*. Presented at the International Conference on AIDS. Paris. (Abstract #S29e)

Snider, W. D., et al. (1983). Neurological complications of acquired immune deficiency syndrome: Analysis of 50 patients. *Annals of Neurology*, 14, 403–418.

Tross, S., et al. (1988). Neuropsychological characterization of the AIDS dementia complex. *AIDS*, 2, 81–88.

A Psychoneuroimmunologic Perspective on AIDS Research: Questions, Preliminary Findings, and Suggestions

14

George F. Solomon
Department of Psychiatry
University of California, Los Angeles
Lydia Temoshok
Department of Psychiatry
University of California, San Francisco

A BIOPSYCHOSOCIAL APPROACH TO AIDS

Acquired immunodeficiency syndrome (AIDS) and AIDS-spectrum disorders have emerged as perhaps the most critical public health problem of the 1980s. While a great deal of effort has been devoted to biomedical research on AIDS etiology and treatment, there is, to date, no known cure and no known vaccine for AIDS. This situation has led to a search for "co-factors" in AIDS onset and progression.

The complexity of interacting variables in the pathogenesis of immune deficiency and consequent vulnerability to a variety of infections and to cancer led the distinguished immunologist Norman Talal (1983) to state, "AIDS teaches us that immunoregulatory diseases are truly multifactorial" (p. 183). The biopsychosocial model of disease, credited to Engel (1960), is multifactoral, taking into account the interaction of genetic, biological (specific and nonspecific), emotional (state and trait), behavioral, situational ("stress"), and cultural factors in the pathogenesis of *all* disease, not just those classically considered "psychosomatic" (cf. e.g., Temoshok, Van Dyke, & Zegans, 1983). Given a particular genetic composition and/or physical exposure to a disease

239

agent, a number of environmental factors can modify the host's basic immunocompetence to produce a temporarily enhanced immunity or acquired immunodeficiency. Perhaps the most prevalent but least understood of the environmental modulators of human immunocompetence are behavioral factors. It is our conviction that a biopsychosocial approach to AIDS research is necessary and that research questions emanating from the fields of health psychology, behavioral medicine, and psychoneuroimmunology may provide critical information for understanding and treating AIDS (Coates, Temoshok, & Mandel, 1984).

Considering that AIDS is under an epidemiologic, clinical, and psychosocial cloud of such uncertainty and bleakness, it is difficult to see a silver lining. One pin point of light, however, is that because of the known immunologic relationships, the increasingly documented neurologic complications (e.g., Levy, Bresdesen, & Rosenblum, 1985a), as well as the relatively rapid disease progression involving infection and/or neoplasia, AIDS may be an ideal laboratory to investigate psychoneuroimmunologic relationships.

BACKGROUND ON PSYCHONEUROIMMUNOLOGY

Since Ader's (1981) edited volume, *Psychoneuroimmunology*, there has been an explosion of research in this area (cf. Fox & Newberry, 1984; Guillemin, Cohen, & Melnechuk, 1985; Locke et al., 1985; Locke & Horning-Rohan, 1983; Plotnikoff, Faith, Murgo, & Good, 1986). and the adjacent area of neuroimmunomodulation (Korneva, Klimenko, & Shkhinik, 1985; Spector, 1985). Psychoneuroimmunology is evolving as a defined multidisciplinary field dealing with the complex bidirectional interactions of psychological factors, such as emotions and behavior, the central nervous system (CNS), and the immune system. Investigators in this new field seek to document mechanisms by which experience, via CNS transduction, can alter resistance to disease.

There is an increasing body of literature on the relationship between behavioral factors and cancer progression or prognosis (e.g., Derogatis, Abeloff, & Melisaratos, 1979; Greer, Morris, & Pettingale, 1979; Levy, Herberman, Maluish, Schlien, & Lippman, 1985b; Pettingale, 1984; Rogentine et al., 1979; Shekelle et al., 1981; Temoshok et al., 1985; Temoshok & Fox, 1984). Further, a number of recent studies in animals and humans have linked stress and/or behavioral factors with immune response (e.g., Bartrop, Luckhurst, Lazarus, Kiloh, & Penny, 1977; Palmblad, Petrini, Wasserman, & Akerstedt, 1979; Schleifer, Keller, Camerino, Thornton, & Stein, 1983; Sklar & Anisman, 1979) and disease outcome (e.g., Borysenko, 1984; Riley, 1981; Temoshok, Peeke, Mehard, Axelssson, & Sweet, 1987; Visintainer, Volpicelli, & Seligman, 1982). There are especially prominent effects on cellular immunity measured by T-lymphocyte proliferation by mitogens (Kiecolt-Glaser et al., 1984b), and natural killer (NK) cell activity (Kiecolt-Glaser et al., 1984a). Probable psychologically conditioned reductions in these crucial defense mechanisms have been related to increased risk of developing cancer and possibly infectious diseases, as well as to cancer progression (Cox & MacKay, 1982). NK cells are particularly important in these situations (Herberman & Holden, 1979; Levy et al., 1985b).

There are only a few studies, however, that examine psychological and immunologic variables in human patients with immunologically implicated diseases (e.g., Glaser, Kiecolt-Glaser, Speicher, & Holliday, 1985; Kemeny, Cohen, & Zegans, 1986; Levy et al., 1985b; Pettingale, Greer, & Tee, 1977; Temoshok, 1985). There are no published studies, of which we are aware, that relate psychological and immunologic variables to disease outcome variables. Possible reasons for this include (a) the expense of conducting adequate immunologic tests, (b) the unknown temporal relationship between an external stressor, behavior, or intrapsychic event and immunologic reaction, (c) the usually unclear causal relationship between immunologic events and disease outcome, and (d) the typically long delays in prospective or longitudinal studies between psychological testing and outcome—disease initiation, progression, or death.

BACKGROUND ON AIDS

Acquired immunodeficiency syndrome (AIDS), first recognized in 1981, is an unusual communicable disease. It is transmitted by cell-containing bodily fluids, especially semen and blood. At present, the two major at-risk groups are homosexual men (about 70% of the cases) and needle-sharing intravenous drug abusers. The incubation period is prolonged; there are documented cases of AIDS after a previous exposure seven years before the appearance of any symptoms. The retroviral (RNA) etiologic agent of AIDS, human immunodeficiency virus (HIV), which was formerly known as HTLV-III, LAV, or ARV, attacks specific components of the immune system, which is responsible for the body's defenses against infections and cancer.

AIDS is defined by the Centers for Disease Control (CDC) by the presence of an opportunistic infection (one caused by an agent not pathogenic in a person with an intact immune system) or an unusual neoplasm (Kaposi's sarcoma or non-Hodgkin's lymphoma) in an immunocompromised host.[1] AIDS is, thus, both an infectious disease and one of immunologic aberration, manifested by an infectious disease and/or cancer. The disordered immune regulation which occurs with AIDS and the "lesser" clinical syndrome result-

---

[1]As of this writing (August 1986), the Centers for Disease Control was expected to expand its definition of AIDS to include diseases of the central nervous system caused by infection with HIV.

ing from HIV infection, often called the AIDS-related complex (ARC), ensues mainly from destruction of a specific "target" of the virus, the helper-inducer T-lymphocyte which carries the CD4 (OKT-4) marker.

PSYCHONEUROIMMUNOLOGIC HYPOTHESES ABOUT AIDS

Soon after the dawn of the concept of "psychoimmunology," Solomon and Moos (1964) posed one "speculative" hypothesis, that "stress can be immuno-suppressive." By 1969, Solomon had demonstrated stress-induced suppression of humoral immunity (primary and secondary antibody response) in rats. In his 1985 review of the field of psychoneuroimmunology, Solomon posed 14 "hypotheses" or corollaries based on the thesis that the immune and central nervous systems are intimately linked, and he presented supporting data. His latest list (Solomon, 1987) of such hypotheses number 31 as research burgeons. Of those 31, no doubt soon to increase, several seem especially relevant to AIDS:

1. Enduring coping style and personality factors (so-called "trait" character-istics) should influence the susceptibility of an individual's immune system to alteration by exogenous events, including reactions to events.

2. Emotional upset and distress (so-called "state" characteristics) should alter the incidence, severity, and/or course of diseases that are immuno-logically resisted (infectious and neoplastic diseases) or are associated with aberrant immunologic function (allergies, autoimmune diseases).

3. Diseases of immunologic aberration should, at times, be accompanied by psychiatric and/or neurologic symptoms.

4. Factors elaborated by the immune system should affect the CNS and substances regulated by it. [While this hypothesis will not be further elaborated in this paper, it is included primarily because alpha interferon, used as an experimental treatment for AIDS, often produces neuropsychiatric side effects, including behavioral, cognitive, affective, and personality changes, particularly suggestive of frontal lobe effects (Adams, Quesada, & Gutterman, 1984).]

5. Behavioral interventions (such as psychotherapy, relaxation techniques, imagery, biofeedback, and hypnosis) should be able to enhance or optimize immune function.

6. Neurotropic virus should also show affinity for lymphocytes, and vice versa.

7. Prenatal hormonal environment may affect both CNS development with behavioral consequences, and immune development with long-lasting altera-tions in the components and function of the immune system. [This hypothesis was originally suggested by Hines (1982).]

8. Thymus hormones regulating immune function should be influenced by the CNS.

PSYCHONEUROIMMUNOLOGIC QUESTIONS AND PRELIMINARY FINDINGS IN AIDS

From these hypotheses, for each of which there is now a varied amount of evidence, we have derived a set of new questions to be addressed in research on AIDS-spectrum disorders from a psychoneuroimmunologic perspective. We shall pose these questions and attempt to address each.

Are Stress and/or Other Psychosocial Factors Related to Vulnerability to HIV Infection?

Another version of this question is: Are psychosocial stressors and pre-existing immune status unique to particular at-risk groups and/or related to vulnerability? Determination of any psychosocial factors related to seroconversion (a change in reaction to an HIV antibody test from negative to positive) requires prospective studies. With the exception of the prospective epidemiologic study being carried out by investigators at the University of California at Berkeley (Winkelstein, Principal Investigator) and in Chicago (Ostrow, Principal Investigator), both as part of the Multicenter AIDS Cohort Study (MACS) funded by NIAID (cf. Kaslow et al., 1987), the prospective studies now under way of gay communities in major metropolitan areas in the United States are notably deficient in psychosocial components. As yet, there are only preliminary reports of relationships of psychosocial variables to immune measures and HIV status in these prospective studies (e.g., Coates, 1986). Psychosocial correlations have been reported, but should be more readily available with further follow-up of the sample.

A recently reported study in New York, using blood samples collected since 1978, cited an annual seroconversion rate among susceptible men ranging from 5.5% to 10.6% (Stevens et al., 1986). This study demonstrated a positive correlation between seropositivity and receptive anal intercourse, and number of partners with whom it is practiced. A prospective Dutch study on seroconversion cited, in addition to those risk factors, the use of nitrites and cannabis (Van Griensven et al., 1986). We await results of studies determining psychological, as well as behavioral, risk factors in seroconversion.

Is an "Immunosuppression-prone" Personality Pattern Similar to Other Constructs in Behavioral/psychosomatic Medicine?

Solomon's (1987) notion of an "immunosuppression-prone" personality pattern shares common features with a "Type C" coping pattern suggested to be predictive of more unfavorable cancer prognosis and, possibly, cancer susceptibility (Morris & Greer, 1980; Temoshok & Fox, 1984; Temoshok & Heller, 1981). Related patterns include psychological profiles of individuals with autoimmune diseases (Solomon & Moos, 1965); McClelland's "inhibited power motivation" (McClelland, Flor, Davidson, & Saron, 1980); and "alexithymia," which is thought to be related to somatic, rather than psychological manifestations of emotional conflict (e.g., Apfel, & Sifneos, 1979). Common to all these proposed patterns are compliance, conformity, self-sacrifice, denial of hostility or anger, and non-expression of emotion.

Measures of most of these constructs are being assessed and related to psychological, as well as physical well-being in two studies of which we are aware: (a) a longitudinal psychosocial study of men with AIDS and ARC conducted by the University of California, San Francisco Biopsychosocial AIDS Project (UCSF-BAP; Temoshok, 1983), and (b) a study of long-term survivors of AIDS (Solomon, Temoshok, O'Leary, & Zich, 1987).

Is Pre-existing Immunosuppression a Necessary or Facilitating Factor for Infection and Seroconversion?

Spermatozoa appear to induce immune dysregulation, apparently via an optiate-mediated mechanism (Fabbri et al., 1985; Mavligit et al., 1984). In intravenous drug abusers, exogenous opiates are immunosuppressive (Brown, Stimmel, Taub, Kochwa, & Rosenfield, 1974). Could emotional distress, probably common (but for different reasons) among gay men, drug abusers, and hemophiliacs, play a role in the increased susceptibility of these groups to AIDS? Gay men are particularly subject to the stress of societal homophobia, which is internalized in some individuals to the detriment of self-esteem (Solomon & Mead, 1987). A variety of severe psychopathologies generally underlie drug addiction, which tends to be characterized by failure to cope with painful affect and by maladaptive use of denial as a defense. Hemophiliacs have a painful, activity-limiting, life-threatening illness, which is certainly stressful. To the extent that these stresses are immunosuppressive, then they may be involved in the increased vulnerability of these groups to AIDS over and beyond what may be accounted for by increased opportunity for exposure to the HIV virus, and/or by drug or spermatozoa-induced immunosuppression.

Perhaps there is an analogy in earlier research concerning another disease of immune dysfunction, the autoimmune disease rheumatoid arthritis. Healthy relatives of rheumatoid arthritis patients with rheumatoid factor (an IgM anti-IgG) and their sera showed less emotional decompensation than those lacking the factor, suggesting that the combination of an immunologic abnormality and emotional distress leads to overt disease (Solomon & Moos, 1965). If an immune system is already compromised (e.g., by semen, opiates, or viral infection), is it not likely that stress would be more immunosuppressive than in an intact, more "resilient" immune system)?

Can Stress Activate HIV from a
Rapidly Replicating State?

It is now known that HIV can exist in a latent, non-replicating form and that activation is related to a gene ("tat") responsible for transacting transcriptional activation (Folks et al., 1985; Sodroski, Rosen, & Haseltine, 1984). Among inducers of latent virus, stimuli such as radiation, infections, chemicals, or stress have been proposed (Sodroski et al., 1984). Such possible stress-induced activation from the latent to active form of HIV, most likely via immunologic mechanisms, would be analogous to stress-induced activation of herpes virus from its latent state (Glaser et al., 1985).

Are Psychosocial Factors Related
to Progression of HIV Disease?

Are psychosocial factors related to (a) post-exposure state of immunity (antibody, no virus), versus (b) asymptomatic carrier states (antibody plus virus), versus (c) constitutional or "lesser AIDS" symptoms (ARC), versus (d) AIDS, versus (e) progression from b to c or d, or from c to d?

In most persons in whom antibodies can be detected, virus can also be isolated (Devita, Hellman, & Rosenberg, 1985). Antibody and virus coexist, probably for life, in most individuals. No detection of virus in HIV antibody-positive individuals may be due to error, variation in quantity of virus present, or elimination of virus in a subset of exposed antibody-positive individuals. (Different tests for virus infectivity can measure either free virus or cell-associated virus.) Greater availability, simplicity, and rapidity, as well as lower cost of virus assays, may make it possible to determine virus neutralization in conjunction with psychosocial-psychoneuroimmunologic research. If neutralization does occur naturally, what characterizes individuals who eliminate virus?

One estimate suggests that the number of adults infected with HIV in the U.S. is 1,765,470 (Sivak & Wormser, 1985). Whatever the true numbers, and bearing in mind the long incubation time for AIDS, those infected but asymptomatic individuals far outnumber the approximately 22,000 cases of AIDS thus far diagnosed (as of August 1986), or the larger number of persons with symptoms of ARC. The existence of a carrier state is also clear from transmission of AIDS to infants by asymptomatic HIV-positive mothers and to blood or blood-product recipients from asymptomatic donors.

Do persons with asymptomatic carrier states differ psychologically from those with ARC, and do asymptomatic HIV-positive persons or those with ARC differ from persons with AIDS? A prospective study found that 10.1% of a cohort who were seropositive as of October 1982 or who seroconverted before August 1985 developed AIDS (Goedert et al., 1986). This study suggested that risk of AIDS development in different populations may depend not only on time, but on "as yet undefined factors." Might some of these factors be psychosocial? Clinicians have long known, for example, that emotional distress is one factor that could activate "dormant" tuberculosis (Day, 1951). Again, we await the results of prospective and longitudinal studies.

Can Psychosocial Variables be Correlated with Specific Alterations in Immune Function Associated with HIV Infection?

Psychoneuroimmunologic studies of AIDS-spectrum disorders with adequate funding to obtain sufficient laboratory data on a variety of immunologic measures are beginning to yield preliminary results (e.g., Solomon et al., 1987; Temoshok et al., 1987; 1988). In a related area, Solomon, Fiatarone, Benton, Morley, Bloom, and Makinoden (1988) are conducting a psychoimmunologic, neuroendocrine, and endorphin study of healthy, aged persons in an attempt to correlate psychosocial factors with specific aspects of variably diminished immune function of the elderly. Because measures were chosen specifically to overlap those used in UCSF-BAP's AIDS/ARC research, any psychological correlates of specific aspects of disordered immune function across studies can be further explored. In mentally and physically healthy elderly persons (over 65), immune functions (lymphocyte blastogenesis induced by PHA and natural killer cell activity) are actually *superior*, on the average, to those of healthy young controls (age 21–40), suggesting that healthy lonevity is correlated with superior immune function and mental well being. Minor mood fluctuations within normal ranges are not reflected by immune changes in young or old. In elderly persons, anticipated life stress is accompanied by decreased natural killer cell stimulability by interleukin-2.

Is Length of Survival Related to Psychosocial Factors Assessed at an Earlier Point in Time?

A corollary question is whether long survival with AIDS and any psychosocial correlates of long survival are related, in turn, to specific aspects of immune function. UCSF-BAP has begun to explore the possible relationship between psychosocial measures assessed within 2–8 weeks of an AIDS or ARC diagnosis and subsequent health outcomes (Solomon et al., 1987; Temoshok et al., 1987, 1988).

Scores on self-report obtained at the time of the initial interview were compared for men who were alive as of March 1986 and those who were deceased. Because most of the variance in outcome is most likely explainable by biological factors, particularly the type of AIDS-associated disorder, we conducted separate analyses for three groups: AIDS subjects with *Pneumocystis carinii* pneumonia (PCP; $n = 21$), AIDS subjects with Kaposi's sarcoma ($n =$

28), and ARC subjects (n = 53). For AIDS-PCP subjects, two psychosocial variables were significantly different between the two outcome groups: (a) Kobasa's "control" subscale (M = 60.0 in the deceased group, M = 65.0 in the alive group; t = 1.99, $p <$ .05, two-tailed), and (b) how often problem-solving help (as assessed by a social-support scale described in Zich & Temoshok, 1987) was used (M = 8.7 in the deceased group, M = 11.0 in the alive group; t = 2.56, $p <$ .02, two-tailed). There were no significant differencs between outcome groups on psychosocial scales for AIDS subjects with Kaposi's sarcoma. For ARC subjects, three psychosocial variables were significantly different between the deceased and alive groups: (a) the Marlowe-Crowne Social Desirability Scale (Crowne & Marlowe, 1964) (M = 12.9 in the deceased group, M = 8.9 in the alive group; $p <$ .009, two-tailed), (b) the anger-hostility sub-scale of the Profile of Mood States Scale (M = 4.2 for the deceased group, M = 7.1 for the alive group; p = .05, two-tailed); and (c) Kobasa's "commitment" subscale (M = 56.4 for the deceased group, M = 53.3 for the alive group; $p <$ .03, two-tailed).

Because of the small sample sizes, group differencs in average length of time in the study at follow-up, and the fact that numerous univariate tests for differences were conducted in this analysis, extreme caution is warranted in interpreting these results. Further, the variables cited above as significant may be only incidentally related to outcome because they are associated with another variable that is causally related to outcome. Thus, these preliminary results are presented to encourage other researchers in posing hypotheses about the possible relationships of psychosical variables to outcome in AIDS.

With these caveats in mind, we will speculate briefly on the possible meaning of these preliminary findings. We view the significant differences between AIDS-PCP outcome groups on Kobasa's "control" subscale as consistent with the literature on helplessness-hopelessness (e.g., Laudenslager, Ryan, Drugan, Hyson, & Maier, 1983; Levy, 1985; Schmale & Ikler, 1966). According to Kobasa (1979), people low in control tend to feel powerless in the face of overwhelming forces. When stressful events occur, such persons have little basis for optimistic cognitive appraisals or decisive actions that could transform events or concerns. As their coping styles provide little or no buffer, stressful events are given free rein to have a debilitating effect on health (Kobasa, Maddi, & Courington, 1980; Kobasa, Maddi, & Kahn, 1982). Items in the social-support measure were categorized as reflecting either emotionally sustaining or problem-solving types of help. The finding that the favorable-outcome group seems to have utilized significantly more problem-solving help is consistent with research at UCLA on the benefits to mental health, at least, of active-behavioral coping (in comparison to active-cognitive and avoidance coping methods) in men with AIDS. Professionally led group interventions with AIDS patients aimed at enhancing problem solving and coping or relaxation led to less depression and anxiety and to more active and less avoidant coping. An unstructured "emotional support group" seemed to engender greater anxiety and had many dropouts (Fawzy, Namir, & Wolcott, in press).

Finding higher social desirability scores in the unfavorable-outcome group for men with ARC is consistent with some reports in the cancer literature about the negative effects of the so-called "Type C" coping style (e.g., Temoshok et al., 1985), and "autoimmune personality" patterns (Solomon, 1981). Other investigators in psychosocial oncology, particularly Greer and his colleagues, have provided evidence for the beneficial effects on cancer outcome of "fighting spirit" as an adjustment style (Greer et al., 1979; Pettingale, 1984). Such work supports the finding that the favorable-ARC-outcome group was initially significantly higher on the POMS anger-hostility subscale than was the unfavorable-outcome group. The finding about Kobasa's "commitment" subscale was unexpected, and we can offer no explanation for it at the present time.

At Any Given Level of Deficient Immune Function, Do Psychological Factors Relate to Presence or Severity of Secondary Disease?

This question, like a number of those critical to the development of psycho-neuroimmunology, arose from a clinical observation. In mid-1983, the first author undertook psychotherapy with a patient diagnosed with ARC (lymphadenopathy syndrome), who agreed to have repeated immunologic tests, in the hope that treatment might result in improved immune status. Unfortunately, however, helper-inducer T-cell numbers and helper-suppressor (CD4/CD8) ratio continued to fall. Prior to undertaking psychiatric treatment (both for dysphoric affect and characterological issues involving difficulty with being in touch with and expressing emotions), the patient was troubled by fevers, night sweats, and severe, frequently recurrent genital herpes. These symptoms ceased after 6–9 months of treatment, in association with dimished depression and increased assertiveness. The patient had renewed vigor and resumed working full-time. Gradually, however, the helper-suppressor ratio worsened until it reached the exceedingly low level of .01–.03 (normal is 1.2–2.0). The patient's treating physician, a prominent clinical researcher, reported that he did not recall any patient with so few helper T-cells who did not have frank AIDS (as defined by opportunistic infection, Kaposi's sarcoma, or non-Hodgkins lymphoma). In late 1985, after only a few days of feeling very ill, an advanced lymphoma with severe hepatomegaly was discovered. Just prior to the institution of chemotherapy, it appeared that the patient had only days or weeks to live. He responded very well to chemotherapy, however, continues to feel relatively well, plans to complete unfinished projects, to see friends and family, to travel, to utilize alternative therapies in addition to chemotherapy, and—perhaps most importantly—to hope.

What enabled this patient to do relatively well (to avoid infection or neoplasia) for so long in the face of such prognostically unfavorable helper T-cell numbers? What enabled his excellent response to chemotherapy for malignancy when CDC-defined AIDS finally ensued? While future research may find that such persons have some genetic or biological attribute which may explain such "hardiness," our current observations support the hypothesis that his superb attitude, determination, "fighting spirit," and social support, and other psychosocial attributes, played a significant role.

Can the Nervous System Mediate Any "Compensating" Mechanisms for the Immunologic Deficiency Induced by HIV?

It would have been instructive to have been able to measure such factors as NK cell activity and interleukin 2, interferon, and thymosin levels in the patient just described. Most persons with AIDS have elevated levels of thymosin alpha 1 (Devita et al., 1985). Thymic hormones may be true neuroendocrines, and there is speculation about the existence of a "thymotropic" hypothalamopituitary substance. Infused thymosin alpha 1 localizes in circumventricular areas of the brain involved in neuroendocrine regulation (Hall & Goldstein, 1983). A component of thymosin fraction 5 is capable of activating the pituitary-adrenal axis. Spangelo, Hall, and Goldstein (1987) proposed that thymosin peptides function as immunotransmitters to modulate functioning of the immune system. Could the elevation of thymosin alpha 1 in AIDS be a compensatory effort at immune stimulation, analogous to the elevation of ACTH found in glandular-based adrenal insufficiency? How would the CNS "know" the immune system is deficient? (Of course, there may be other factors contributing to the increase in thymosin.)

Does Both the Lymphotropic and Neurotropic Nature of HIV Imply Underlying Commonalities Between the CNS and the Immune System?

The retrovirus etiologic agent of AIDS, human immunodeficiency virus, is neurotropic as well as lymphotropic. In up to 10% of cases of AIDS, the first manifestation of ARC/AIDS may be neurological signs and symptoms, which ultimately occur in 30-75% of AIDS patients (Lowenstein & Sharfstein, 1983-1983). Up to 65% have manifestations of an organic brain syndrome ranging from subtle recent memory loss to full-blown dementia. HIV and antibody to it can be isolated from cerebrospinal fluid of most patients with neurological symptoms (Ho et al., 1985; Resnick et al., 1985). There is growing concern that HIV-induced CNS damage may progress in the absence of marked immunodeficiency or clinical manifestations of disease. Viral infectivity is related to specific surface-membrane molecular configuration. Thus, the dual neural-lymphocytic tropism of HIV does appear to imply structural cellular relatedness between the nervous and immune systems. Measles virus, which can cause subacute sclerosing panencephalitis, can also be detected both in nerve cells and in lymphocytes (Fournier et al., 1985).

Can Prenatal Endocrine Environment Affect
Both Subsequent Sexual Orientation and Immune Competence?

The causes of the range of homosexualities and bisexualities are unknown and likely represent a complex interplay of biological, cultural, and psychodynamic-developmental influences (Tripp, 1975). Among biological theories, an influence of prenatal endocrine environment on the organization of the developing CNS is one controversial speculation for which there is some evidence, at least in the female. It is claimed that women exposed to diethylstiblestrol (DES) in utero have a higher incidence of homosexuality and bisexuality, as well as aggressivity (Ehrhardt, Mayer-Bahlburg, Feldman, & Ince, 1984). More convincingly, in-utero endocrine environment appears to have lasting effects of immunity. Proportions of T-cell subpopulations, particularly reduction in T-cell helper cells, and of B-cells are altered in adult mice whose mothers were treated with DES during pregnancy (Blair, 1981). Such animals show long-lasting effects on ability to respond to antigenic stimuli. Classical psychoanalytic theory, as well as more recent developmental psychology, emphasizes the importance of early life experience in later gender-related behaviors and sexual object choice (Freud, 1953; Tripp, 1975). Early life experience may also play a role in level of immune competence. Rat pups handled for three minutes a day from birth until weaning (21 days) have a more vigorous primary and secondary antibody response to a novel antigen as adults than do unhandled rats (Solomon, Levine, & Kraft, 1968).

Can Psychological Interventions Ameliorate Distress
Associated with AIDS and ARC?

This question suggests two more. If so, are there consequent beneficial effects on immune function, clinical status, and length of survival? Can specific techniques enhance immunity in HIV infections?

Higher levels of distress assessed soon after diagnosis of malignant melanoma distinguished those patients who had an unfavorable outcome by 28-month follow-up from those with no evidence of disease, even when the two groups were matched initially on seven important biological prognostic factors (Temoshok, 1985). Decreased lymphocyte function in major depressive disorder remits when illness responds to treatment (Schleifer et al., 1984). A single study showed immune enhancement by hypnotic imagery in young, highly hypnotizable subjects (Hall, 1983). Even if psychological interventions can be immune enhancing in a person with an intact immune system, it is an empirical question whether such would be the case in a person with AIDS/ ARC. To the extent that group interventions with AIDS patients are successful in reducing depression and anxiety and in enhancing active behavioral coping (Fawzy et al., in press), such interventions may also have positive immunologic effects, and, potentially, may influence survival.

The UCSF-Biopsychosocial AIDS Project is currently engaged in an intensive immunologic and psychological study of factors associated with long-term survival of AIDS (Solomon, Temoshok, O'Leary, & Zich, 1987). Immune studies comprise an extensive array of cellular subsets, and NK cell activity. Psychological measures are designed to assess 21 hypothetical dimensions of adaptive coping which are derived from exploratory interviews with very-long AIDS survivors. Two examples of these hypotheses are: having a sense of humor and having a personalized means of active coping believed by the subject to have beneficial health effects. If this study finds that certain behaviors, emotional proclivities, or coping methods characterize those persons with AIDS who are or who become relatively long-term survivors, then psychosocial interventions can be designed to enhance these behaviors and/or to change health-damaging behaviors in persons with HIV infection.

PROBLEMS AND SUGGESTIONS FOR PSYCHONEUROIMMUNOLOGIC RESEARCH

Problems

Certain underlying uncertainties affect all research which attempts to explore relationships between psychosocial and immune variables. Problems are compounded by effects of disease processes themselves on the immune system, particularly in the case of a disease whose agent is "lympholethal." Certain diseases, including cancer, and infections (particularly viral) are both immunosuppressive and psychologically distressing. How can one sort out "direct" from indirect, psychologically mediated effects?

A major problem is the timing of assessment of immune variables in relationship to the psychosocial variables. What is the "lag" between the presence of a psychological state and its influence on an immune function; or, conversely, what is the "lag" between a particular immunologic aberration and psychological state? Does it seem likely that such lags vary among specific aspects of immune function? In a single case of a patient with rheumatoid arthritis receiving dynamically oriented psychotherapy, who was followed by the first author years ago, there seemed to be a clear relationship between stressful life events about two weeks prior—sometimes already resolved—and clinical exacerbation, accompanied by an increase in erythrocyte sedimentation rate. On the other hand, this patient had no significant changes in titer of rheumatoid factor (an IgM anti-IgG autoantibody), regardless of psychological or medical state.

Our knowledge of the vastly complex nature and functions of the immune system advances exponentially. "New" subsets of lymphocytes and lympho-kines are making increasingly frequent "debuts." (The 1951 textbook on medical microbiology which introduced the first author to immunology offered the single sentence, "The function of lymphocyte is unknown.") The adage "the more we know, the more aware we become of what we don't know" seems ever more relevant. What specific aspects of immune function are most relevant to health? What homeostatic adjustments may compensate for insults or defects?

Suggestions

We need to apply the existing state of knowledge of immunity to some basic issues in order to understand the psychosocial correlates of immunopathology and disease, and to be convinced that these associations are meaningful. We need to ascertain the timing and sequence of immunologic consequences of experiential events. Immune correlates of psychosocial factors in healthy persons under natural conditions should be followed. For example, the normal distribution curve of helper-inducer T-cell numbers has about a fourfold range between the 5th and 95th percentiles. Does a healthy person at the 5th percentile differ psychologically from one at the 95th, and is he or she significantly more susceptible to disease? Are there immune correlates of "hardiness," as defined by Kobasa, in terms of commitment, control, and challenge (Kobasa, 1979)?

In addition to "effector" functions such as mitogen response or NK cell activity, the "central compartment" of the immune system—neuroendocrine, neuropeptide, and lymphokine processes—should be investigated. The functional capacity, as well as numbers of specific cell types, should be assessed (e.g., the influence of a specific immunomodulator on cellular function, and how this may be related to psychosocial processes). An area of great promise, but no research to date, concerns the experiential influences on specific receptor site numbers and functions.

Above all, prospective and/or longitudinal studies are in order. Such studies are particularly feasible in the case of HIV infection and disease because of the predominance of infection among particular at-risk groups, the existence of latent and subclinical infection, the relatively rapid course of HIV disease, and the range of clinical manifestations and outcome (cf. Temoshok & Heller, 1984).

CONCLUSIONS

On a final and philosophical note, we can look back at the rapid emergence of psychoneuroimmunology from a vision of a few isolated investigators in different parts of the world to a defined interdisciplinary field pursued by established behavioral scientists, neuroscientists, and immunologists. The field can now be characterized as sailing between the Scylla of pseudoscience (e.g., an advertisement for "The Immune Power Diet") and the Charybdis of "molecularization" that ignores thoughts, feelings, and behaviors, as well as the clinical medical psychology from which the field arose.

As the field dealing with the complex bidirectional CNS-immune system interactions, psychoneuroimmunology can provide specific testable hypotheses with regard to HIV diseases or AIDS-spectrum disorders. At this point in psychoneuroimmunologic research on AIDS, there are many questions and virtually no answers. We believe, however, that by posing some of these questions in the context of previous work in psychoneuroimmunology and our own preliminary findings, other researchers may be stimulated to approach this research frontier. Further, we believe that HIV/AIDS as a multifactoral disease offers a unique opportunity to explore the relationships among psychological, immunologic, neurologic, and health-outcome variables.

ACKNOWLEDGMENTS

The psychoimmunologic AIDS research reported here was supported by NIMH Grant #MH 39344 (Lydia Temoshok, Principal Investigator). We wish to acknowledge the members of the University of California Biopsychosocial AIDS Project who have been involved in this research formally since 1983.

Please send reprint requests and all correspondence to: George F. Solomon, M.D., Veterans Administration Medical Center, 116A-10, 16111 Plummer Street, Sepulveda, CA 91343.

REFERENCES

Adams, F., Quesada, J. R., & Gutterman, J. U. (1984). Neuropsychiatric manifestations of human leukocyte interferon therapy in patients with cancer. *Journal of the American Medical Association, 252,* 938-941.

Ader, R. (Ed.). (1981). *Psychoneuroimmunology.* New York: Academic Press.

Apfel, R., & Sifneos, P. (1979). Alexithymia: Concept and measurement. *Psychotherapy and Psychosomatics, 32,* 180-190.

Bartrop, R. W., Luckhurst, L., Lazarus, L. G., Kiloh, R., & Penny, R. (1977). Depressed lymphocyte function after bereavement. *Lancet, 1,* 343-836.

Blair, P. B. (1981). Immunologic consequences of early exposure of experimental rodents to diethylstibestrol and steroid hormones. In A. L. Herbst & H. A. Berm (Eds.), *Developmental effects of diethylstilbestrol in pregnancy* (pp. 167-178). New York: Thieme-Stratton.

Borysenko, M. (1984, June). *Immunological alterations underlying tumor growth promoting effects of stress in mice.* Paper presented at the Joint Symposium of the European Working Group for Psychosomatic Cancer Research and the R. E. Kavetsky Institute of Oncolony Problems. Kiev, U.S.S.R.

Brown, S. M., Stimmel, B., Taub, R. N., Kochwa, S., & Rosenfield, R. E. (1974). Immunologic dysfunction in heroin addicts. *Archives of Internal Medicine, 134,* 1001–1006.

Coates, T. J. (1986, March). *Preliminary results of a prospective psychosocial study of men at risk for AIDS.* Paper presented at the 7th Annual Scientific Sessions of the Society for Behavioral Medicine, San Francisco, CA.

Coates, T. J., Temoshok, L., & Mandel, J. S. (1984). Biopsychosocial research is essential to understanding and treating AIDS. *American Psychologist, 39,* 1309–1314.

Cox, T., & MacKay, C. (1982). Psychosocial factors and psychophysiological mechanisms in the aetiology and development of cancers. *Social Science in Medicine, 16,* 381–396.

Crowne, D. P., Marlow, D. (1964). *The approval motive: Studies in evaluative dependence.* NY: Wiley.

Day, G. (1951). The psychosomatic approach to pulmonary tuberculosis. *Lancet,* May 12, 1025–1028.

Derogatis, L. R., Abeloff, M. D., & Melisaratos, N. (1979). Psychological coping mechanisms and survival time in metastatic breast cancer. *Journal of the American Medical Association, 242,* 1504–1508.

Devita, V. T., Jr., Hellman, S., & Rosenberg, S. A. (1985). *AIDS: Etiology, diagnosis, treatment, and prevention.* Philadelphia: J. B. Lippincott.

Ehrhardt, A. A., Meyer-Bahlburg, H. F., Feldman, J. F., & Ince, S. E. (1984). Sex-dimorphic behavior in children subsequent to prenatal exposure to exogenous progestogens and estrogens. *Archives of Sexual Behavior, 13,* 457–477.

Engel, G. (1960). A unified concept of health and disease. *Perspectives on Medical Biology, 3,* 459–485.

Fabbri, A., Gnessi, L., DeSanctis, G., Moretti, C., DeCarolis, C., Fontana, L., Isidori, A., & Fraioli, F. (1985). Human semen inhibits T rosette formation through an opiate-mediated mechanism. *Journal of Clinical Endocrinology and Metabolism, 60,* 807–809.

Fawzy, F. Namir, S., & Wolcott, D. (in press). Group intervention with newly diagnosed patients. *Psychiatric Medicine.*

Folks, T., Powell, D. M., Lightfoote, M. M., Benn, S., Martin, M. A., & Fauci, A. S. (1985). Induction of HTLV/LAV from a non-virus-producing T-cell line: Implications for latency. *Science, 231,* 600–602.

Fournier, J. G., Tardieu, M., Lebon, P., Robain, D., Ponset, G., Mozenblatt, S., & Bouteille, M. (1985). Detection of measles virus RNA from peripheral-blood and brain perivascular infiltrates of patients with subacute sclerosing panencephalitis. *New England Journal of Medicine, 315,* 910–915.

Fox, B. H., & Newberry, B. H. (Eds.). (1984). *Impact of psychoendocrine systems in cancer and immunity.* Toronto: C. J. Hogrefe, Inc.

Freud, S. (1953). Three essays on the theory of sexuality. In J. Strachey (Ed. & Trans.), *The standard edition of the complete psychological works of Sigmund Freud* (Vol. 7, pp. 125–143). London: Hogarth Press. (Original work published 1905.)

Glaser, R. J., Kiecolt-Glaser, J., Speicher, C. E., & Holliday, J. E. (1985). Stress, loneliness and changes in herpes virus latency. *Journal of Behavioral Medicine, 8,* 249–260.

Goedert, J. J., Biggar, R. J., Melye, M., Mann, D. L., Wilson, S., Gail, M. H., Grossman, R. J., DiGiora, R. A., Sanchez, W. C., Weiss, S. H., Blattner, W. A. (1987). Effect of T4 count and cofactors on the incidence of AIDS in homosexual men infected with the human immunodeficiency virus. *Journal of the American Medical Association, 257,* 331–334.

Greer, S., Morris, T., & Pettingale, K. W. (1979). Psychological response to breast cancer: Effect on outcome. *Lancet, 13,* 785–787.

Guillemin, R., Cohn, M., Melnechuk, T., Eds. (1985). *Neural modulation of immunity.* New York: Raven Press.

Hall, N. R. (1983). Hypnosis and the immune system: A review with implications for cancer and the psychology of healing. *American Journal of Clinical Hypnosis, 25*, 92-103.

Hall, N. R., & Goldstein, A. L. (1983). The thymus-brain connection: Interactions between thymosin and the neuroendocrine system. *Lymphokine Research, 2*, 1-6.

Herberman, R., & Holden, H. (1979). Natural killer cells as antitumor effector cells. *Journal of the National Cancer Institute, 62*, 441-445.

Hines, M. (1982). Prenatal gonadal hormones and sex differences in human behavior. *Psychological Bulletin, 92*, 56-80.

Ho, D. D., Rota, R. R., Schooley, R. T., Kaplan, J. C., Allan, J. D., Groopman, J. E., Resnick, L., Felsenstein, D., Andrews, C. A., & Hirsch, M. S. (1985). Isolation of HTLV-III from cerebrospinal fluid and neural tissues of patients with neurologic syndromes related to acquired immune deficiency syndrome. *New England Journal of Medicine, 313*, 1493-1497.

Kaslow, R. A., Ostrow, D. G., Detels, R., Phair, J. P., Polk, B. F., & Rinaldo Jr., C. R. (1987). The Multicenter AIDS Cohort Study: Rationale, organization, and selected characteristics of the participants. American Journal of Epidemiology, *126*, 310-318.

Kemeny, M., Cohen, F., & Zegans, L. S. (1986, June). *Stress, mood, immunity and genital herpes recurrence.* Poster presented at the Second International Workshop on Psychoneuroimmunomodulation. Dubrovnik, Yugoslavia.

Kiecolt-Glaser, J. K., Garner, W., Speicher, C., Penn, C. M., Holliday, J., & Glaser, R. (1984a). Psychosocial modifiers of immunocompetence in medical students. *Psychosomatic Medicine, 46*, 7-14.

Kiecolt-Glaser, J. K., Ricker, D., George, J., Messick, G., Speicher, C. E., Garner, W., & Glaser, R. (1984b). Urinary cortisol levels, cellular immunocompetency, and loneliness in psychiatric inpatients. *Psychosomatic Medicine, 46*, 15-23.

Kobasa, S. C. (1979). Stressful life events, personality and health: An inquiry into hardiness. *Journal of Personality and Social Psychology, 37*, 1-11.

Kobasa, S. C., Maddi, S. R., & Courington, S. (1980). Personality and constitution as mediators in the stress-illness relationship. *Journal of Health and Social Behavior, 22*, 368-378.

Kobasa, S. C., Maddi, S. R., & Kahn, S. (1982). Hardiness and health: A prospective study. *Journal of Personality and Social Psychology, 42*, 168-177.

Korneva, E. A., Klimenko, V. M., & Shkhinek, E. K. (1985). *Neurohumoral maintenance of immune homeostasis.* Chicago: University of Chicago Press.

Laudenslager, M. D., Ryan, S. M., Drugan, R. C., Hyson, R., & Maier, S. (1983). Coping and immunosuppression: Inescapable but not escapable shock suppresses lymphocyte proliferation. *Science, 221*, 568-580.

Levy, R. M., Bresdesen, D. E., & Rosenblum, M. L. (1985a). Neurological manifestations of the acquired immuno-deficiency syndrome (AIDS): Experience at UCSF and review of the literature. *Journal of Neurosurgery, 62*, 475-479.

Levy, S. M. (1985). Behavior as a biological response modifier: The psychoimmunoendocrine network and tumor immunology. *Behavioral Medicine Abstracts, 6*, 1-4.

Levy, S. M., Herberman, R. B., Maluish, A. M., Schlien, B., & Lippman, M. (1985b). Prognostic risk assessment in primary breast cancer by behavioral and immunological parameters. *Health Psychology, 4*, 99-113.

Locke, S., Ader, R., Besedovsky, H., Hall, N., Solomon, G., & Strom, T. (Eds.). (1985). *Foundations of psychoneuroimmunology.* New York: Aldine.

Locke, S., & Horning-Rohan, M. (Eds.). (1983). *Behavioral immunity: Mind and immunity. An annotated bibliography, 1976-1982.* New York: Institute for the Advancement of Health.

Lowenstein, R. J., & Sharfstein, S. S. (1983-1984). Neuropsychiatric aspects of acquired immune deficiency syndrome. *International Journal of Psychiatry in Medicine, 13*, 255-260.

Mavligit, G. M., Talpaz, M., Hsia, F. T., Wong, W., Lichtiger, B., Mansell, P. W. A., & Mumford,

D. M. (1984). Chronic immune stimulation by sperm alloantigens. *Journal of the American Medical Association, 251,* 237-241.

McClelland, D., Flor, E., Davidson, R. J., & Saron, C. (1980). Stressed power motivation, sympathetic activation, immune function, and illness. *Journal of Human Stress, 1,* 11-19.

McNair, D., Lorr, M., & Doppleman, L. F. (1971). *Edits manual: Profile of Mood States.* San Diego: Educational and Industrial Testing Service.

Morris, Y. Greer, S. (1980). A "Type C" for cancer? Low trait anxiety in the pathogenesis of breast cancer. *Cancer Detection and Prevention, 3,* Abstract No. 102.

Palmblad, J., Petrini, B., Wasserman, J., & Akerstedt, T. (1979). Lymphocyte and granulocyte reactions during sleep deprivation. *Psychosomatic Medicine, 41,* 273-278.

Pettingale, K. W. (1984). Coping and cancer prognosis. *Journal of Psychosomatic Research, 28,* 363-364.

Pettingale, K. W., Greer, S., & Tee, D. E. H. (1977). Serum IgA and emotional expression in breast cancer patients. *Journal of Psychosomatic Research, 21,* 395-399.

Plotnikoff, N. P., Faith, R. E., Murgo, A. J., & Good, R. A. (Eds.). (1986). *Enkephalins and endorphins: Stress and the immune system.* New York: Plenum Press.

Resnick, F., di Marzo-Veronese, F., Schupbach, J., Tourtellotte, W. W., Ditto, D., Muller, F., Shapshak, P., Vogt, M., Groopman, J. E., Markham, P. D., & Gallo, R. C. (1985). Intra-blood brain barrier synthesis of HTLV-III specific Ig-G in patients with neurological symptoms associated with AIDS or AIDS-related complex. *New England Journal of Medicine, 313,* 1498-1504.

Riley, V. (1981). Psychoneuroendocrine influences on immunocompetence and neoplasia. *Science, 212,* 1100-1109.

Rogentine, S., Boyd, S., Bunney, W., Doherty, J., Fox, B., Rosenblatt, J., & Van Kammen, D. (1979). Psychological factors in the prognosis of malignant melanoma. *Psychosomatic Medicine, 41,* 647-658.

Schleifer, S. J., Keller, S. E., Camerino, M., Thornton, J. C., & Stein, M. (1983). Suppression of lymphocyte stimulation following bereavement. *Journal of the American Medical Association, 250,* 374-377.

Schleifer, S. J., Keller, S. E., Meyerson, A. T., Raskin, M. J., Davis, K. L., & Stein, M. (1984). Lymphocyte function in major depressive disorder. *Archives of General Psychiatry, 41,* 484-486.

Schmale, A. H., & Iker, H. P. (1966). The affect of hopelessness and the development of cancer. *Psychosomatic Medicine, 28,* 714-721.

Shekelle, R. B., Raynar, W. J., Ostfield, A. M., Garron, D. C., Bieliauskas, L. A., Liu, S. C., Maliza, C., & Paul, O. (1981). Psychological depression and 17-year risk of death from cancer. *Psychosomatic Medicine, 43,* 117-125.

Sivak, S. L., & Wormser, G. P. (1985). How common is HTLV-III infection in the United States? *New England Journal of Medicine, 313,* 1352.

Sklar, L., & Anisman, H. (1979). Stress and coping factors influence tumor growth. *Science, 205,* 513-515.

Sodroski, J. G., Rosen, C. A., & Haseltine, W. A. (1984). Trans-acting transcription of the long terminal repeat of human lymphocyte viruses in infected cells. *Science, 225,* 381-385.

Solomon, G. F. (1969). Stress and antibody response in rats. *International Archives of Allergy, 35,* 97-104.

Solomon, G. F. (1981). Emotional and personality factors in the onset and course of autoimmune disease, particularly rheumatoid arthritis. In R. Ader (Ed.), *Psychoneuroimmunology* (pp. 159-182). New York: Academic Press.

Solomon, G. F. (1985). The emerging field of psychoneuroimmunology with a special note on AIDS. *Advances, 2,* 6-19.

Solomon, G. F. (1987). Psychoneuroimmunology: Interactions between central nervous system and immune system. *Journal of Neuroscience Research, 18*, 1-9.

Solomon, G. F. (1987). Psychoneuroimmunology. In G. Adelman (Ed.), *The encyclopedia of neuroscience* (pp. 1001-1004). Cambridge, MA: Birkhauser.

Solomon, G. F., Fiatrone, M. A. Benton, D., Morley, J. E. Bloom, E., & Makinoden, T. (1988). Psychoimmunologic and endorphin function in the aged *Annals of the New York Academy of Sciences, 521*, 43-58.

Solomon, G. F., Levine, S., & Kraft, J. K. (1968). Early experience and immunity. *Nature, 220*, 821-822.

Solomon, G. F., & Mead, C. W. (1987). Considerations in the treatment of gay patients with AIDS or ARC. *Humane Medicine, 3*, 10-19.

Solomon, G. F., & Moos, R. H. (1964). Emotions, immunity and disease: A speculative theoretical integration. *Archives of General Psychiatry, 11*, 657-764.

Solomon, G. F., & Moos, R. H. (1965). The relationship of personality to the presence of rheumatoid factor in asymptomatic relatives of patients with rheumatoid arthritis. *Psychosomatic Medicine, 27*, 350-360.

Solomon, G. F., Temoshok, L., O'Leary, A., & Zich, J. (1987). An intensive psychoimmunologic study of long-surviving persons with AIDS: Pilot work, background studies, hypotheses, and methods. *Annals of the New York Academy of Science, 496*, 647-655.

Spangelo, B. L., Hall, N. R., & Goldstein, A. L. (1987). Biology and chemistry of thymosin peptides: Modulators of immunity and neuroendocrine circuits. *Annals of the New York Academy of Science, 496*, 196-204.

Spector, H. N. (Ed.). (1985). Neuroimmunomodulation. *Proceedings of the First International Workshop on Neuroimmunomodulation, 1984*. Bethesda, MD: National Working Group on Neuroimmunomodulation.

Stevens, L. E., Taylor, P. E., Zang, E. A., Morrison, J. M., Harley, E. J., de Cordoba, S. R., Bacino, L., Ting, R. C. J., Bodner, A. J., Sarngadharan, M. G., Gallo, R. C., & Rubinstein, P. (1986). Human T-cell lymphotropic virus type III in a cohort of homosexual men in New York City. *Journal of the American Medical Association, 225*, 2167-2171.

Talal, N. (1983). A clinician and a scientist looks at acquired immune deficiency syndrome (AIDS): A validation of immunology's theoretical foundation. *Immunology Today, 4* (Supplement), 180-183.

Temoshok, L. (principal investigator). (1983). *A longitudinal psychosocial (psychoimmunologic) study of AIDS (ARC)* (funded grant). Bethesda, MD: National Institute of Mental Health, Grant No. MH 39344.

Temoshok, L. (1985). Biopsychosocial studies on cutaneous malignant melanoma: Psychosocial factors associated with prognostic indicators, progression, psychophysiology and tumor-host response. *Social Science and Medicine, 20*, 833-840.

Temoshok, L., & Fox, B. H. (1984). Coping styles and other psychosocial factors related to medical status and to prognosis in patients with cutaneous malignant melanoma. In B. H. Fox & B. H. Newberry (Eds.), *Impact of psychoendocrine systems in cancer and immunity* (pp. 258-287). Toronto: C. J. Hogrefe.

Temoshok, L., & Heller, B. W. (1981, August). *Stress and "Type C" versus epidemiological risk factors in melanoma*. Paper presented at the 89th Annual Convention of the American Psychological Association. Los Angeles.

Temoshok, L., & Heller, B. W. (1984). On comparing apples, oranges, and fruit salad. In C. L. Cooper (Ed.), *Psychosocial stress and cancer* (pp. 231-260). Chichester, Great Britain: John Wiley.

Temoshok, L., Heller, B. W., Sagebiel, R. W., Blois, M. S., Sweet, D. M., DiClemente, R. J., & Gold, M. L. (1985). The relationship of psychosocial factors to prognostic indicators in cutaneous malignant melanoma. *Journal of Psychosomatic Research, 29*, 139-153.

Temoshok, L., Peeke, H. V. S., Mehard, C. W., Axelsson, R., & Sweet, D. M. (in press). Stress-behavior interactions in hamster tumor growth. *Annals of the New York Academy of Sciences, 496*, 501-509.

Temoshok, L., Solomon, G. F., Sweet, D. M., Jenkins, S., Zich, J., Straits, K., Pivar, I., Moulton, J. M., & Stites, D. P. (1988, June). Psychoimmunologic studies of men with AIDS and ARC. Paper presented at the IV International Conference on AIDS, Stockholm, Sweden.

Temoshok, L., Van Dyke, C., & Zegans, L. S. (Eds.). (1983). *Emotions in health and illness: Theoretical and research foundations.* New York: Grune & Stratton.

Temoshok, L., Zich, J., Solomon, G. F., & Stites, D. P. (1987, June). An intensive psychoimmunologic study of long-surviving persons with AIDS. Paper presented at the III International Conference on AIDS, Washington, DC.

Tripp, C. A. (1975). *The homosexual matrix.* New York: McGraw-Hill.

Van Griensven, G. J. P., Goudsmit, J., van der Noordaa, J., de Wolf, F., de Vroome, E. M. & Coutinho, R. A. (1987). Risk factors and prevalence of HIV antibodies in homosexual men in the Netherlands. *American Journal of Epidemiology, 125*, 1048-1057.

Visintainer, M. A., Volpicelli, J. R., & Seligman, M. E. (1982). Tumor rejection in rats after inescapable or escapable shock. *Science, 216*, 1100-1109.

Zich, J., & Temoshok, L. (1987). *Perceptions of social support in persons with AIDS and ARC. Journal of Applied Social Psychology, 17*, 193-215.

Aerobic Exercise Training and Psychoneuroimmunology in AIDS Research

15

Arthur LaPerriere
Neil Schneiderman
Michael H. Antoni
Mary Ann Fletcher
Center for Biopsychosocial Study of AIDS
University of Miami

Relationships among behavior, immunological functioning, and human immunodeficiency virus (HIV-1) progression are not well understood, but there are reasons to believe that such relationships exist. First, both naturally occurring (Baum, McKinnon, & Silvia, 1987; Glaser et al., 1987; Irwin, Daniels, Bloom, Smith, & Weiner, 1987; Kiecolt-Glaser et al., 1987; Patterson, Grant, & McClurg, 1988) and experimentally induced stressors (Borysenko & Borysenko, 1982; Monjan & Collector, 1977; Shavit & Martin, 1987) have been linked to immune function. Second, behavioral interventions, such as relaxation training (Gruber, Hall, Hersh, & Dubois, in press; Kiecolt-Glaser et al., 1985, 1986) and aerobic exercise (Watson et al., 1986), have also been related to changes in immune parameters. Third, suggestive evidence has accrued associating psychosocial stress with the progression of HIV-1 infection (Cecchi, 1984; Coates, Temoshok, & Mandel, 1984; Donlou, Wolcott, Gottlieb, & Landsverk, 1985; Solomon & Temoshok, 1987). With these findings in mind, it appears reasonable to assess the extent to which behavioral interventions enhance immune function in subjects at high risk for acquired immunodeficiency syndrome (AIDS), and thereby either prevent seroconversion or retard the progression of HIV-1 infection from an asymptomatic stage to AIDS-related complex (ARC) and/or AIDS symptomatology.

The etiologic agent of AIDS is HIV-1, a retrovirus of the human T-cell leukemia/lymphoma line. The HIV-1 infection involves an asymptomatic phase that may last as long as 15 years (Munoz et al., 1988), during which time immune functioning is compromised (Fletcher er al., 1988) and the infected individual is capable of transmitting the virus (Stevens, Taylor, & Zang, 1986). As HIV-1 disease progresses, an overall loss in immunocompetence leaves th HIV-1 seropositive individual susceptible to opportunistic infections including candidiasis, herpes simplex, and *Pneumocystis carinii* pneumonia (Kalplan, Wofsky, & Volberding, 1987). Because the HIV-1 infection is associated with decrements in immunological functioning and involves disease progression that occurs over a long period of time, the HIV-1 syndrome should be viewed as a chronic disease. Because an enhancement of immune functioning is likely to decrease susceptibility to opportunistic infection among HIV-1 infected individuals, there is a clear need for interventions that can enhance immune functioning. Unfortunately, the pharmacologic interventions that have thus far been developed (e.g., interferon; azidothymidine, AZT) have been only mildly successful and have major side effects (Fischl et al., 1987). With these considerations in mind, we have been assessing the effects of behavioral interventions on immune function, susceptibility to the HIV-1 infection, and disease progression in an AIDS high-risk group (gay males) comprising HIV-1 seropositive and seronegative individuals (Laperriere et al., 1988).

In this chapter, we provide a brief overview of the immune system and the nature of the HIV-1 infection. We then briefly review some of the data relating psychological and behavioral factors to immune system functioning and provide a rationale for the use of behavioral interventions in AIDS research. This is followed by a brief outline of the strategies we have adopted for an aerobic exercise intervention study and a description of the exercise intervention and some preliminary outcomes.

OVERVIEW OF IMMUNE SYSTEM

Immunity is a complex and dynamic process through which an individual defends against foreign invasion by exogenous pathogens such as bacteria, viruses, and parasites, as well as by endogenous mutant cells (e.g., neoplasia). The immune system has classically been subdivided into two broad components: (1) cell-mediated, and (2) humoral immunity (Calabrese, Kling, & Gold, 1987; Ehrlich, 1906; Katz, 1987; Rodgers, Dubey, & Reich, 1979). Recently, however, the functional boundaries between cellular and humoral immunity have been found to be less distinct. In fact, several aspects of immunity have been shown to be intimately dependent on one another, requiring a balance of structural components and communicating soluble factors (e.g., lymphokines).

Cell-mediated Immunity

Thymus-derived or T-lymphocytes (T-cells), the major component of cell-mediated immunity, confer immunity by direct cell-antigen interaction. Two major subsets of T-cells have been identified by the presence of unique cell-surface antigens (measured by monoclonal antibody techniques). These are the T4-helper/inducer and T8-cytotoxic/suppressor cells, recently designated CD4+ and CD8+ (Bernard & Boumsell, 1984). The names "helper/inducer" and "cytotoxic/suppressor" refer to their functional roles in the immune system.

CD4+ cells can be considered the "turn-on" mechanism for the immune response. These cells confer their immunological effects by producing and releasing lymphokines that act as "immunohormones," regulating other T cell lines and macrophages. Recent work has identified subpopulations of helper/inducer cells with specific functions. For example, a subset of CD4+ cells (2H4+T4+) are thought to activate T-cytotoxic/suppressor cells (DeMartini et al., 1988).

Although CD4+ cells are considered to up-regulate the immune response, a subset of CD8+ cells (I2+T8+), which have been ascribed a predominant suppressor function, down-regulates or suppresses the immune response once the pathogenic challenge is contained (DeMartini et al., 1988). A second subset of CD8+ cells (I2–T8+) is thought to have a predominant cytotoxic function (DeMartini et al., 1988) and is thereby able to destroy virally infected cells and tumor cells—a function which is promoted by lymphokines such as interleukin-II (IL–II) and interferon (Cerrottini & Brunner, 1974).

Another structural component of cell-mediated immunity is the natural killer (NK) cell, often characterized as a large granular lymphocyte. This effector cell has been shown to destroy virally infected cells and certain kinds of tumor cells without the prior antigen interaction required of I2–T8+ cells (Herberman & Ortaldo, 1981), but this cytotoxic activity is augmented by CD4+ release of IL–II. NK cells secrete interferon, which is believed to confer and perpetuate their direct cytotoxic properties (Krim, 1980).

Humoral Immunity

Although it has been seen that cell-mediated immunity is capable of mounting a complex response to antigenic challenge, these cellular responses are only a prelude to the precise and repetitive antibody responses comprising humoral immunity. Humoral immunity relies on B cells (Bursa equivalent or B-lymphocytes), which have been activated by a lymphokine (B-cell growth and differentiation factor) released by CD4+ cells (Kehrl, Muraguchi, Butler, Falkoff, & Fauci, 1984). Activated B-cells then differentiate into either mature antibody-secreting "plasma" cells or memory B-cells. Plasma cells secrete specific antibodies that circulate and combine with antigens to form an inactive complex. The antibodies secreted from plasma cells are found in globulin fraction of plasma; hence, the term immunoglobulins (Ig), used to refer to these substances. Immunoglobulins are divided into 5 classes: IgG, IgA, IgM, IgE, and IgD, with additional designation by subclasses (Spiegelberg, 1974). Memory B-cells, which do not produce Igs, remain at rest until a second exposure to the same antigen initiates a rapid differentiation into antigen-specific plasma cells (Kehrl et al., 1984).

Humoral immunity is thought to confer protection against antigens, extracellular viruses, and to engage immediate allergic reactions, such as anaphylaxis and asthma (Rosen, Cooper, & Wedgewood, 1984). Intracellular bacteria and viruses, on the other hand, are not susceptible to the antibodies' effects, because antibodies are unable to penetrate cell membranes (Bellanti & Artenstein, 1964).

Other Immune Components

Additional immune components not traditionally classified as a part of cell-mediated or humoral immunity include macrophages and the complement system. Macrophages are bone-marrow-derived monocytes found in connective tissue that display a wide range of functions. One of these funtions is phagocytosis, a process of nonspecific ingestion of most inert particles. Additionally, once a macrophage has been activated by a certain lymphokine, macrophage-arming factor (MAF), it may attain tumoricidal capacity (Roitt, Brostoff, & Male, 1985). The most important function of macrophages is, however, the trapping, processing, and presentation of antigen to CD4+ cells, initiating both cell-mediated and humoral immunity (Borysenko, 1987).

The complement system is composed of approximately 20 circulating proteins that can be stimulated by either IgG or IgM. Once activated, this system promotes several recognition and effector functions, including attraction of phagocytes to the site of infection (chemotaxis), coating the antigen for easier recognition (opsonization), as well as direct lysis of antigen (Porter & Reid, 1978).

Immune Response

The first line of bodily defense is the prevention of virus or antigen from entering the body. Most invaders are repelled at the body surface by the skin, mucous membranes, mechanical reflexes (i.e., sneezing), production of oral-nasal lysozymes, and increases in gastric acidity. Although the immune system is thought to play a minor role in these primary functions, IgA is found in mucous secretions of both the nasopharynx and gastrointestinal tract (Hanson,

Ahlstedt, & Anderson, 1980) and may, therefore, provide a front-line defense against some airborne and ingested pathogens.

The relatively few antigens that are able to penetrate the body's outer shell encounter the phagocytic activity of macrophages, the initial phase of the immune response. If the entire antigen is phagocytized, the immune response stops with no accompanying symptoms of disease (e.g., fever). It is only when macrophages are unable to completely eliminate the antigen, accompanied by a concurrent host cell infection and manifest symptomatology, that the classical immune response is activated. This response consists of a cascade of cell-mediated and humoral events that result in an escalating mobilization of complex, interdependent, and redundant mechanisms (Calabrese et al., 1987). This reactive process begins when the macrophages, overwhelmed by antigen, display a portion of the antigen on their surface for presentation to CD4+ cells (Pierce, 1980). These CD4+ cells then initiate the previously described cell-mediated and humoral functions of the immune system via lymphokine production and release. Now activated cellular and humoral components attempt to eliminate the antigen by a variety of mechanisms, including target-cell lysis, phagocytosis, and opsonization. If successful, the immune response if "turned-off" by the CD8+ cells, and a memory of the invading antigen is maintained in the event of a subsequent attack. It can thus be seen that the immune system is, indeed, a complex dynamic process requiring a precise balance of structural ingredients (cells) and regulatory soluble factors (lymphokines).

In the past decade, investigators have begun to understand the important contribution of the central and autonomic nervous systems to this delicate balance. A subspecialty of immunology and the neurosciences, focusing on the interations of these systems, has recently crystallized under the rubric of neuro-immunology or neuroimmunomodulation. Perhaps most relevant to our work with stress-attenuating behavioral interventions are neuroimmunologic findings which provide a mechanism for the translation of stressful stimuli and stress responses into alterations in immune-system structural and functional properties. What follows is a brief review of those soluble factors in the nervous system (autonomic, neuroendocrine, and peptidergic substances) that are known to characterize stress responses. This section is followed by a synopsis of neuroimmunologic findings that help to explain the relationship between stress-associated changes in these soluble factors and immune-system alterations.

NEUROIMMUNOLOGY

Stress-related Humors

An organism's perception of the nature of a stressor and/or the availability of a coping response to that stressor has been found to trigger a series of physiological events leading to specific autonomic, neuroendocrine, and neuropeptide changes (McCabe & Schneiderman, 1985). A specific pattern of autonomic nervous system (ANS) activation, referred to as coping, occurs when coping responses are available and adequate to meet stressful demands. The sympathoadrenomedullary system (SAM), activated during active coping responses, releases norepinephrine (NE) and epinephrine (E), which prepare the organism for stressor confrontation. In stressful situations characterized as unpredicatable, uncontrollable, and/or unrelenting, another physiological pattern appears to be dominant. This pattern, characterized by hypervigilance, lack of adequate coping resources, and conservation-withdrawal, is believed to be associated with behavioral inhibition and is accompanied by activation of the hypothalamico-pituitary adrenocortical (HPAC) system. Mobilization of the HPAC system is associated with adrenocorticotropin hormone (ACTH) and cortisol release following signaling from hypothalamic corticotropin-releasing factor (CRF; McCabe & Schneiderman, 1985). Some investigators have noted that in prolonged, distressing affective states such as clinical depression, the accompanying hypercortisolemia may be due to decreased central noradrenergic tone and consequent disinhibition of CRF secretion in the hypothalamus (Sachar, 1976).

A large collection of animal and human studies has indicated that catecholamine and corticosteroid secretion patterns in response to stress can occur as a function of ambiguous, upredictable, and uncontrollable contexts in which coping opportunities are absent or not evident (Mason, 1975; Selye, 1956; Weiss, Stone, & Harrell, 1980). It is also known that glucocorticoids regulate E synthesis in the adrenal medulla and the E stimulates ACTH release from the pituitary via β_2-adrenergic receptors and cyclic AMP (cAMP) second messenger effects (Axelrod & Reisine, 1984). It is not surprising therefore, that patients treated with glucocorticoids show an increase in receptor number and enhanced receptor-adenyl cyclase coupling, resulting in increased β-adrenergic reactivity (Davies & Lefkowitz, 1984). Consequently, it becomes necessary to consider these two stress response systems (autonomic and endocrine) as integrated, not only due to the concomitant release of catecholamines and corticosteroids during stressful situations, but for the potentiated reactivity responses that can be induced by these hormones.

Stress Hormones and Immune Function

Recent findings suggest that elevations in both catecholamines and cortisol are primarily associated with a decrease in cell-mediated immunity. Elevations in peripheral E and NE have been shown to down-regulate immune functioning, presumably via β-adrenergic receptors on lymphocytes (Felten, Felten, Carlson, Olschawka, & Livnat, 1985; Plaut, 1987). Sympathetic noradrenergic fibers innervate the parenchymal and vascular regions of lymphocytes and other immune cells in several lymphoid organs where NE terminals are generally directed into zones rich in T-lymphocytes (Felten et al., 1985). In electrophysiologic studies of the ANS and immune system, Besedovsky et al. (1983) found altered electrical activity in specific hypothalamic nuclei and altered NE metabolism across the hypothalamus following in-vivo antigen challenge. Further work has isolated the paraventricular nucleus of the hypothalamus as the key area experiencing NE depletions following immune challenge (Carlson, Felten Livnat, & Felten, 1987). These findings have relevance for our work in view of the fact that the paraventricular nucleus is regarded as a central locus in the initiation of HPAC activity. An immunoneural feedback model of HPAC control has been proposed by Carlson and colleagues (Carlson et al., 1987). Accordingly, NE depletion following immune challenge is posited to play a role in down-regulating subsequent immune responses. Here noradrenergic depletion may disinhibit CRF production with resulting HPAC activation, ACTH and cortisol elevations, and corticosteroid-induced inhibition of immune functioning. Exogenous stressors that trigger hypothalamic NE depletion may contribute to compromised immunity by creating an imbalance in this regulatory loop in favor of immunosuppression.

Lymphocytes are known to have receptors for many neurotransmitter/neurohormones including β-adrenergic and cholinergic agonists, as well as serotonin (Plaut, 1987). The administration of β-adrenergic agonists has been associated with decreases in mouse and human NK-cell-lysing capabilities and decreased T-lymphocyte proliferation. Both of these effects might be mediated by increases in intracellular cAMP levels (Plaut, 1987). In-vivo human studies have shown a decrease in leukocyte number and impaired lymphocyte mitogen responsivity following E infusion (Crary et al., 1983; Livnat, Felten, Carlson, Bellinger, & Felten, 1985). These immunomodulatory effects are believed to be mediated by cyclic nucleotide action as well.

Whereas β-adrenergic stimulation has been associated with impaired lymphocyte proliferation and cytotoxic activity, cholinergic stimulation has been associated with enhancement of these two cellular immune responses (Plaut, 1987), possibly via elevation in lymphocyte intracellular cyclic GMP (cGMP) levels. Other work indicates that agents such as isoproterenol and prostaglandin E, which increase lymphocyte cAMP, can impair lymphocyte proliferation and lysis of target cells, whereas agents such as carbamylcholine, which increase lymphocyte cGMP levels, may enhance lymphocyte proliferative and killing abilities (Livnat et al., 1985). Muscarinic (cholinergic) agonists (e.g., carbamylcholine) enhance cytotoxic T-cell activity in rats (Strom, Sytkowski, Carpenter, & Merrill, 1974) and are believed to have these stimulating effects via adenylate cyclase inhibition or guanylate cyclase activation. All of these enhancing effects are blocked by muscarinic antagonists, providing further support for receptor mediation. One study helps to explain the mechanism by which cholinergic agents bring about these changes in immune function. In this work, acetylcholine was shown to induce interferon-γ production from antigen stimulated mouse spleen cells (Johnson, 1985). Such increases in production of this lymphokine (most likely by CD4+ cells) could account for the cholinergic-induced enhancement of T-lymphocyte and NK cell cytotoxic activities previously noted.

A different body of literature indicates that adrenal cortical hormones may impair T-lymphocytes (Cupps & Fauci, 1982; Felten et al., 1985), macrophages (Hall & Goldstein, 1981; Monjan, 1981), and NK cell activity (Levy, Herberman, Lippman, & d'Angelo, 1987). Corticosteroids have also been shown to decrease numbers of certain T-cell subpopulations (Stites, Stobo, Fudenberg, & Wells, 1982) and retard production of IL–II (Cupps & Fauci, 1982) in response to antigen (e.g., tentanus toxoid). Recent research has confirmed the existence of cortisol receptors on lymphocytes, indicating the possibility of a built-in inhibitory role for this stress-related hormone in the immune system (see Antoni, 1987, for review).

In addition to catecholamines and corticosteroids, pituitary and adrenal peptide stress hormones such as methionine (MET)-enkephalin, β-endorphin, and substance P have been shown to stimulate T-lymphocyte and NK cell responses (Hadden, 1987; Kusnecov, Husband, King, Pang, & Smith, 1987; Mandler, Biddison, Mander, & Serrate, 1986; Mathews, Froelich, Sibbit, & Bankhurst, 1983; Williamson, Knight, Lightman, & Hobbs, 1987), γ-interferon production (Brown & vanEpps, 1986), as well as macrophage functioning (for review, see Sibinga & Goldstein, 1988). The synthesis and release of β-endorphin is inhibited by glucocorticoids, thus providing a further immunosuppressive role for substances such as cortisol (Simantov, 1979). However, it should also be noted that ACTH and subsequent cortisol release is suppressed by β-endorphin (Reid, Hoff, Yen & Li, 1981), thereby completing the peptide-endocrine regulatory loop.

In summary, substantial evidence now exists for immunomodulatory effects of autonomic and neuroendocrine agents on several aspects of cellular immunity, including lymphocyte, macrophage, and NK-cell functioning. Because psychological variables are known to influence the stress hormones as well, it is a natural extension to consider them in relation to immune system functioning. The area of work focusing on the association between psychological processes, neuroendocrine/neuropeptide mediators, and immune functioning has been termed psychoneuroimmunology.

Psychoneuroimmunology

Several psychological variables have recently been associated with impaired immune functioning. These include environmental stressors, anticipation of stressful events, perceived loss of control and feelings of helplessness, restraint immobility, and depression. The experience of chronic environmental stressors characterized by a loss of personal control (e.g., being a resident of Three Mile Island during the nuclear reactor accident) resulted in increased reports of psychological distress, such as anxiety and depression (Baum et al., 1987). These distress reports were accompanied by elevated levels of uninary catecholamines and decreases in total T-lymphocytes, CD4+ cells, and macrophages (Baum et al., 1987). In similar studies with animals, uncontrollable stressors or learned-helplessness regimens also increased peripheral catecholamine release (Mason, 1975), as well as elevating plasma corticosteroids and depleting brain NE levels (Pericic, Manev, Boranic, Poljak-Blazi, & Lakic, 1987; Weiss et al., 1981). Immune function was also found to be impaired in studies using similar paradigms, as evidenced by decreases in the CD4+/CD8+ cell ration (Teshima et al., 1987) and NK-cell cytotoxicity (Shavit & Martin, 1987).

A sustained stressful anticipatory period (e.g., studying for medical school examinations in normal healthy individuals) has been associated with decreased NK-cell number and T-lymphocyte cytotoxic functioning, impaired lymphokine production and activity, and increased levels of intracellular cAMP in peripheral blood lymphocytes (Glaser et al., 1987; Glaser, Rice, Speicher, Stout, & Kiecolt-Glaser, 1986). Glaser et al. (1987) suggested that a peak in β-adrenergic catecholamines during the anticipatory period may explain the cyclic nucleotide elevations. These studies seem to provide evidence for immunomodulatory effects of either uncontrollable or sustained anticipatory stressors.

Mental depression has also been associated with impaired cellular immune functioning (Calabrese, Skwerer, & Barna, 1986; Kronfol et al., 1983; Schleifer, Keller, Siris, Davis, & Stein, 1985) and a decreased percentage of CD4+ cells (Krueger, Levy, & Cathcart, 1984). An explanatory mechanism for these immune alterations noted among depressed individuals may operate via chronic activation of the HPAC system with subsequent persistent cortisol elevations. Additionally, depressed individuals have been shown to display high basal levels of plasma catecholamines (Louis, Doyle, & Anavekar, 1975), which may also contribute to immunosuppression by way of lymphocyte β-adrenreceptor stimulation.

In summary, both cellular and humoral immunity have been shown to be influenced by behavioral variables. This association appears to be mediated, in large part, by neuropeptide and neuroendocrine activity. The accumulation of research findings relating behavior, nervous system function, neuroendocrine activity, and immunologic function has given rise to an area of study referred to as psychoneuroimmunology. Several investigators (e.g., Antoni et al., in press; Coates et al., 1984; Solomon, 1987) have pointed out that research on AIDS is well suited to a psychoneuroimmunological framework because of likely relationships that may exist between behavior and immunomodulation in this disease process.

NATURE OF HIV-1 INFECTION

The immunologic abnormalities of AIDS have been well established (Fauci, 1984; Fauci, Macher, & Longo, 1983). Evidence for psychosocial and behavioral immunomodulation in HIV-1-infected individuals is beginning to accumulate (Cecchi, 1984; Coates et al., 1984; Ironson et al., 1988; Laperriere et al., 1988; Solomon & Temoshok, 1987). The possibility that this immunomodulation may play a role in disease progression needs to be investigated.

Immune Effects

AIDS, as its name implies, is primarily a syndrome of widespread immunologic defects derived through infection by HIV-1. These pervasive defects precede and contribute to an inability to initiate and sustain an effective response to pathogenic challenge. Thus, the likelihood of numerous subsequent opportunistic infections is dramatically increased. The global magnitude of immunologic deficiencies suggests that the HIV-1 infection amounts to a profuse assault upon the entire immune system. However, as Fauci (1984) reports, virtually every defect in the various components of the immune system could be considered secondary to the primary quantitative and qualitative defect of the CD4+ cells. The central role of CD4+ cells in the up-regulation of the immune response has been presented previously. It is now known that the CD4+ cell is directly infected by way of HIV-1 attachment to a surface-membrane receptor (Fauci et al., 1983). Infected CD4+ cells are not immortalized by HIV-1, but growth is actually slowed, cloning efficiency is reduced, regulatory and effector functions are impaired (Fauci, 1984), and these cells soon die. The loss of CD4+ cells in significant numbers has several consequences, not the least of which is a reversal of the CD4+/CD8+ ratio (Fletcher, Baron, Ashman, Fischl, & Klimas, 1987) from the normal two-to-one balance found among peripheral blood T-cells (Fauci et al., 1983). This abnormal deviation from immunologic homeostasis not only retards initiation of immune responses, but the higher than normal percentage of CD8+ cells (many of which are suppressor cells) may act to dampen subsequent immune responsivity, thereby, in effect, rendering the immune system in a refractory state (Fletcher et al., 1988).

Also, the cell-mediated cytotoxic function of CD8+ cells is decreased with HIV-1 infection (Fauci, 1984). One possible explanation for diminished cytotoxicity could be the reduction of the 2H4+T4+ subset of CD4 cells (Raise et al., 1988), resulting in failure to induce cytotoxic DC8+ cells. Low levels of 2H4+T4+ has been associated with a decreased prospective clinical status (DeMartini et al., 1988).

B-cells of AIDS patients, although hyperactive and spontaneously releasing Ig (Lane, Masur, & Edgar, 1983), respond with diminished stimulation to the

T-cell-dependent B-cell mitogen (Pokeweed, PWM; Fletcher et al., 1987). The observed early reduction in the 4B4+T4+ subset of CD4+ cells (Raise et al., 1988) may reflect decreased humoral immunocompetence to a secondary response of CD4+-infected cells.

Psychological Effects

Several of the immunomodulatory psychosocial variables previously noted may be salient for HIV-1-infected individuals. These include, among others, mild to severe affective reactions to the diagnosis of seropositivity, excessive demands on coping resources for dealing with the uncertainty of the disease's clinical course, and the psychosocial disruption brought about by the need for drastic behavior change (e.g., employment of safer-sex techniques; cessation of IV drug abuse). Such affective, cognitive, and behavioral parallels provide an impetus for psychoneuroimmunologic research targeted at these specific issues with the HIV-1 disease spectrum population.

Solomon and Mead (in press) have noted that AIDS patients' emotional reactions to their diagnoses are similar to those of newly diagnosed cancer patients. Such reactions include sadness, anger, and depression, as well as fear of serious illness, dependency, death, loss of bodily control, pain, and disfigurement. Although anxiety and depression are common sequelae to the diagnosis of AIDS, it is noteworthy that persons with ARC have been shown to be a more distressed group than those with AIDS (Temoshok, Zich, Mandel, & Moulton, 1986). Utilizing general and AIDS-specific measures of distress, others have found that gay men with ARC score at least as high or higher than those with AIDS on parameters of depression and anxiety (Tross, Hirsch, Rabin, Berry, & Holland, 1987). In addition, Tross (1987) found that 50% of an AIDS group and 75% of an ARC group developed adjustment disorders in response to their diagnosis. These differences were attributed to the greater degree of uncertainty present in the lives of ARC patients.

It seems reasonable, based on these preliminary results, to postulate that asymptomatic HIV-1 seropositive patients may report similar levels of distress as do ARC patients, even though they are free from physical symptoms. In one study, about half of a seropositive sample reported elevated depression and anxiety, as well as a preoccupation with AIDS (Frigo et al., 1986). In our ongoing investigation of asymptomatic high-risk individuals (gay males), we have found that during a five-week anticipation period before diagnosis, those individuals who ultimately receive a positive HIV-1 antibody diagnosis consistently report higher levels of both depression and anxiety (Ironson et al., 1988). The psychological impact of receiving a positive HIV-1 diagnosis has been investigated by Morin, Charles, and Malyon (1984) who note guilt, fear of infecting others, lowered self-esteem, and fear of decreased social support from significant others, as well as isolation and stigmatization by society as salient psychological responses. In our research, we have observed an increase (from baseline) in depression and anxiety as a result of the impact of a positive HIV-1 diagnosis, whereas individuals receiving a negative HIV-1 diagnosis decreased on both of these measures (Ironson et al., 1988).

The uncertain future for HIV-1 infected individuals, who are at present asymptomatic and relatively healthy, may itself increase unmanageable anxiety (Morin et al., 1984). This additional anxiety may further suppress an already compromised immune system. Therefore, these individuals may benefit both psychologically and immunologically from behavioral interventions designed to reduce anxiety and stress. Relaxation training and biofeedback have been suggested by Morin and Batchelor (1984) as potential stress-management techniques for this population. We are currently investigating the effects of aerobic exercise training and cognitive stress management/relaxation training programs on psychological and immunological endpoints among seropositive and seronegative gay males.

Immune-behavior Interaction

Investigations that have associated psychosocial stress with disease progression in HIV-1-infected individuals have been reported (Cecchi, 1984; Coates et al., 1984; Donlou et al., 1985; Solomon & Temoshok, 1987), and these relationships have been posited as a possible underlying mechanism to explain stress-triggered transformation of latent HIV-1 virus to an active state capable of replication (Glaser & Kiecolt-Glaser, 1987; Sodroski, Rosen, & Haseltine, 1984). Although these specific mechanisms have not yet been elucidated, associations between psychosocial stress and suppression of cellular immunity, which may in turn account for HIV-1-related disease progression, have been shown (Fletcher et al., 1988; Ironson et al., 1988).

Psychosocial stress in the form of a 5-week anticipation period prior to receiving an HIV-1 diagnosis has been associated with significant immune enhancement for individuals receiving news of seronegativity (Ironson et al., 1988). These effects included increases in the 2H4+T4+ subset of CD4+ cells, and in lymphocyte proliferative responses to phytohemmagglutinin (PHA) and PWM as well as in NK cytotoxicity (Ironson et al., 1988). The NK cytotoxicity then returned to original levels in the HIV-1 negative individuals. Thus, mobilization of defenses during the anticipatory period appears to be followed, at least on this parameter, by a return to baseline upon learning of seronegativity.

In contrast, individuals receiving a positive HIV-1 diagnosis showed neither immunoenhancement during the anticipation period nor immunosuppression following diagnosis. Because compromise of the immune system due to the HIV-1 infection itself is already evident in these subjects (Fletcher et al., 1988), the immune system of these individuals may be insensitive to psychosocial factors such as anxiety. Hence, antibody status may interact with psychosocial-immune relationships despite a lack of overt physical symptomatology. The empirical findings provide a preliminary basis for beginning to understand the interaction between behavior and immune function in an HIV-1 infected population and suggest the importance of studying psychoimmunological relationships in both HIV-1 seropositive and seronegative subjects.

RATIONALE FOR BEHAVIORAL INTERVENTIONS
IN AIDS RESEARCH

AIDS is characterized by a long symptomatic phase after seroconversion, which may last as long as 10 to 15 years (Munoz et al., 1988). HIV-1 infected individuals are capable of transmitting the disease during the entire period (Stevens et al., 1986). Even though the infected individuals are asymptomatic and relatively healthy, as previously noted, several immune parameters are already suppressed (Fletcher et al., 1988). The clinical course of disease progression in HIV-1 infected subjects is typically associated with a progressive decrement in immunological functioning over an extended period of time. Therefore, HIV-1 can be viewed as a long-term chronic disease culminating with AIDS as a late-stage manifestation, reflecting a major loss in immune function associated with increased vulnerability to secondary opportunistic diseases.

The suppressed immunological functioning found in very early stage HIV-1-infected individuals suggests that interventions specifically designed to enhance immune competence at early stages of infection may provide a means for increasing resistance to opportunistic infections. At these initial stages, the apparent sluggishness of immunological functioning may be most amenable to interventions that enhance effector functions and communication between CD4+ cells, macrophages, and NK and B cells via increases in lymphokine production. Recently, immunomodulatory pharmacological treatments have been developed for HIV-1-infected individuals, including interferon and AZT regimens. Although these pharmacological treatments can produce improvements in cellular immunity (Fischl et al., 1987), they often do so at the cost of undesirable physiological (e.g., bone-marrow suppression, anemia, neutropenia; Richman et al., 1987) and psychological (Solomon & Mead, in press) side effects.

Because pharmacological treatments, thus far, have proven to be less than optimal, we have reasoned that behavioral stress-management techniques, such as relaxation and/or aerobic exercise training, may provide immunological benefits without adverse side effects. Relaxation training, for example, has been shown to increase NK cytotoxic activity in a geriatric population (Kiecolt-Glaser et al., 1985). A similar protocol increased IL–II production, mitogen responsivity to PHA, and NK cytotoxic activity among metastic cancer patients (Gruber et al., in press). Both of these study samples, which prior to training most likely consisted of immunocompromised individuals, benefited immunologically from a relaxation protocol. Preliminary results from our study of relaxation training with an HIV-1 high-risk group awaiting diagnosis indicate that frequency of relaxation practice may buffer the effects of anticipatory anxiety on immune function (Baggett et al., in press).

Aerobic exercise training, the highlighted behavioral intervention of this chapter, has been associated with enhanced self-esteem (Morgan, 1982), reductions in anxiety (Morgan, 1984a, 1984b), increased perceptions of psychological well-being (Morgan, 1985), and decreases in depression (Greist et al., 1979), as well as an increase in the percentage of T-lymphocytes (Watson et al., 1986). Survival time of HIV-1 infected males and several markers of immune functioning have recently been related to aerobic fitness level by Temoshok, Zich, Solomon, Stites, and O'Leary (1987).

We have investigated both the psychological and immunomodulatory effects of an aerobic exercise training program among very early stage asymptomatic HIV-1 seropositive and seronegative gay males. Before describing this work, we shall briefly summarize the available evidence for mechanistic links between aerobic exercise and immunomodulatory consequences.

AEROBIC EXERCISE TRAINING

Increases in physical fitness are often associated with improvements in health status and disease prevention (Fox, Naughton, & Haskell, 1971; Kannel & Sorlie, 1979). It is well established than an exercise training program of vigorous physical exertion, performed on a routine basis, improves functioning of the cardiovascular system and is inversely related to coronary heart disease (Leon, 1985). Recent evidence has also linked aerobic exercise to enhancement of the immune system and reduced risk for cancer. In a longitudinal study of 17,000 Harvard alumni, exercise was associated with longevity and reduced deaths from cancer as well as heart diseae (Paffenbarger, Hyde, Wing, & Hsieh, 1986). Eichner (1987) has presented a summary of findings suggesting that exercise, or the exerciser's lifestyle, may interact with immune function to help prevent cancer. Temoshok et al. (1987) have reported that physical activity is related to survival time for those infected with the AIDS virus, and our exercise intervention study has revealed that an increase in aerobic fitness is accompanied by potentially beneficial increases in T-lymphocyte subsets among HIV-1 seropositive individuals (Laperriere et al., 1988).

Although the specific components of aerobic exercise that mediate these immune changes are not yet fully understood, aerobic exercise has been shown to impact several physiological mechanisms known to affect the immune system. For instance, aerobic exercise has been associated with attenuated physiological responses to psychological stress (Brooke & Long, 1987; Kobasa, Maddi, Puccetti, & Zola, 1985), increased release of endogenous opioids (Pargman & Baker, 1980; Ransford, 1982), alterations in ANS functioning (Ekblom, Astrand, Saltin, Stenberg, & Wallstrom, 1968; Frick, Elovainio, & Somer, 1967) and plasma lipoprotein concentration (Seals et al., 1984; Williams, Wood, Haskell, & Vranizan, 1982). In addition, recent studies have noted immunomodulatory effects from an aerobic exercise training program implemented among healthy males (Watson et al., 1986), as well as asymptomatic HIV-1 seropositive males (Laperriere et al., 1988). Collectively, these recent findings suggest mechanistic links that provide a rationale for the use of aerobic exercise training as an immunomodulatory behavioral intervention.

Exercise and Stress

Aerobic exercise has been proposed as an important resistance resource against illness, which may act by decreasing or buffering organismic strain produced by stressful events (Kobasa et al., 1985). Increasing an individual's aerobic fitness level may provide one means for reducing the effects of unavoidable stress, thereby attenuating the stress-illness relationship (Roth & Holmes, 1985). In fact, aerobic exercise training has been used as a relaxation technique (Morgan, Horstman, Cymerman, & Stokes, 1980).

A decreased heart rate at rest (Frick, Kottinen, & Sarajas, 1963; Winder, Hagberg, Hickson, Ehsani, & McLane, 1978) and in response to the physiologic challenge of submaximal exercise (Ekblom et al., 1968; Frick et al., 1967) is the most robust and consistent physiological adaptation produced by aerobic exercise training. This pronounced bradycardia is the result of a synergistic decrease in sympathetic (β-adrenergic) activity coupled with an increase in parasympathetic influence evidenced by enhanced vagal tone (Frick et al., 1967; Moore, Riedy, & Gollnick, 1982). In view of the previously noted decrease in T-lymphocyte proliferation and NK cell lysing capability observed in association with increased sympathetic activity, it is reasonable to postulate that aerobic exercise training may counteract this stress-related immune suppression by its action upon the ANS. Recently, aerobic exercise training has been shown to decrease β-adrenergic myocardial responses to physical and behavioral challenges (Light, Obrist, James, & Strogatz. 1987). Such training could enable individuals to display lowered sympathetic reactivity, faster ANS recovery, and, hence, an attenuated immune response to stressful events.

Improvements in autonomic reactivity and recovery may also allow the aerobically trained individual to cope more effectively with psychosocial stressors (Keller & Seraganian, 1984). There is now substantial evidence suggesting that both a single episode of aerobic exercise and maintained improvements in aerobic fitness level are associated with anxiety reduction (Bahrke & Morgan, 1978; Goldwater & Collis, 1985; Morgan, 1979, 1984a,

1984b; Morgan et al., 1980) and increased perceptions of psychological well-being (Goldwater & Collis, 1985; Morgan, 1985). In addition, a 6-to-20-week aerobic exercise training program was found to be associated with a reduction in depression (Greist, 1979; Morgan, Roberts, Brand, & Feinermem, 1970) and an elevation in self-esteem (Morgan, 1981, 1982, 1984a, 1984b). In our own research, we have observed that depression and anxiety are associated with immune suppression and have provided evidence that aerobic exercise training can attenuate these affective factors and enhance immune function (Laperriere et al., 1988). In view of the reported increases in anxiety and depression among persons with ARC and AIDS, it therefore seems appropriate to suggest that implementation of an aerobic exercise training program as a stress-management technique might reduce psychosocial stress, while possibly providing beneficial immunomodulation for HIV-1-infected individuals.

Exercise and Endogenous Opioids

It has been hypothesized that the affective benefits associated with aerobic exercise may be produced, in part, by release of endogenous opiate-like substances that mimic the euphoric "high" produced by injection or ingestion of various opiate-containing drugs (Pargman & Baker, 1980; Ransford, 1982; Sachs, 1984). It is well established that increases in serum concentrations of several of these endogenous opiates or neuropeptides including β-lipotropin, β-endorphin, and MET-enkephalin occur in response to aerobic exercise (Grossman & Sutton, 1985; see Harber & Sutton, 1984, for review).

The role of intensity ion aerobic exercise (an important element of the exercise prescription) and its relation to plasma concentrations of endogenous opioids is not as well elucidated. One study, however, reported that only 45% of trained long-distance runners studied increased β-lipotropin and β-endorphin levels in response to a low-intensity "easy" run, whereas 80% showed increases in these opioids following a high-intensity "strenuous" run of the same distance (Colt, Wardlaw, & Frantz, 1981). These findings indicate that the intensity of exercise may be a critical component in determining the release of endogenous opioids and suggest the possibility of an intensity-related threshold for their release. However, these intensity-augmented release differentials failed to replicate (Farrell, Gates, Morgan, & Maksud, 1982), a disparity which might be, in part, attributable to the substantial differences between exercise protocols and study designs. The inconsistencies presented by these preliminary studies highlight the need for standardized exercise protocols in psychoneuroimmunologic research.

One additional aspect to the exercise and endogenous opioid relationship that may be important is the reported augmented release of endorphin by more aerobically fit individuals. Aerobic training was reported to augment β-

endorphin release in seven women who participated in a rigorous 8-week protocol consisting of conditioning exercises involving cycling and running (Carr et al., 1981). These results suggest that aerobically fit individuals who continue to exercise and maintain their aerobic fitness may release more endogenous opioids than their less-fit counterparts, and thus may derive greater and more sustained health benefits.

Exercise and Lipoproteins

The relationship between aerobic exercise and lipoprotein fractions has been well established in animal and human work. Four weeks of aerobic exercise training reduced one class of lipoproteins (low density lipoprotein, VLDL) to a significantly lower level in rats (Papadopoulos, Bloor, & Standefer, 1969). The uptake of VLDL from plasma is dependent on the enzyme lipoprotein lipase (LPL; Robinson, 1970). Again, using rats, LPL activity was shown to increase in response to a 12-week program of treadmill running (Borensztajin, Rone, Babirak, McGarr, & Oscai, 1975). These latter findings suggest that aerobic exercise training may improve clearance of VLDL by stimulating LPL activity.

Individuals who engage in regular aerobic exercise are not only leaner and more physically fit than generally sedentary individuals, but are reported to have plasma that is higher in high-density liproproteins (HDL) while lower in total cholestrol, low-density liproproteins (LDL), and VLDL concentrations than the plasma of sedentary control subjects (Enger, Herbjornsen, Eriksen, & Fretland, 1977; Hartung, Foreyt, Mitchell, Vlasek, & Gotto, 1980; Lehtonen & Viikari, 1978; Wood & Haskell, 1979). Williams et al. (1982) found that with a minimum of 5 miles of running per week, at an intensity of 75% to 85% of maximal heart rate, fitness level increased and percentage of body fat decreased after only 3 months of training. In contrast, however, 10 miles of running per week, at a similar intensity, for at least 9 months, was required for an increase in HDL and decrease in LDL plasma concentrations to be realized.

Although the dynamic role that lipoproteins play in regulating immune function is just beginning to be investigated, initial results indicate that VLDL specifically inhibits the initiation of protein and DNA synthesis in lymphocytes, and a subset of LDL reduces blastogenesis of T-cells (Stites et al., 1982). Furthermore, a cholesterol enrichment of lymphocyte and macrophage membranes can greatly reduce their responsivity and tumoricidal capacity (Stites et al., 1982). Thus, aerobic exercise training may have immunomodulatory effects by both a chronic increase in parasympathetic vagal tone and improved lipid metabolism. Such lipoprotein-associated immunomodulatory effects of aerobic exercise may require a sustained training program and attainment of a "good" fitness level.

Exercise and Immunomodulation

It is well documented that acute aerobic exercise results in both cellular and humoral immune changes (see Simon, 1984, for review). These include a transient granulocytosis and lymphocytosis, as well as an enhancement of lymphocyte function accompanied by increases in both T-and B-cell numbers. Enhancement of cytotoxic action following acute bouts of exercise has been noted as well. In one study, 5 minutes of moderate aerobic augmented NK-cell cytotoxity, presumably by recruiting a "new" population of active cytotoxic NK cells (Targan, Britvan, & Dorey, 1981). A challenge of maximum aerobic exercise (i.e., exercise to exhaustion) in both trained and untrained healthy men increased NK cytotoxic activity immediately following exercise; however, this activity decreased to a low point 2 hours later and returned to pre-exercise levels within 20 hours (Brahmi, Thomas, Park, & Dowdeswell, 1985). Well-conditioned runners showed an increase in antibody-dependent cellular cyto-toxicity in response to a "moderate" 8-mile run (75% intensity); these increased levels remained for 24 hours. Finally, a study that evaluated the immune effects of an aerobic exercise training program on young, healthy, previously inactive men found an increase in the percentage of T-lymphocytes (Watson et al., 1986).

Collectively, the studies just described indicate that immunomodulatory effects of aerobic exercise enhance both cellular and humoral immunity by increasing the number of immune cells, as well as intensifying their functions. All of the investigations, however, used healthy subjects with apparently intact immune systems, whereas in our research we have been contrasting such individuals with asymptomatic HIV-1-infected subjects having significantly impaired immune functioning. Thus, a major question addressed by our research is whether HIV-1-infected individuals with already compromised immune functioning can show immune enhancement in response to a program of aerobic exercise.

MIAMI EXERCISE INTERVENTION STUDY

At the University of Miami, we are currently investigating the efficacy of an aerobic exercise training program as a psychoneuroimmunologic intervention for individuals infected with the AIDS virus. This study has shown that individuals who are simply at risk for AIDS or already infected and at a very early asymptomatic stage in the HIV-1 disease process (having fulfilled our exclusion criteria) can benefit both physiologically and psychologically from regular moderate exercise.

The study sample included 46 gay males who were unaware of their HIV status at entry. Each subject completed an informed consent and indicated his willingness to receive an HIV diagnosis as part of the study. In addition, a complete physical examination, including an aerobic fitness evaluation and a medical history questionnaire, was administered. Exclusion criteria were: (1) having a diagnosis of AIDS or ARC; (2) unexplained weight loss of greater than 10% or 15 lbs. within the previous 3 months; (3) mucocutaneous oral candidiasis; (4) lymphadenopathy other than inguinal or anterior cervical; (5) fever of unexplained origin; (6) unexplained night sweats or diarrhea; (7) herpes zoster within 3 months; (8) drug or ethanol abuse; (9) use of anabolic steroids; (10) regular use of antihistamines; (11) being younger than 18 or older than 40; (12) regular aerobic exercise, either as a participant in a group exercise program or on an individual basis; and (13) a pre-test estimated maximum oxygen consumption ($VO_{2\ max}$) greater than 53 ml/kg/min if age 18 to 29 or 49 ml/kg/min if age 30 to 40. Subjects meeting these requirements were thus asymptomatic and relatively healthy, although of average and below-average fitness. Because these subjects were asymptomatic, they were presumed to be very early in the disease process and could potentially derive maximum benefit from the behavioral intervention.

Aerobic Exercise Protocol

Subjects were randomly assigned to either an aerobic exercise training or a control group. The aerobic exercise training group were exercised (bicycle ergometer) during 45-minute sessions, 3 times per week for 10 weeks at approximately 80% of their age-predicted maximum heart rate (i.e., 220 minus each subject's age).

Manipulation-check questionnaires, designed to assess potential confounds (e.g., sleep, physical activity), were administered at weeks 0, 5, 5.5, 7, 8, and 10. Several questions, for example, were included to ensure that members of the control group were not exercising on their own. These questions were empirically verified by aerobic fitness evaluations at weeks 1, 5, and 10. These aerobic-fitness evaluations consisted of 5 min of bicycle exercise, producing a fifth-minute submaximal heart rate. This heart rate was then substituted into the Fox equation to yield a predicted $VO_{2\ max}$ (Fox, Billings, Bartels, Bason, & Mathews, 1973). $VO_{2\ max}$ is considered to be the best overall indicator of aerobic fitness level (Saltin & Astrand, 1967).

In addition to the aerobic-fitness evaluation, immunological and psychological data were collected at weeks 0, 5, 5.5, 7, 8, and 10. Cellular immune measures included enumerations of total T-cells, B-cells, T-helper/suppressor cell ratio, T-helper cell subsets, NK cells, coexpression and antigen density surface markers for T-cell activation, B-cell activation markers, monocyte activation markers, lymphocyte proliferative responses to PHA and PWM, and NK cytotoxic activity. Humoral measures included serum immunoglobulins (IgG, IgA, and IgM) and HIV antibodies (ELISA plus confirmation by Western blot). A detailed explanation of the methods used to determine these immune

measures can be found in our report of baseline differences between HIV positive and negative individuals (Fletcher et al., 1988). To evaluate alternative
explantions of immune effects, nutritional status was assessed by albumin determination, and changes in blood volume were derived by hematocrit. Psychological outcome measures included several indices of coping skills/styles, affective
measures, such as the Profile of Mood States (POMS) and the State-Trait Anxiety Inventory (STAI); behavioral measures of sexual and health functioning; and
cognitive/attitudinal measures of optimism, hardiness, and self-efficacy.

Subjects in the exercise protocol showed a significant improvement in
$VO_{2\ mac}$ after week 5, an increase which they maintained at week 10. Controls
showed no similar changes in their fitness levels. Subjects did not differ in
measures of albumin or hematocrit, which remained unchanged during the
study.

Aerobic exercise training was shown to enhance cellular immunity by
increasing a number of specific T-lymphocyte subsets for both HIV-1 negative
and positive subjects relative to controls. CD4+ cells (those cells greatly
reduced by the AIDS virus, although not significantly attenuated in our early
stage HIV-1 positive exercisers) increased from 960 cpm to 1180 cpm for
HIV-1 negative and from 905 cpm to 1020 cpm for HIV-1 positive subjects
when measured pre- to post-training. In addition, the subset of CD4+ cells
(2H4+T4+)—low levels of which are associated with declining clinical course
of disease—increased from 4.6% to 6.2% among seronegative individuals.
Humoral immunity was also enhanced in HIV-1 negative subjects, as evidenced by a significant increase in mature B-cells (7.8% to 20.0%) across the
intervention period.

Aerobic exercise training also appears to act as a buffer for anxiety and
depression among seropositives. HIV-1-infected contol subjects showed a significant increase in mean scores on the Tension-Anxiety (10.7 to 18.2),
Depression (9.3 to 26.8), and Confusion-Bewilderment (5.3 to 11.8) scales of
the POMS in response to their diagnosis. Seropositive exercisers, however, did
not show such increases on any of these POMS scales (Tension-Anxiety 11.8
to 12.6; Depression 10.4 to 14.0; Confusion-Bewilderment 7.2 to 8.7) following news of diagnosis. In fact, HIV-1-infected exercisers' POMS scale
scores resembled those observed in subjects receiving an HIV-1 negative
diagnosis. This buffering effect of the exercise intervention on psychosocial
variables accompanied a similar buffering of cellular immune impairment in
response to diagnosis. Whereas controls showed a significant 170 mm^3
decrease in NK cells in response to receiving a positive HIV-1 diagnosis,
seropositive exercisers showed only a nonsignificant 38 mm^3 drop.

Summary of Results

Our data offer evidence that HIV-1 negative subjects clearly show beneficial
immunologic effects of aerobic exercise training by an increase in B-cells,

CD4+ cells and the 2H4+T4+ subset. HIV-1 positive subjects also show some immunologic enhancement, although to a lesser extent, by an increase in CD4+ cells only. The attenuated immunologic augmentation seen in HIV-1 positive subjects may indicate that their already compromised immune system is less responsive to exercise training. However, the increase in CD4+ cells shown by HIV-1 positive subjects is comparable to the magnitude of increase seen in studies of AZT administration (Yarchoan et al., 1988a, 1988b), but without the accompanying side effects. Furthermore, the buffering effect of aerobic training displayed in HIV-1 positive subjects appears to indicate that aerobic exercise training may prove to be an appropriate stress-management technique yielding immunologic (i.e., attenuated NK cell decrease to a stressor) and psychosocial benefits in this population. It would thus appear that HIV-1 can be viewed as a chronic disease for which early immunomodulatory behavioral interventions, such as aerobic exercise training, may have important physical and psychological impact, including the slowing of disease progression, reduction of opportunistic infections, and improved quality of life.

REFERENCES

Antoni, M. (1987). Neuroendocrine influences in psychoimmunology and neoplasia: A review. *Psychology & Health, 1*, 3-24.

Antoni, M. H., Schneiderman, N., Laperriere, A., Baggett, H. L., August, S., & Fletcher, M. (in press). Stress management and immunce function. *Proceedings of NIMH conference on Priorities in Stress Research*, Washington, DC: U.S. Government Printing Office, National Institute of Mental Health.

Axelrod, J., & Reisine, T. (1984). Stress hormones: Their interaction and regulation. *Science, 224*, 452-459.

Baggett, L. A., Antoni, M. H., August, S. M., Laperriere, A., Schneiderman, N., Ironson, G., & Fletcher, M. A. (in press). *Frequency of relaxation practice, state anxiety, and immune markers in a HIV-1 high risk group*. Submitted to the tenth annual scientific meetings of the Society of Behavioral Medicine, San Francisco.

Bahrke, M. S., & Morgan, W. P. (1978). Anxiety reduction following exercise and meditation. *Cognitive Therapy & Research, 2*, 323-333.

Baum, A., McKinnon, W., & Silvia, C. (1987, March). *Chronic stress and the immune system*. Paper presented at the eighth annual scientific meetings of the Society of Behavioral Medicine, Washington, DC.

Bellanti, J. A., & Artenstein, M. S. (1964). Mechanisms of immunity to virus infection. *Pediatric Clinics of North America, 11*, 558-569.

Bernard, A., & Boumsell, L. (1984). The clusters of differentiation (CD) defined by the First International Workshop of Human Leukocyte Differentiation Antigens. *Human Immunology, 11*, 1-10.

Besedovsky, H., del Rey, A., Sorkin, E., DaPrada, M., Burri, R., & Honegger, C. (1983). The immune responses evokes changes in brain noradrenergic neurons. *Science, 221*, 564-565.

Borensztajin, J., Rone, M., Babirak, S., McGarr, J., & Oscai, L. (1975). Effects of exercise on lipoprotein lipase activity in rat heart and skeletal muscle. *American Journal of Physiology, 229*, 394-397.

Borysenko, M. (1987). The immune system: An overview. *Annals of Behavioral Medicine, 9*(2), 3-10.

Borysenko, M., & Borysenko, J. (1982). Stress, behavior, and immunity: Animal models and mediating mechanisms. *General Hospital Psychiatry, 4*, 56–67.

Brahmi, Z., Thomas, J., Park, M., Park, M., & Dowdeswell, I. R. G. (1985). The effect of acute exercise on natural killer-cell activity of trained and sedentary human subjects. *Journal of Clinical Immunology, 5*, 321–328.

Brooke, S. T., & Long, B. C. (1987). Efficiency of coping with a real-life stressor: A multimodal comparison of aerobic fitness. *Psychophysiology, 24*, 173–180.

Brown, S., & VanEpps, D. (1986). Opioid peptides modulate production of interferon-γ by human mononuclear cells. *Cellular Immunology, 103*, 19.

Calabrese, J., Kling, M., & Gold, P. (1987). Alterations in immunocompetence during stress, bereavement, and depression: focus on neuroendocrine regulation. *American Journal of Psychiatry, 144*, 1123–1134.

Calabrese, J., Skwerer, R., & Barna, B. (1986). Depression, immunocompetence, and prostaglandins of the E series. *Psychiatric Research, 17*, 41–47.

Carlson, S., Felten, D., Livnat, S., & Felten, S. (1987). Alterations of monamines in specific central autonomic nuclei following immunization in mice. *Brain, Behavior, and Immunity, 1*, 52–63.

Carr, D. B., Bullen, B. A., Skrinan, G. S., Arnold, M. A., Rosenblatt, M., Beitins, I. Z., Martin, J. B., & McArthur, J. W. (1981). Physical conditioning facilitates the exercise-induced secretion of β-endorphin and β-lipotropin in women. *New England Journal of Medicine, 305*, 560–563.

Cecchi, R. L. (1984). Stress: Prodrome to immune deficiency. *Annals of the New York Academy of Sciences, 437*, 286–289.

Cerrottini, J. C., & Brunner, K. T. (1974). Cell mediated cytotoxicity, allograft rejection and tumor immunity. *Advanced Immunology, 18*, 67–132.

Coates, T. J., Temoshok, L., & Mandel, J. (1984). Psychosocial research is essential to understanding and treating AIDS. *American Psychologist, 39*, 1039–1314.

Colt, E. W. D., Wardlaw, S. L., & Frantz, A. G. (1981). The effect of running on plasma β-endorphin. *Life Sciences, 28*, 1637–1640.

Crary, B., Borysenko, M., Sutherland, D., Kutz, I., Borysenko, J., & Benson, H. (1983). Decrease in mitogen responsiveness of mononuclear cells from peripheral blood after epinephrine administration in humans. *Journal of Immunology, 130*, 694–697.

Cupps, T., & Fauci, A. (1982). Corticosteroid-mediated immunoregulation in man. *Immunology Review, 65*, 133–155.

Davies, A., & Lefkowitz, R. (1984). Regulation of β-adrenergic receptors by steroid hormones. *Annual Review of Physiology, 46*, 119–130.

DeMartini, R. M., Turner, R. R., Formenti, S. C., Boone, D. C., Bishop, P. C., Levine, A. M., & Parker, J. W. (1988). Peripheral blood mononuclear cell abnormalities and their relationship to clinical course in homosexual men with HIV infection. *Clinical Immunology and Immunopathology, 46*, 258–271.

Donlou, J. N., Wolcott, M. S., Gottlieb, M. S., & Landsverk, J. (1985). Psychosocial aspects of AIDS and AIDS-related complex: A pilot study. *Journal of Psychosocial Oncology, 3*(2), 39–55.

Ehrlich, P. (1906). On immunity with special reference to cell life. *Proceedings of the Royal Society of London (Biology), 66*, 424–430.

Eichner, E. R. (1987). Exercise, lymphokines, calories, and cancer. *The Physician and Sports Medicine, 5*, 109–116.

Ekblom, B., Astrand, P., Saltin, B., Stenberg, J., & Wallstrom, B. (1968). Effect of training on circulatory response to exercise. *Journal of Applied Physiology, 24*, 518–528.

Enger, S., Herbjornsen, K., Eriksen, J., & Fretland, A. (1977). High density lipoproteins (HDL) and physical activity: The influence of physical exercise, age and smoking on HDL-cholesterol and the HDL/total cholesterol ratio. *Scandinavian Journal of Clinical Laboratory Investigations, 37*, 251–255.

Farrell, P. A., Gates, W. K., Morgan, W. P., & Maksud, M. G. (1982). Increases in plasma B-EP and B-LPH immunoreactivity after treadmill running in humans. *Journal of Applied Physiology: Respiratory, Environmental and Exercise Physiology, 52*, 1245–1249.

Fauci, A. S. (1984). Immunologic abnormalities in the acquired immunodeficiency syndrome (AIDS). *Clinical Research, 32*, 491–499.

Fauci, A. S., Macher, A. M., & Longo, D. L. (1983). Acquired immunodeficiency syndrome: Epidemiologic, clinical, immunologic, and therapeutic considerations. *Annals of Internal Medicine, 100*, 92–106.

Felten, D., Felten, S., Carlson, S., Olschawka, J., & Livnat, S. (1985). Noradrenergic and peptidergic innervation of lymphoid tissue. *Journal of Immunology, 135*, (2 Supplement),755s–765s.

Fischl, M. A., Richman, D., Grieco, M., Gottlieb, M., Volberding, P., Laskin, O., Leedom, J., Groopman, J., Mildvan, D., Schooley, R., Jackson, G., Durack, D., & King, D. (1987). The efficacy of azidothymidine (AZT) in the treatment of patients with AIDS and AIDS-related complex. *New England Journal of Medicine, 317*, 185–191.

Fletcher, M. A., Baron, G. C., Ashman, M. R., Fischl, M. A., & Klimas, N. G. (1987). Use of whole blood methods in assessment of immune parameters in immunodeficiency states. *Diagnostic and Clinical Immunology, 5*, 69–81.

Fletcher, M. A., Caralis, P., Laperriere, A., Ironson, G., Klimas, N., Perry, A., Ashman, M., & Schneiderman, N. (1988). Immune function and aerobic training as a function of anti-HIV status in healthy gay males. *Proceedings of the Fourth International Conference on AIDS, 1*, 469.

Fox, E., Billings, C., Bartels, R., Bason, R., & Mathews, D. (1973). Fitness standards for male college students. *International Zeitschrift Fuer Angewandte Physiologie Einschliesslich Arbeitsphysiologie, 31*, 231–236.

Fox, S. M., Naughton, J. P., & Haskell, W. L. (1971). Physical activity and prevention of coronary heart disease. *Annals of Clinical Research, 3*, 404–432.

Frick, M., Elovainio, R., & Somer, T. (1967). The mechanism of bradycardia evoked by physical training. *Cardiologia, 51*, 46–54.

Frick, M., Kottinen, A., & Sarajas, S. (1963). Effects of physical training on circulation at rest and during exercise. *American Journal of Cardiology, 12*, 142–147.

Frigo, M. A., Zones, J. S., Beeson, D. R., Rutherford, G. W., Echenberg, D. F., & O'Malley, P. M. (1986). *The impact of structured counseling in acute adverse psychiatric reactions associated with LAV/HTLV-III antibody testing.* Proceedings of the 114th annual meeting of the American Public Health Association, Las Vegas.

Glaser, R., & Kiecolt-Glaser, J. (1987). Stress-associated depression in cellular immunity: Implications for acquired immune deficiency syndrome (AIDS). *Brain, Behavior, and Immunity, 1*, 107–112.

Glaser, R., Rice, J., Sheridan, J., Fertel, R., Stout, J., Speicher, C., Pinsky, D., Kotur, M., Post, A., Beck, M., & Kiecolt-Glaser, J. (1987). Stress-related immune suppression: Health implications. *Brain, Behavior, and Immunity, 1*(1), 7–20.

Glaser, R., Rice, J., Speicher, C., Stout, J., & Kiecolt-Glaser, J. (1986). Stress depresses interferon production and natural killer cell activity in humans. *Behavioral Neurosciences, 100*, 675–678.

Goldwater, B. C., & Collis, M. L. (1985). Psychologic effects of cardiovascular conditioning: A controlled experiment. *Psychosomatic Medicine, 47*, 174–181.

Greist, J. H., Klein, M. H., Eischens, R. R., Faris, J., Gurman, A. S., & Morgan, W. P. (1979). Running as treatment for depression. *Comparative Psychiatry, 20*, 41–53.

Grossman, A., & Sutton, J. R. (1985). Endorphins: What are they? How are they measured? What is their role in exercise? *Medicine and Science in Sports and Exercise, 17*, 74–81.

Gruber, B., Hall, N., Hersh, S., & Dubois, P. (in press). Immune system and psychologic changes in metastatic cancer patients while using ritualized relaxation and guided imagery. *Scandinavian Journal of Behavior Therapy.*

Hadden, J. (1987). Neuroendocrine modulation of the thymus-dependent immune system. *Annals of the New York Academy of Sciences, 496,* 39-48.

Hall, N., & Goldstein, A. (1981). Neurotransmitters and the immune system. In R. Ader (Ed.), *Psychoneuroimmunology* (pp. 521-538). New York: Academic Press.

Hanson, I. A., Ahlstedt, T. S., Anderson, B. (1980). The biological properties of secretory IgA. *Journal of Reticuloendothelial Society, 28* (Supplement), 15-95.

Harber, V. J., & Sutton, J. R. (1984). Endorphins and exercise. *Sports Medicine, 1,* 154-171.

Hartung, G. H., Foreyt, J. P., Mitchell, R. E., Vlasek, I., & Gotto, A. M. (1980). Relation of diet to high-density lipoprotein cholesterol in middle-aged marathon runners, joggers and inactive men. *New England Journal of Medicine, 307,* 357.

Herberman, R. B., & Ortaldo, J. R. (1981). Natural killer cells: Their role in defense against disease. *Science, 214,* 24-30.

Ironson, G., O'Hearn, P., Laperriere, A., Antoni, M., Ashman, M., Schneiderman, N., & Fletcher, M. (1988, April). *News of HIV antibody status and immune function in healthy gay males.* Paper presented at the ninth annual scientific meetings of the Society of Behavioral Medicine, Boston.

Irwin, M., Daniels, M., Bloom, E., Smith, T., & Weiner, H. (1987). Life events, depressive symptoms, and immune function. *American Journal of Psychiatry, 144,* 437-441.

Johnson, H. (1985). Mechanism of interferon γ production and assessment of immunoregulatory properties. *Lymphokines, 2,* 33-46.

Kannel, W. B., & Sorlie, P. (1979). Some health benefits of physical activity: The Framingham Study. *Archives of Internal Medicine, 139,* 857-861.

Kaplan, L. D., Wofsky, C. B., & Volberding, P. A. (1987). Treatment of patients with acquired immunodeficiency syndrome and associated manifestations. *Journal of the American Medical Association, 257,* 1367-1376.

Katz, H. (1987). The immune system: An overview. In D. P. Stites, J. D. Stobo, H. H. Fudenberg & J. V. Wells (Eds.), *Bacis and clinical immunology* (6th ed, pp. 13-20). Los Altos, CA: Lange Medical Publications.

Kehrl, J. H., Muraguchi, A., Butler, J. L., Falkoff, R. J., & Fauci, A. S. (1984). Human B-cell activation, proliferation, and differentiation. *Immunological Reviews, 78,* 75-96.

Keller, S., & Seraganian, P. (1984). Physical fitness level and autonomic reactivity to psycho-social stress. *Journal of Psychosomatic Research, 28,* 279-287.

Kiecolt-Glaser, J., Fisher, L., Ogrocki, P., Stout, J., Speicher, C., & Glaser, R. (1987). Marital quality, marital disruption, and immune function. *Psychosomatic Medicine, 49,* 13-34.

Kiecolt-Glaser, J., Glaser, R., Strain, E., Stout, J. C., Tarr, K. L., Holliday, J. E., & Speicher, C. E. (1986). Modulation of cellular immunity in medical students. *Journal of Behavioral Medicine, 9,* 311-320.

Kiecolt-Glaser, J., Glaser, R., Williger, D., Stout, J., Messick, G., Sheppard, S., Ricker, D., Romisher, S. C., Briner, W., Bonnell, G., & Donnerberg, R. (1985). Psychosocial enhancement of immunocompetence in a geriatric population. *Health Psychology, 4,* 25-41.

Kobasa, S., Maddi, S., Puccetti, M., & Zola, M. (1985). Effectiveness of hardiness, exercise, and social support as resources against illness. *Journal of Psychosomatic Research, 29,* 525-533.

Krim, M. (1980). Towards tumor therapy with interferons (parts 1 and 2). *Blood, 5,* 711-721, 875-884.

Kronfol, Z., Silva, J., Greden, J., Dembinski, S., Gardener, R., & Carroll, B. (1983). Impaired lymphocyte function in depressive illness. *Life Science, 33,* 241-247.

Krueger, R., Levy, E., & Cathcart, E. (1984). Lymphocyte subsets in patients with major depression: Preliminary findings. *Advances, 1,* 5-9.

Kusnecov, A., Husband, A., King, M., Pang, G., & Smith, R. (1987). In vivo effects of β-endorphin or lymphocyte proliferation and interleukin-2 production. *Brain, Behavior, and Immunity, 1*(1), 88-97.

Lane, H., Masur, H., & Edgar, L. C. (1983). Abnormalities of B cell activation and immuno-regulation in patients with acquired immunodeficiency syndrome. *New England Journal of Medicine, 309*, 453-458.

Laperriere, A., O'Hearn, P., Ironson, G., Caralis, P., Ingram, F., Perry, A., Klimas, N., Schneiderman, N., & Fletcher, M. (1988, April). *Exercise and immune function in healthy HIV antibody negative and positive gay males.* Paper presented at the ninth annual scientific meetings of the Society of Behavioral Medicine, Boston.

Lehtonen, A., & Viikari, J. (1978). Serum triglycerides and cholesterol and serum high-density lipoprotein cholesterol in highly physically active men. *Acta Medical Scandinavia, 204*, 111.

Leon, A. S. (1985). Physical activity levels and coronary heart disease. *Medical Clinics of North America, 69*, 3-17.

Levy, S., Herberman, R., Lippman, M., & d'Angelo, T. (1987). Correlation of stress factors with sustained depression of natural killer cell activity and predicted prognosis in patients with breast cancer. *Journal of Clinical Oncology, 5*, 348-353.

Light, K. C., Obrist, P. A., James, S. A., & Strogatz, D. S. (1987). Cardiovascular responses to stress: Relationships to aerobic exercise patterns. *Psychophysiology, 24*, 79-86.

Livnat, S., Felten, S., Carlson, S., Bellinger, D., & Felten, D. (1985). Involvement of peripheral and central catecholamine systems in neural immune interactions. *Journal of Neuro-immunology, 10*, 5-30.

Louis, W., Doyle, A., & Anavekar, S. (1975). Plasma noradrenalin concentrate and blood pressure in essential hypertension, pheochromocytoma, and depression. *Clinical Science and Molecular Medicine, 48* (Supplemental Issue 2), 239S-242S.

Mandler, R., Biddison, W., Mander, R., & Serrate, S. (1986). Beta-endorphin augments the cytolytic activity and interferon production of natural killer cells. *Journal of Immunology, 136*, 934-939.

Mason, J. (1975). A historical view of the stress field. I. *Journal of Human Stress, 1*, 6-12.

Mathews, P., Froelich, C., Sibbit, W., & Bankhurst, A. (1983). Enhancement of natural cyto-toxicity by β-endorphin. *Journal of Immunology, 130*, 1658-1662.

McCabe, P. M., & Schneiderman, N. (1985). Psychophysiologic reactions to stress. In N. Schneiderman & T. J. Tapp (Eds.), *Behavioral medicine: The biopsychosocial approach* (pp. 99-131). Hillsdale, NJ: Lawrence Erlbaum Associates.

Monjan, A. (1981). Immunologic competence in animals. In R. Ader (Ed.), *Psychoneuro-immunology* (pp. 185-228). New York: Academic Press.

Monjan, A., & Collector, M. (1977). Stress-induced modulation of the immune response. *Science, 196*, 307-308.

Moore, R. Riedy, M., & Gollnick, P. (1982). Effect of training on beta-adrenergic receptor number in rat heart. *Journal of Applied Physiology: Respiration, Environment, Exercise, and Physiology, 52*, 1133.

Morgan, W. P. (1979). Anxiety reduction following acute physical activity. *Psychiatric Annals, 9*, 36-45.

Morgan, W. P. (1981). Psychological benefits of physical activity. In F. S. Nagle & H. J. Montoye (Eds.), *Exercise in health and disease* (pp. 299-314). Springfield, IL: Charles C. Thomas, Co.

Morgan, W. P. (1982). Psychological effects of exercise. *Behavioral Medicine Update, 4*, 25-30.

Morgan, W. P. (1984a). *Coping with mental stress: The potential and limits of exercise intervention* (final report). Bethesda, MD: NIMH.

Morgan, W. P. (1984b). Physical activity and mental health. In H. Eckert & H. J. Montoye (Eds.), *Exercise and health* (pp. 132-145). Champaign, IL: Human Kinetics Publishers.

Morgan, W. P. (1985). Affective benefits of vigorous physical activity. *Medicine and Science in Sports and Exercise, 17*, 94-100.

Morgan, W. P., Horstman, D. H., Cymerman, A. R., & Stokes, J. D. (1980). Exercise as a relaxation technique. *Primary Cardiology, 6*, 48-57.

Morgan, W., Roberts, J., Brand, F., & Feinerman, A. (1970). Psychological effect of chronic physical activity. *Medicine and Science in Sports and Exercise, 2*, 213-217.

Morin, S. F., & Batchelor, W. F. (1984). Responding to the psychological crisis of AIDS. *Public Health Reports, 99*, 4-9.

Morin, S., Charles, K., & Malyon, A. (1984). The psychological impact of AIDS on gay men. *American Psychologist, 39*, 1288-1293.

Munoz, A., Wang, M. C., Good, R., Detels, H., Ginsberg, L., Kingsley, J., Phair, J., & Polk, B. F. (1988, June). *Estimation of the AIDS-free times after HIV-1 seroconversion.* Paper presented at the fourth meeting of the International Conference on AIDS, Stockholm, Sweden.

Papadopoulos, N. M., Bloor, C. M., & Standefer, J. C. (1969). Effect of exercise and training on plasma lipids and lipoproteins in the rat. *Journal of Applied Physiology, 26*, 760-763.

Paffenbarger, R. S., Hyde, R. T., Wing, A. L., & Hsieh, C. (1986). Physical activity, all-cause mortality, and longevity of college allumni. *New England Journal of Medicine, 314*, 605-613.

Pargman, D., & Baker, M. C. (1980). Running high: Enkephalin indicated. *Journal of Drug Issues, 10*, 341-349.

Patterson, T., Grant, I., & McClurg, J. (1988, April). *Relationship between immune status and stressful events in an elderly population.* Paper presented at the ninth annual scientific meetings of the Society of Behavioral Medicine, Boston.

Pericic, D., Manev, H., Boranic, M., Poljak-Blazi, M., & Lakic, N. (1987). Effect of diazepam on brain neurotransmitters, plasma cortisol, and the immune system of stressed rats. *Annals of the New York Academy of Sciences, 496*, 450-458.

Pierce, C. W. (1980). Macrophages: Modulators of immunity. *American Journal of Pathology, 98*, 10-28.

Plaut, M. (1987). Lymphocyte hormone receptors. *Annual Review of Immunology, 5*, 621-669.

Porter, R. R., & Reid, K. B. M. (1978). The biochemistry of complement. *Nature, 275*, 699-704.

Raise, E., Gritti, F. M., Sabbatani, S., Schiattone, M. L., Pulsatelli, L., Di Pede, B., & Martuzzi, M. (1988). Reduction of T helper/inducers of B lymphocytes and increase of T suppressors as an early pattern of HIV infection. *Proceedings of the Fourth International Conference on AIDS, 1*, 171.

Ransford, C. P. (1982). A role for amines in the antidepressant effect of exercise: A review. *Medicine and Science in Sports and Exercise, 14*, 1-10.

Reid, R. L., Hoff, S. D., Yen, S. S. C., & Li, C. H. (1981). Effects of exogenous β-endorphin on pituitary hormone secretion and its disappearance rate in normal human subjects. *Journal of Clinical Endocrinology and Metabolism, 52*, 1179-1184.

Richman, D. D., Fischl, M., Grieco, M., Gottlieb, M., Volberding, P., Laskin, O., Leedom, J., Groopman, J., Mildvan, D., Hirsch, M., Jackson, G., Durack, D., & Nusinoff-Lehrman, S. (1987). The toxicity of azidothymidine (AZT) in the treatment of patients with AIDS and AIDS-related complex. *New England Journal of Medicine, 317*, 192-197.

Robinson, D. S. (1970). The function of the plasma triglycerides in fatty acid transport. In M. Florkin & E. H. Stotz (Eds.), *Comprehensive biochemistry* (Vol. 18, pp. 51-116). Amsterdam: Elsevier.

Rodgers, M. P., Dubey, D., & Reich, P. (1979). The influence of the psyche and the brain on immunity and disease susceptibility: A critical review. *Psychosomatic Medicine, 41*, 147-164.

Roitt, I., Brostoff, J., & Male, E. (1985). *Immunology.* London: Gower.

Rosen, F. S., Cooper, M. D., & Wedgewood, R. J. (1984). The primary immunodeficiencies, 1. *New England Journal of Medicine, 811*, 235-242.

Roth, D., & Holmes, D. (1985). Influence of physical fitness in determining impact of stressful life events in physical and psychological health. *Psychosomatic Medicine, 47*, 164-173.

Sachar, E. J. (1976). Neuroendocrine abnormalities in depressive illness. In E. J. Sachar (Ed.), *Topics in psychoendocrinology.* New York: Grune & Stratton.

Sachs, M. J. (1984). The runner's high. In M. L. Sachs, & G. W. Buffone (Eds.), *Running as therapy: An integrated approach* (pp. 273-287). Lincoln: University of Nebraska Press.

Saltin, B., & Astrand, P. (1967). Maximal oxygen uptake in athletes. *Journal of Applied Physiology*, *23*, 353-358.

Schleifer, S., Keller, S., Siris, S., Davis, K., & Stein, M. (1985). Depression and immunity: Lymphocyte function in ambulatory depressed patients, hospitalized schizophrenic patients, and patients hospitalized for herniorrhaphy. *Archives of General Psychiatry*, *42*, 129-133.

Seal, D. R., Allen, W. K., Hurley, B. F., Dalsky, G. P., Ehansi, A. A., & Hagberg, J. M. (1984). Elevated high-density lipoprotein cholesterol levels in older endurance athletes. *American Journal of Cardiology*, *54*, 390-391.

Selye, H. (1956). *The stress of life*. New York: McGraw-Hill.

Shavit, Y., & Martin, F. (1987). Opiates, stress, and immunity: Animal studies. *Annals of Behavioral Medicine*, *9*(2), 11-15.

Sibinga, N., & Goldstein, A. (1988). Opioid peptides and opioid receptors in cells of the immune system. *Annual Review of Immunology*, *6*, 219-249.

Simantov, R. (1979). Glucocorticoids inhibit endorphin synthesis by pituitary cells. *Nature*, *280*, 684-685.

Simon, H. (1984). The immunology of exercise: A brief review. *Journal of the American Medical Association*, *252*, 2735-2738.

Sodroski, J. G., Rosen, C. A., & Haseltine, W. A. (1984). Transacting transcription of the long terminal repeat of human T lymphotropic viruses in infected cells. *Science*, *225*, 381-385.

Solomon, G. F. (1987). Psychoneuroimmunologic approaches to research on AIDS. *Annals of the New York Academy of Sciences*, *496*, 628-636.

Solomon, G. F., & Mead, C. W. (in press). Psychosocial and human considerations in the treatment of the gay patient with AIDS or ARC. *Journal of Humanistic Medicine*.

Solomon, G. F., & Temoshok, L. (1987). A psychoneuroimmunologic perspective on AIDS research: Questions, preliminary findings and suggestions. *Journal of Applied Social Psychology*, *17*, 286-308.

Spiegelberg, H. L. (1974). Biological activities of immunoglobulins of different classes and subclasses. *Advanced Immunology*, *19*, 259-270.

Stevens, C. E., Taylor, P. E., & Zang, E. A. (1986). Human T-cell lymphotropic virus Type III in a cohort of homosexual men in New York City. *Journal of the American Medical Association*, *225*, 2167-2171.

Stites, D., Stobo, J., Fudenberg, H., & Wells, J. (1982). *Basic and clinical immunology* (4th ed.). Los Altos, CA: Lange.

Strom, T., Sytkowski, A., Carpenter, C., & Merrill, J. (1974). Cholinergic augmentation of lymphocyte-mediated cytotoxicity. A study of the cholinergic receptor of cytotoxic T lymphocytes. *Proceedings of the National Academy of Sciences, U.S.A.*, *71*, 1330-1333.

Targan, S., Britvan, L., & Dorey, F. (1981). Activation of human NKCC by moderate exercise: Increased frequency of NK cells with enhanced capability of effector-target lytic interactions. *Clinical Experimental Immunology*, *45*, 352-360.

Temoshok, L., Zich, J. M., Mandel, J. S., & Moulton, J. M. (1986). *Research and clinical impressions from psychosocial investigations of AIDS in San Francisco*. Unpublished manuscript. University of California, San Francisco, Department of Psychiatry and Langley Porter Institute.

Temoshok, L., Zich, J., Solomon, G. F., Stites, D. P., & O'Leary, A. (1987, June). *An intensive psychoimmunologic study of men with AIDS*. Paper presented at the Third International Conference on the Acquired Immune Deficiency Syndrome, Washington, DC.

Teshima, H., Sogawa, H., Kihara, S., Nagata, S., Ago, Y., & Nakagawa, T. (1987). Changes in populations of T cell subsets due to stress. *Annals of the New York Academy of Sciences*, *496*, 459-466.

Tross, S. (1987). *Psychological response to AIDS and HIV disease*. Proceedings of conference on "Current concepts in psycho-oncology and AIDS." New York: Memorial Sloan-Kettering Cancer Center.

Tross, S., Hirsch, D. A., Rabkin, B., Berry, C., & Holland, J. C. (1987, June). *Determinants of current psychiatric disorder in AIDS spectrum patients.* Proceedings of the III International Conference on Acquired Immunodeficiency Syndrome (AIDS). Washington, DC.

Watson, R. R., Moriguchi, S., Jackson, J. C., Werner, L., Wilmore, J. H., & Freund, B. J. (1986). Modification of cellular immune functions in humans by endurance exercise training during β-adrenergic blockade with antenolol or propranolol. *Medicine and Science in Sports and Exercise, 18,* 95–100.

Weiss, J. M., Goodman, P. A., Losito, B. G., Corrigan, S., Charry, J. M., & Bailey, W. H. (1981). Behavioral depression produced by an uncontrollable stressor: Relationship to norepinephrine, dopamine, and serotonin levels in various regions of rat brain. *Brain Research, 3,* 167–205.

Weiss, J., Stone, E., & Harrell, N. (1980). Coping behavior and brain norepinephrine level in rats. *Journal of Comparative Physiology and, 72,* 153–160.

Williams, P. T., Wood, P. D., Haskell, W. L., & Vranizan, K. (1982). The effects of running mileage and duration on plasma lipoprotein levels. *Journal of the American Medical Association, 247,* 2674–2679.

Williamson, S., Knight, R., Lightman, S., & Hobbs, J. (1987). Differential effects of β-endorphin fragments on human natural killing. *Brain, Behavior, and Immunity, 1,* 329–335.

Winder, W., Hagberg, J., Hickson, R., Ehsani, A., & McLane, J. (1978). Time course of sympathoadrenal adaption to endurance exercise training in man. *Journal of Applied Physiology, 45,* 370–374.

Wood, P. D., & Haskell, W. L. (1979). The effects of exercise on plasma high density lipoproteins. *Lipids, 14,* 417–427.

Yarchoan, R., Pluda, J. M., Thomas, R. V., Perno, C. F., McAtee, N., Myers, C. E., & Broder, S. (1988a). Long-term treatment of AIDS and AIDS-related complex (ARC) with alternative weekly regimen of AZT and 2′, 3′-Dideoxycytide (DDC). *Proceedings of the Fourth International Conference on AIDS, 1,* 257.

Yarchoan, R., Surbone, A., Pluda, J. M., McAtee, N., Blum, M. R., Maha, M., Myers, C. E., & Broder, S. (1988b). Pharmacokinetics and long-term therapy of AIDS and ARC with AZT and acyclovir. *Proceedings of the Fourth International Conference on AIDS, 1,* 254.

Psychosocial Responses of Hospital Workers to Acquired Immunodeficiency Syndrome (AIDS)*

16

Lydia O'Donnell
Education Development Center
Newton, Massachusetts
Carl R. O'Donnell
Department of Medicine
New England Deaconess Hospital
Joseph H. Pleck
Wheaton College
John Snarey
Northwestern University
Evanston, Illinois
Richard M. Rose
Department of Medicine
New England Deaconess Hospital

As the first group of service providers to come into regular, intimate, and prolonged contact with individuals who have acquired immunodeficiency syndrome (AIDS), hospital workers are in a unique position to influence the mental as well as physical health of those with AIDS. In addition, they are, at times, called upon to educate others in the community. Assessment of their responses to AIDS will facilitate the development of strategies for improving the quality of medical care delivered to AIDS patients, reducing the job-related stress experienced by health-care providers, and facilitating dissemination of information about the disease to the public.

Since the number of AIDS cases is projected to double annually for the next several years (Centers for Disease Control, 1985), a growing proportion of hospital workers will become AIDS-care providers. It is estimated that in 1991, 80% of the 145,000 people needing treatment will be found outside New York and San Francisco, which currently harbor 40% of all cases (Cen-

*This chapter was originally published in *Journal of Applied Social Psychology*, 1987, Vol. 17, No. 3, pp. 269–285. Copyright 1987 by V. H. Winston & Sons, Inc. Reprinted with permission.

ters for Disease Control, 1986). Therefore, many hospital workers who currently have little or no experience with the disease will be called upon to provide AIDS-related care. Evaluation of the difficulties experienced by staff, to date, will enable institutions less familiar with AIDS treatment to prepare for the future. Thus, understanding the perceptions of hospital workers about AIDS, as well as the difficulties they experience when providing care, will be increasingly important if patients are to receive optimum treatment.

The physical and neuropsychiatric manifestations of AIDS, the medical and infection-control procedures required in care, and negative public attitudes about the disease may combine to make the delivery of AIDS care particularly stressful. The epidemic nature of the disease, its lethality, and potential transmissibility via body fluids contribute to situations in which staff may perceive themselves to be at risk for developing the disease by virtue of direct contact with patients or clinical specimens. This could lead to fear when caring for AIDS patients and anger at having to do so (Furstenberg & Olson, 1984; Golin, 1978; Halloran, 1984; Klein & Pfeffer, 1985; Marshall, 1980). As documented with cancer patients, fear of contracting a disease may interfere with the ability of health-care workers to objectively evaluate evidence that the disease is not transmitted from patient to provider (Wortman & Dunkel-Schetter, 1979). In addition, hospitalized AIDS patients are often gravely ill, at times suffering either from Kaposi's sarcoma, which can be disfiguring, or from neuropsychiatric complications. Both of these conditions may interfere with normal social interactions. Furthermore, due to the lack of successful treatments, staff have little control over their patients' conditions and little hope to offer. The relatively young age of patients heightens feelings of futility, and may make it difficult for staff to cope with patients and with their own grief. Such factors have previously been shown to contribute to the stress experienced by health-care providers, as well as to avoidance and rejection of the patient (Wortman & Dunkel-Schetter, 1979).

Cultural differences between patient and health-care provider have also been shown to be a source of stress for both parties (Graham & Reeder, 1972). The two major risk groups in this country, male homosexuals and intravenous drug abusers, comprise subcultures which are frequently stigmatized. Thus, the attitudes of staff may create barriers to communication, imposing additional limitations on the care-giving process. To what extent public attitudes about AIDS and individuals with AIDS affect hospital workers is unclear (Altman, 1986). Clinical and impressionistic reports relate examples of "AIDS anxiety" and other difficulties among hospital workers ("AIDS: A time bomb..," 1986; Foreman, 1985; Mather, 1985; Phillips, 1983; Wachter, 1986). Yet, the extent of the problem and the amount and types of educational intervention needed in the hospital setting are not documented. In the following, we report on the psychosocial responses of hospital staff to caring for AIDS patients and suggest directions for the development of educational and management strategies.

METHODS

Questionnaires were administered to professional and technical-level health-care workers at the major AIDS patient-care facility in Massachusetts, a 500-bed, university-affiliated referral hospital which provides care to a diverse patient population. By the time of the study (spring 1985), the hospital had admitted approximately 60 patients, or 28% of AIDS cases reported in the state.

We identified seven medical units where virtually all AIDS patients had received care. We also identified hospital departments (e.g., respiratory therapy) which routinely provide services to this patient population. We focused on professional and technical-level employees because their behavior affects patient care most directly (Freidson, 1970; "Notes of a dying professor," 1972).

All members of the identified groups were asked to participate in the study, including those having no experience with AIDS patients. Personal interviews were administered to 150 employees. An additional 87 staff members returned self-administered questionnaires. This latter group consisted of those unable to donate the time to complete a personal interview. The self-administered and personal interviews were comparable. The resulting sample ($N = 237$) represents a response rate of 60%. However, this figure is deceptively low, since nurses in one area, the intensive care unit (ICU), account for 43% of all refusals. Shortly before interviewing began, there was a sharp decline in AIDS patient admissions to the ICU, reflecting changes in clinical decisions regarding terminal care. As a result, only 10 of 79 nurses from this group participated, several of whom had recently rotated from other floors providing AIDS care. Exclusion of ICU nurses from the sample would increase the response rate to 71%. The response rate was considerably more uniform among employees in other areas.

Seventy-six percent of the sample were women, 59% had completed college, and respondents had worked at the hospital for an average of 5.4 years ($sd = 4.6$). The average age of respondents was 31.3 years ($sd = 7.6$). Forty-eight percent ($n = 114$) were registered nurses; 19% ($n = 44$) technicians; 14% ($n = 32$) house officers; 11% ($n = 27$) LPNs and orderlies; and 8% ($n = 20$) social workers and clergy.

Data were collected on four dimensions. First was the frequency and nature of contact with AIDS patients. We collected objective information (e.g., number of patients seen) and more subjective information (e.g., perception of time spent providing AIDS care). We also gathered information on the frequency of specific kinds of physical and social interactions (e.g., contact with blood, conversations about AIDS).

Second, we assessed the accuracy of respondents' factual knowledge of the clinical and epidemiological characteristics of AIDS, as well as their sources of information about AIDS. Questions on the number of cases reported and risk groups, for example, were chosen since these are facts most frequently reported in the media and in medical briefs. Questions on disease transmission were developed based on the types of exposures most frequently experienced by hospital workers. For some of these exposures (e.g., CPR), it is impossible to assign a "correct" answer, given the limitations of available knowledge. However, a variety of such exposures were included to reflect the range of potential modes of transmission, from improbable to highly possible, as well as a range of staff concerns.

Third, we measured attitudes about AIDS and about homosexuality. A self-administered "AIDS Phobia" questionnaire was developed. On a seven-point Likert scale, respondents indicated the extent to which they agreed with statements of specific interest to hospital workers and statements depicting more general fears and perceptions about AIDS. Attitudes about homosexuality were assessed using items drawn from scales previously developed by Smith (1974) and Gartrell, Kramer, and Brodie (1974). Respondents' perceptions of homosexuality as abnormal and pathological, as well as their personal comfort with homosexuals and their attitudes about gay rights, were tabulated.

Finally, respondents were asked about personal difficulties and stresses they experienced. For example, subjects reported their perceived job-related risk of contracting AIDS and assessed their comfort and performance with AIDS patients. They also compared AIDS care with other types of care.

The questionnaire was reviewed by a team of consultants experienced in health-care delivery and evaluation research, as well as several individuals with AIDS. Pretests were conducted on an independent sample of health-care workers.

Descriptive statistics were computed, and selected items were cross-tabulated by job category. Indices were developed for analysis of responses in four areas: AIDS-Contact, AIDS-Phobia, Homophobia, and AIDS-Stress. Indices were derived empirically from larger pools of items, and index reliability was measured using Cronbach's alpha. Items not contributing to alpha were deleted.

AIDS-Contact contained 15 items (alpha = 0.83). These included: over the past year, the number of AIDS patients seen; the percentage of time spent with such patients; and the approximate number of interactions with the families and friends of AIDS patients; over the past month, the average number of hours spent with AIDS patients; and estimates of how frequently respondents interact with AIDS patients. More specifically, regarding patient-care duties, there were estimates of how often respondents work in the same room with AIDS patients, come into direct physical contact, handle their bedclothes, obtain and/or handle blood, handle other body fluids, and handle equipment that has come into contact with their body fluids. Finally, there were three estimates of social contact: how often respondents have general conversations with AIDS patients, talk about physical or emotional problems related to the disease with patients, and talk with their families and friends of AIDS patients.

TABLE 16.1
AIDS-Phobia: Distribution of Items

Item	Response (% agree)[a]		
1. A hospital worker should not be required to work with AIDS patients.	42.0		
2. AIDS patients have as much right to quality medical care as anyone else.	94.3		
3. AIDS makes my job a high-risk occupation.	53.9		
4. AIDS is God's punishment for immorality.	5.0		
5. Dealing with AIDS patients is different than dealing with other types of patients.	71.3		
6. The high cost of treating AIDS patients is unfair to other people in need of care.	13.0		
7. AIDS patients offend me morally.	16.0		
8. If I learned that someone I knew had AIDS, it would be hard for me to continue my relationship with him or her.	16.9		
9. Having a co-worker with AIDS would not bother me.	35.7		
10. If I got AIDS, I would worry that other people would think I was a homosexual.	43.5		
11. Working with AIDS patients can be a rewarding experience.	54.8		
12. It's important to go out of your way to be helpful to a patient with AIDS.	49.3		
	% yes	% no	% don't know
13. Do you think that people with AIDS should be allowed to work in public schools?	42.4	36.9	20.8
14. Do you think that people with AIDS should be allowed to handle food in restaurants?	15.2	74.7	10.1
15. Do you think that people with AIDS should be allowed to work with patients in hospitals?	27.8	59.1	13.1
16. Has the growing number of AIDS cases made you more tolerant, less tolerant, or not changed your attitude at all about homosexuality?			
% more tolerant	17.8		
% no change	62.7		
% less tolerant	19.5		

[a]Items 1–12 used a 7-point agree-disagree scale; 1 = very strongly agree, 7 = very strongly disagree. % agree = proportion of respondents answering in the 1–3 range.

TABLE 16.2
Homophobia: Distribution of Items

Item	Response (% agree)[a]
1. Men and women deserve equal status in society, regardless of their sexual orientation or behavior.	86.1
2. Homosexuality is a natural expression of love and affection.	36.2
3. It would be upsetting for me to find out I was alone with a homosexual.	10.4
4. Homosexuals should be allowed to hold government positions.	80.1
5. My concept of mental health includes the possibility of a well-adjusted homosexual.	62.1
6. Homosexuality is usually a pathological state, rather than one of the many ways of loving and relating.	17.3
7. I find the thought of homosexual acts disgusting.	47.6
8. I would be afraid for a child of mine to have a teacher who was homosexual.	20.9
9. A homosexual could be a good president of the United States.	55.9
10. If a child of mine showed homosexual tendencies, I would want him or her to get psychiatric treatment.	43.0
11. If a homosexual sat next to me on a bus, I would get nervous.	6.5

[a]Items 1–11 used a 7-point agree-disagree scale; 1 = very strongly agree, 7 = very strongly disagree. % agree = proportion of respondents answering in the 1–3 range.

AIDS-Phobia contained 16 items (alpha = 0.76), including the "AIDS Phobia" scale as well as 4 additional items regarding the social acceptability and activities of individuals with AIDS. Table 16.1 lists these items.

Homophobia was assessed using 11 items (alpha = 0.86). Four items focused on personal comfort with homosexuals; three on their civil rights; and four on perceptions of the abnormality/pathology of homosexuality. These items can be found in Table 16.2.

AIDS-stress contained 8 items (alpha = 0.66). These included perceptions of personal risk and stress experienced due to interactions with AIDS patients, comfort around AIDS patients and their loved ones, how good a job respondents felt they did in dealing with physical and emotional needs of patients, and whether they felt it would be difficult to deal with more such patients in the future (see Table 16.3).

Correlations between the separate indices were computed and an analysis of vriance was performed to assess the effect of job category and AIDS-Contact on AIDS-Stress, controlling for age, gender, and religion.

TABLE 16.3
AIDS-Related Stress and Difficulties: Selected Items

Item	Response
1. How much risk do you think you have of getting AIDS because of your job? (% high risk)[a]	23.9
2. Is working with AIDS one of the more stressful parts of your job? (% yes)	48.0
3. How comfortable are you with AIDS patients? (% *not* comfortable)	35.5
4. Is your knowledge sufficient to deal with AIDS patients' physical needs? (% no or maybe)	38.4
5. Is your knowledge sufficient to deal with AIDS patients' emotional problems? (% no or maybe)	58.0
6. Is your knowledge sufficient to deal with the needs of AIDS patients' families and friends? (% no or maybe)	60.3
7. How comfortable are you with the friends and families of AIDS patients? (% not comfortable)	35.6
8. Do you think that it will be hard for you to deal with a larger number of AIDS patients in the future? (% yes)	65.2
9. Assess the job your fellow workers do in dealing with AIDS patients' physical needs. (% not good)[b]	54.5
10. Assess the job your fellow workers do in dealing with AIDS patients' emotional needs. (% not good)[b]	42.7
11. Assess the job your fellow workers do in dealing with AIDS patients' family and friends. (% not good)[b]	34.1

[a] value of 3 or 4 on a 4-point scale.
[b] value of 1 or 2 on a 4-point scale; these were not included in the AIDS-Stress Index

RESULTS

Respondents had seen an average of 11 AIDS patients over the past year, although this number was highly variable ($sd = 11.7$), as was the percentage of time respondents estimated they spent with AIDS patients ($\bar{x} = 8.1\%$, $sd = 10.7\%$). Sixty-six percent reported that they interacted with patients either sometimes or often.

Technicians had seen the most patients ($n = 18$). Nurses and aides saw fewer than the average number of patients, but reported spending the most time with patients and the highest number of interactions with families and friends.

Estimates of the percentage of time spent with AIDS patients were greater than might be expected, based on the reported numbers seen. For example,

LPNs/aides had seen an average of 9 patients during the year, but estimated that caring for these patients consumed 15% of their time. While the degree of physical contact with AIDS patients reported by technicians was comparable to the overall sample, they reported less social contact both with AIDS patients and with their families and friends.

Respondents were most likely to have received their information about AIDS either from news media accounts or from hospital in-service education programs. Approximately 60% felt that they had sufficient knowledge to deal with the physical needs of AIDS patients, while only 42% felt that they had sufficient knowledge to deal with their emotional needs, and 40% felt equipped to deal with the needs of families and friends. One third (33.6%) felt that they had insufficient knowledge about infection-control procedures.

The accuracy of respondents' knowledge about AIDS is reported in Table 16.4.

TABLE 16.4
Knowledge About AIDS: Selected Items

	Epidemiology	
	Response	Correct
1. How many cases of AIDS have been reported in the United States?	modal response = 5,001–10,000	approx. 10,000 (as of 4/85)
2. What percentage of male homosexuals have AIDS?	mean = 13.5%	approx. 0.2%
3. What percentage of male homosexuals have the AIDS virus in their blood?	mean = 29.9%	approx. 2%
4. What percentage of persons with AIDS are male homosexuals?	mean = 73.7%	approx. 73%

Modes of Transmission Can AIDS be transmitted in the following ways?	% yes	% possibly	% no
1. by blood transfusion	92.8	6.8	0.4
2. being stuck with a needle from AIDS patient	68.7	30.9	0.4
3. giving CPR	57.6	34.2	8.2
4. kissing an individual with AIDS	44.2	47.8	8.0
5. sharing eating utensils	38.1	48.9	13.0
6. airborne transmission	26.1	51.3	22.6
7. emptying bedpans	20.4	56.6	23.1
8. changing bed linens	13.6	47.4	39.0
9. shaking hands with an AIDS patient	5.3	28.4	66.2
10. being in the same room with an AIDS patient	4.6	21.7	73.7

Although there was a considerable range, on the average, the sample correctly estimated the number of AIDS cases identified in the United States at the time of the interviews, as well as the percentage of individuals with AIDS who are male homosexuals ($\bar{x}$ = 73.7%). Similarly, major risk groups were accurately identified. However, respondents considerably overestimated that 13.5% of the male homosexual population currently has AIDS, with house officers estimating a low of 6.1% and LPNs/aides a high of 21.9%. Even using the conservative estimate that 5% of the total male population is exclusively homosexual, this would result in well over one-half million hypothetical AIDS cases (Kinsey, Pomeroy, & Martin, 1948). Thus, the size of the homosexual population was underestimated by approximately 100-fold. Not surprisingly, accuracy of information about cases and risk groups varied by job category, undoubtedly reflecting differences in amount of education. For example, house officers and social workers, the most highly educated groups, were least likely to grossly mis-estimate the total number of cases in the U.S.

Although there are few definitive answers to questions about modes of transmission, research suggests that the virus associated with AIDS is not spread through casual contact and that health-care workers, if they follow accepted infection-control procedures, are at very low risk of contracting the disease through occupational exposure ("Update: Evaluation of human T-lymphotropic virus..., 1985"). Table 16.4 also contains the number of respondents who believe that AIDS can be transmitted in various ways. Close to 70% felt that AIDS can be transmitted through an accidental needle stick. Similarly, 57.6% reported that it could be transmitted while giving CPR. In most cases, there were not significant differences by job category. However, no house officers felt that there was a risk of airborne transmission, in contrast to 26.1% of nurses and 38% of technicians ($p < 0.05$). House officers, along with social-service staff, were also least likely to think that there was a risk of transmission through sharing eating utensils ($p = .0357$).

Table 16.1 presents responses to items included in the AIDS-Phobia index.

Forty-two percent agreed that hospital workers should not be required to work with AIDS patients, although 94.3% agreed that "AIDS patients have as much right to quality medical care as anyone else." Even though three-quarters of those sampled were women and, therefore, currently at very low risk for sexual transmission of the disease, 43.5% agreed with the statement that "If I got AIDS, I would worry that other people would think that I was a homosexual." Nearly half (48.3%) said that having a co-worker with AIDS would bother them.

A majority (73.3%) reported that AIDS had made them think more about homosexual lifestyles, although the percentage who say that they have become more tolerant as a result (17.8%) is roughly equal to the percentage of those who say that it has made them less so (19.5%). The most homophobic responses were recorded on issues of personal comfort with homosexuality (only 36.2% agreed that homosexuality is a natural expression of love and affection), while the least phobic scores were recorded on issues of civil rights (86% agreed that homosexuals should be allowed to hold government positions). Only 5 respondents reported that over 5% of their friends were gay. Homophobia items are reported in Table 16.2.

The final set of items incorporated into an index concerned the possible stresses and difficulties staff may encounter when providing AIDS care. About one-quarter of respondents (23.9%) felt that they had a relatively high risk of getting AIDS because of their job (score of 3 or 4 on a 1 to 4 scale). Almost half (48%) reported that working with AIDS was one of the more stressful parts of their duties. Over a third (35.5%) reported that they were not comfortable with AIDS patients, and 41% said no disease concerned them more than AIDS (see Table 16.3).

Reported stress differed significantly by job category for all but one of the items included in the AIDS-Stress index. For example, 79.5% of technicians rated how their fellow workers dealt with patients' physical needs as "not good," compared with 40.7% of house officers and 38.5% of social-service workers (sample $\bar{x}$ = 54.5%, $p < .001$). Technicians also felt at greatest risk of getting AIDS because of their jobs. Thirty-six percent felt at relatively high risk, in contrast to 3.1% of house officers and no social-service workers ($p < .001$).

TABLE 16.5
Index Scores by Job Category

| Index (possible range) | Sample Average (range of individual scores) | RN | Hospital Staff Subgroups | | | | F | p |
			Technical Services	House Officers	LPN/ Aides	Social Services		
AIDS-CONTACT (10–40)	27.7 (10–38)	25.5	23.0	24.3	23.6	14.4	9.71	< .0001
HOMO-PHOBIA (10–70)	29.5 (10–65)	30.0	32.4	26.5	32.0	22.2	3.21	.0138
AIDS-PHOBIA (30–90)	62.0 (45–86)	62.8	64.2	60.4	63.3	53.3	6.85	< .0001
AIDS—STRESS (10–40)	18.1 (10–30)	17.8	20.0	16.2	19.9	16.3	7.54	< .0001

Twenty percent of the overall sample, and a high of 37.1% of the technicians, felt that recommended infection-control procedures were not adequate. Eighty percent were concerned that it will be difficult for the hospital to deal with more AIDS patients, and 65.2% felt that they personally would have difficulty.

Scores were calculated both for individuals and by job category for the four indices (AIDS-Contact, AIDS-Phobia, Homophobia, and AIDS-Stress). For each index, scores varied significantly by job category (one-way ANOVA, see Table 16.5).

Interrelationships between individual index scores were examined using correlational analysis. Results are reported in Table 16.6. The strongest correlations were between Homophobia and AIDS-Phobia ($r = 0.62$), and AIDS-Phobia and AIDS-Stress ($r = 0.55$). There was also a significant correlation between Homophobia and AIDS-Stress ($r = 0.42$). Both AIDS-Phobia and AIDS-Stress were negatively correlated with AIDS-Contact ($r = -0.18$ and $r = 0.25$, respectively). AIDS-Contact was not significantly correlated with Homophobia.

We performed an analysis of variance which examined AIDS-Stress in relation to both AIDS-Contact and job category, controlling for age, gender, and religion. As shown in Table 16.7, higher amounts of contact with AIDS patients were significntly associated with lower reported stress. The interaction between job category and degree of contact on stress was not significant.

TABLE 16.6
Index Correlation Matrix[a]

	AIDS-Contact	AIDS-Phobia	Homophobia	AIDS-Stress
AIDS-Contact	1.00	—	—	—
AIDS-Phobia	-0.18	1.00	—	—
Homophobia	-0.11	0.62	1.00	—
AIDS-Stress	-0.25	0.55	0.42	1.00

[a]All reported correlations, except for AIDS-Contact by Homophobia, are significant at the .01 level.

TABLE 16.7
Analysis of Variance:
Stress Index by Hospital Staff Subgroup and Contact Index

Contact Index	Hospital Staff Subgroup				
	RN	Technical services	House officers	LPNs/Aides	Social Services
High	17.1	20.6	15.0	18.7	15.4
Low	19.8	20.0	17.4	22.5	17.1

Note: Hospital staff subgroup, $F_{(4,220)} = 7.8$, $p < 0.0001$. Contact index, $F_{(1,220)} = 14.8$, $p < 0.0001$. Subgroup × contact index, $F_{(4,220)} = 1.7$, NS.

In a supplementary analysis, with job category dichotomized as technicians versus all others, the interaction between job category and contact on reported stress was significant $[F(1, 226) = 4.0, p < .05]$. The data indicate that greater contact with AIDS patients is associated with lower AIDS-Stress for all groups except technicians.

DISCUSSION

Caring for individuals with AIDS was a source of concern for the hospital workers surveyed. Staff exaggerated the proportion of time spent in AIDS-related care, and considered this to be among the more stressful aspects of their work. Overall, they were dissatisfied with how they and their colleagues responded to patients' emotional needs. For a substantial minority of individuals, job-related exposure to AIDS patients was perceived as a personal health threat. In part, this fear can be explained by an inaccurate understanding of how AIDS is transmitted. For example, those in job categories most likely to overestimate the possibility of contracting AIDS through casual contact also felt at greatest risk of contracting the disease.

Social factors clearly play a role in shaping the attitudes of staff toward AIDS patients and, in turn, the difficulties and stresses staff experience when providing such care. AIDS-Phobia, including fears of contagion, was positively correlated with Homophobia and AIDS-Stress. Although these correlations do not imply causality, it is likely that AIDS-Phobia and ultimately AIDS-Stress are heightened by negative attitudes about homosexuality. Given the lack of correlation between AIDS-Contact and Homophobia, it does not appear that individuals who were more homophobic avoided AIDS-patient contact. Therefore, the observed negative correlations of AIDS-Phobia and AIDS-Stress with AIDS-Contact do not appear to result from the influence of homophobia on patient-care assignments.

These findings have implications for hospitals providing care to individuals with AIDS, since we interpret them to mean that staff will have the greatest difficulties in the transitional period when AIDS is new to them, and that these difficulties will subside as they become more experienced. Thus, we would expect AIDS to present the greatest difficulties in those places where it is still relatively unfamiliar. Since the number of patients seen in such locations will increase at a faster rate than the rate where AIDS is currently most prevalent, AIDS education efforts should be directed to these areas.

The nature of staff-patient interactions influenced the relationship between amount of direct AIDS-patient contact and stress. Employees who had more opportunity to engage in social interactions with patients experienced reduction in stress with increased patient contact. However, high frequency of contact coupled with brief and impersonal interactions, as was the case with technicians, negated this effect.

Additional research is indicated to characterize the psychosocial dynamics of AIDS care longitudinally, to assess institutional differences in employees' responses to AIDS, and to evaluate the difficulties of AIDS care among more diverse patient populations. Continuing widespread media accounts and new clinical evidence on AIDS may have improved health-care workers' accuracy of knowledge about the disease since the time of the survey, but how this new information has affected staffs' perceptions of the risks and stresses associated with care-giving is an open question. On the one hand, it is possible that new evidence about the difficulties of HIV transmission might have eased their concerns about occupational exposure. On the other hand, the larger number of AIDS patients served by the hospital in the past year may have increased perceptions of the difficulties and stresses associated with AIDS-patient care.

In summary, while they are probably more knowledgeable than the general public about health issues, hospital workers are not immune to AIDS fears. However, close contact with AIDS patients allows them to come to terms with their fears. Our survey suggests that most will benefit from special education and support in this process. The current generation of hospital workers often has little training or experience to prepare them for dealing with a disease such as AIDS, one which is epidemic, infectious, usually lethal, and as yet untreatable. For this reason, it is justified to devote special resources to AIDS education.

Despite the availability of infection-control education at this institution, a substantial number of individuals were still uncertain about the risk of AIDS transmission during routine patient care. This represents a major area of concern for hospital workers and requires that the value of infection-control measures in reducing the risk of disease transmission be reinforced and updated through ongoing series of staff-training sessions.

In addition, the inverse relationship of both AIDS-Stress and AIDS-Phobia with AIDS-Contact suggests the need to target new employees and those whose patient interactions are primarily technical in nature. Programs should emphasize the importance of establishing social interactions with patients. Such interactions would apparently reduce employee stress and should, ultimately, improve delivery of care.

Furthermore, programs should provide not just facts, but should offer support for coping with the unknowns about the disease. Employees need time to accept the low level of risk imposed by AIDS and to place it in the context of the various other uncertainties they deal with routinely. They also need to be sensitized to issues of homosexuality, as well as to psychosocial issues relevant to other risk groups, particularly intravenous drug users.

It is the responsibility of health-care workers to respond professionally and compassionately to patients' needs, irrespective of their own attitudes and fears. Our data suggest that to provide the best quality of care to individuals with AIDS and to assure that such care is not delivered at the expense of employee well-being, concerted efforts must be made to implement AIDS educational and support programs at the institutional level. An informed hospital work force can then be expected to help disseminate accurate information about AIDS and to reduce AIDS anxiety in the community.

ACKNOWLEDGMENTS

This research was supported in part by a grant from the Massachusetts Department of Public Health. The authors thank Health Research Associates for their assistance in data collection and members of the AIDS Action Committee for their comments and suggestions.

Please send reprint requests to Lydia N. O'Donnell, Ed.D., Associate Director, Education Development Center, 55 Chapel Street, Newton, MA 02160.

REFERENCES

AIDS: A time bomb at hospitals' door. (1986). *Hospitals*, January 5, 54-61.

Centers for Disease Control, (1985). Update: Acquired immunodeficiency syndrome—United States. *Morbidity and Mortality Weekly Report, 34* (18), 245-248.

Centers for Disease Control, (1986). Press release, June 12.

Foreman, J. (1985). In epidemic proportion, public fear of AIDS is spreading across U.S. *Boston Globe*, September 25, p. 1.

Freidson, E. (1970). *Profession of medicine: A study of the sociology of applied knowledge.* New York: Dodd-Mead.

Furstenberg, A. L., & Olson, M. M. (1984). Social work and AIDS. *Social Work in Health Care, 9* (4), 45-62.

Gartrell, N., Kraemer, H., & Brodie, H. H. (1974). Psychiatrists' attitudes toward female homosexuality. *Journal of Nervous and Mental Disorders, 159,* 141-144.

Golin, G. B. (1978). MDs assess problems in treating gays. *American Medical News*, October 27, *21,* 2.

Graham, S., & Reeder, L. G. (1972). Social factors in chronic illnesses. In *Handbook of medical sociology* (pp. 63-107). Englewood Cliffs, NJ: Prentice-Hall.

Halloran, L. G. (1984). AIDS: Risk of transmission to medical care workers. *Journal of the American Medical Association, 251,* 397.

Kinsey, A. C., Pomeroy, W. B., & Martin, C. E. (1948). *Sexual behavior in the human male.* Philadelphia: W. B. Saunders.

Klein, M., & Pfeffer, D. (1985). Homosexuality and the physician. *New Physician, 34* (6), 43-48.

Marshall, J. (1980). Stress among nurses. In C. L. Cooper & J. Marshall (Eds.), *White collar and professional stress* (pp. 19-62). New York: John Wiley.

Mather A. D. (Ed.). (1985). AIDS update: Halting the "epidemic of fear." *Infection Reports, 2,* 1-3.

Notes of a dying professor. (1972). *Pennsylvania Gazette*, March.

Phillips, J. L. (1983). As a nurse, I want to find out what the facts are on AIDS. *Critical Care Update, 10* (9), 37.

Sande, M. A. (1986). Transmission of AIDS: The case against casual contagion. *New England Journal of Medicine, 334,* 380-302.

Smith, K. (1974). Homophobia: A tentative personality profile. *Psychology Reports, 29,* 1091–1094.

Update: Evaluation of human T-lymphotropic virus types III/lymphadenopathy-associated virus infection in health-care personnel—United States. (1985). *Morbidity and Mortality Weekly Report, 34,* 575–577.

Wachter, R. M. (1986). The impact of the acquired immunodeficiency syndrome on medical residency training. *New England Journal of Medicine, 314,* 177–179.

Wortman, C. B., & Dunkel-Schetter, C. (1979). Interpersonal relationships and cancer: A theoretical analysis. *Journal of Social Issues, 35,* 120–155.

The Worried Well: Phenomenology, Predictors of Psychological Vulnerability, and Suggestions for Management

17

David Miller
The Middlesex Hospital Medical School
London, England

> ... here in this unfortunate extreme, if but a pimple appears or any slight ache is felt, they distract themselves with terrible apprehensions.... And so strongly are they for the most part possessed with this notion that any honest practitioner generally finds it more difficult to cure the imaginary evil than the real one. (Friend, 1727, p. 385)

Recent surveys of psychiatric and psychological disturbance among patients within sexually transmitted disease (STD) or genitourinary medicine (GUM) clinics have shown high rates of morbidity in these populations (Catalan, Bradley, Gallwey, & Hawton, 1982, Fitzpatrick, Frost, & Ikkos, 1986; Ikkos Fitzpatrick, Frost, & Nazeer, 1987; Mayou, 1975; Pedder & Goldberg, 1970). With the exception of the study by Mayou, rates of 30–43% psychiatric morbidity were found using the General Health Questionnaire (GHQ; Goldberg, 1978). Mayou (1975) found 20% morbidity using the Standardised Psychiatric Interview (SPI; Goldberg, Cooper, Eastwood, Kedword, & Shepherd, 1970), and recognized significant psychiatric morbidity in up to 45% of patients surveyed. Examples of disorders revealed in these surveys include affective disorders (e.g., depression and anxiety), personality disorders, psychosexual dysfunctions and disorders associated with physical symptoms (e.g., primary hypochondriasis, dysmorphophobia, obsessive-compulsive and monosymptomatic hypochonriacal psychotic states; Ikkos, 1987).

An important subset of these patients has somatic symptoms misattributed by them to some form of STD. Macalpine (1957) described 24 patients suffering from "syphilophobia," in which the patient presents with a wide spectrum of physical symptoms which "are expressions of their morbid fear or conviction of being infected" (p. 92), yet with no objective evidence of infection or disease upon examination. Frost (1985) described 36 patients suffering from hypochondriasis whose presentations featured morbid bodily concern (with disease phobia, psychongenic pain, and misperception and misinterpretation of physical symptoms), and abnormal illness behavior (failure to be reassured by medical staff and demand for further investigation, affective distress, and psychological defensiveness). Other studies (Bhanji & Mahoney, 1978; Kite & Grimble, 1963; Miller, Green, Farmer, & Carroll, 1985; Oates & Gomez, 1984) have described similar conditions associated with STDs, variously referred to as "hypochondriasis," "nosophobia," "venereophobia," and "pseudo-AIDS," which seem to characterize over 30% of patients referred to psychiatrists from an STD or GUM clinic setting.

This particular chapter describes the presenting and background phenomenology of patients suffering with the conviction that they have symptoms of infection associated with human immunodeficiency virus (HIV), the causative agent of acquired immuneodeficiency syndrome (AIDS), despite remaining infection-free as verified by (often repeated) serological testing and clinical assessment (Forstein, 1984; Miller, 1986b; Miller et al., 1985). This patient group is known as the "worried well." They may present for a variety of reasons—they may have had sex with a bisexual or drug-injecting man or woman in the past; they may be homosexual or have a history of (periodic) homosexual activity (frequently involving only low-risk activity); they may be psychologically vulnerable personalities responding to media reports or advertising about AIDS (the public anxiety about AIDS appears to act as a vehicle for the expression of their sexual guilt or anxiety, or of their general vulnerability; Miller, 1987).

This population is significant for the following reasons:

1. There appears to be a remarkable consistency in both presenting and background features of patients within this group, irrespective of sexuality or gender;

2. patients are often suicidal and involve considerable amounts of clinical time in investigation and management;

3. it appears to represent an expression of vulnerability in previously described populations which, in the context of rapidly increasing public awareness of AIDS and routes of HIV transmission, have "latched on" to this present major public health issue; and

4. it provides a "window" through which a form of heterosexual (and homosexual) reaction to the HIV pandemic can be assessed. To the present time, studies of psychosocial morbidity associated with AIDS have concentrated on the social subgroups most directly affected, that is, homosexual men (e.g., Christ & Wiener, 1985; Dilley, Ochitill, Perl, & Volberding, 1985; Miller, Green, & McCreaner, 1986; Temoshok, Mandel, & Moulton, 1986), hemophiliacs (e.g., Kernoff & Miller, 1986), and intravenous drug users (e.g., Des Jarlais & Friedman, 1987).

PATIENTS AND METHODS

Patients assessed for this phenomenological review were randomly selected from those referred to the author at St. Mary's and the Middlesex Hospitals for counseling over a period of 16 months. Referrals came from physicians and counselors in the GUM and Medicine Departments. All patients were assessed according to the following protocols:

1. Sexual history—patients were asked about their psychosexual adjustment from adolescence, together with the nature and context of all subsequent sexual experience. Issues monitored included level of sexual contact providing risk of HIV infection, overt/covert sexual identification/activity, and levels of stress and/or guilt associated with sexual activities leading to fears of HIV and other sexually transmitted diseases (STDs). History of previous STDs was assessed, and any "bargaining" toward a patient-perceived future low-risk sexuality or form of sexual expression was noted.

2. Clinical and laboratory examination—comprising full physical assessment, including examination of signs and symptoms suggested by patients as indicative of HIV disease. Any intercurrent disease was recorded and, if possible, treated. Laboratory assessment of HIV antibody status was facilitated (competitive ELISA) only with patient consent after precounseling (Glover & Miller, 1987) and other routine markers of immunological functioning were routinely performed. In cases of suspected non-HIV viral infection, relevant assays were performed.

3. Psychiatric history and examination—comprising assessment of previous personal and family psychiatric history, together with full psychiatric/psychological assessment (Miller, 1987). Psychosocial vulnerability was measured according to frequency of attendance to HIV physicians/counselors—and attendance for assessment of somatic phenomena at other sites (e.g., generalpractice clinics)—within the past 12 months; psychosocial isolation and dependence within current stable relationships; and numbers of prior negative HIV antibody tests or requests for testing.

All assessments were conducted by physicians, psychologists, and psychiatrists within GUM and liaison-psychiatry out patient clinics. As most patients presented with somatic complaints, and psychological and psychosexual distrubances, it was felt unhelpful to attempt separate subcategorizations of patient groups according to these and other previously applied groupings (Frost, 1985).

In some cases, HIV antibody testing had been previously facilitated and negative results obtained. In only two cases, however, were there any sexual activities reported that may have led to possible HIV infection in the previous six years. In these, antibody tests were given as part of the pre-referral intervention. In cases where the sexual history involved activities that would not lead to transmission of HIV infection (Green, 1986), antibody testing was only provided with patient consent after precounseling.

Patients were excluded from this study where they showed a maintained response to appropriate health education and counseling after presenting with anxieties over their possible antibody status. In this respect, a distinction is made between "AIDS anxiety," in which cognitive preoccupations and somatic indices of anxiety relating to recognition of risk-group membership or sensationalistic media reports may have provided transient concerns over personal health; and "the worried well," in which patients are chronically ruminative about their possible exposure to infection, despite informed and sympathetic counseling, clinical physical examination, and negative antibody screening.

RESULTS

Phenomenological features of 19 cases are presented in Table 17.1. Of the 19 subjects studied, eight were exclusively heterosexual, three bisexual, and eight

TABLE 17.1
Demographic Data

	Number	Mean age	Single	Married	Divorced	Widowed
Heterosexuals						
Male	6	40	2	3	1	0
Female	2	35	0	2	0	0
Bisexuals:	3	41	2	1	0	0
Homosexuals:	8	30	6	2*	0	0

*Where homosexual men were co-habiting in a stable, loving relationship by mutual assent for over 12 months, they were classified as "married."

exclusively homosexual. Two of the heterosexual subjects were female. The mean age of heterosexual subjects was 39 years; bisexuals, 41 years; and homosexuals, 30 years. Most cases showed considerable consistencies in both their presenting and background features.

PRESENTING FEATURES

Almost all of the subjects showed an unshakable and anxiety-laden conviction that they had HIV infection or disease, as indicated to them by the presence of physical anxiety-based features that they had misinterpreted as signs of HIV disease. Such confirmatory symptoms included fatigue, sweating, skin rashes, muscle pains, intermittent diarrhea, slight intermittent lymphadenopathy, sore throats, slight weight loss, minor mouth infections, and dizziness. In many cases, the misattribution of such features to HIV disease resulted from reading popular newspapers and magazines featuring descriptions of AIDS-related symptoms, many of which are mimicked by chronic anxiety symptoms (Miller, 1987). Ten of the 19 cases also suffered panic attacks, triggered by the appearance of anxiety symptoms, by media coverage of AIDS, by social discussion of the subject, or by involuntary thoughts or associations (e.g., of disease or deaths from HIV, or otherwise, in friends).

A further consistent presenting feature was the appearance of obsessive or obsessive-compulsive disorders associated with chronic rumination about HIV disease. Ruminations concerned images and/or thoughts of HIV disease and death, past "high-risk" sexual practices, punishment (moral or legal) for high-risk behavior, loss of loved ones as a consequence of personal high-risk activities, threates of infection to the spouse/lover/family/children, and dirtiness of infectivity of bodily fluids (e.g., semen, saliva, urine).

Obsessive-compulsive disorders involved responses to ruminative or obsessive thoughts, such as described above, including checking the body for Kaposi's sarcoma (KS) lesions (usually involving the counting of moles, freckles, and skin blemishes), and palpating specific bodily areas (glands, lymph nodes, sinus regions, veins) to "confirm" a swelling or pathology. Not surprisingly, this palpation would often result in pain and swelling, which added further confirmation to suspicions held by the patient. Other compulsions included washing sources of potential contamination, including clothes, shared bathrooms and lavatories, books, etc., and repeatedly scrutinizing the body or bodily areas (including mouth and genitals) of spouses/lovers and questioning them for signs of HIV-related disease. The rituals associated with such phenomena were primarily anxiety-reducing, and not of an avoidance type: washing, palpating, etc., were associated with a temporary reduction in the subjective tension concerning HIV infection.

In all but five cases, obsessive-compulsive symptoms were associated with a primary diagnosis of depression. Where this is not the case, an obsessive disorder was diagnosed (two patients subsequently developed a delusional state regarding their supposed infection). Depressive phenomena were associated with fears or feeling of the "inevitability" of exposure and HIV-related disease and decline; effects of fears on relationships and loved ones; and guilt at having placed oneself "at risk" in the past and at having done the same to the loved one. Depression was frequently associated with a full somatic and cognitive symptomatology and a declining sufficiency at work and in general.

The high proportion of suicidal subjects ($n = 10$) necessitated very close clinical monitoring and acute psychiatric admission in some cases. This, and the high level of expressed anxiety, resulted in such cases requiring inordinate levels of clinical time and intervention, both active and supportive, for the subjects and their loved ones. In most cases where suicidal activity was a presenting feature, the patient had made advanced plans for the facilitation of suicide, such as storing prescribed medications for overdosage or making detailed arrangements for suicide in cars or on public transportation.

Related to this was a significant degree of substance abuse in many patients, typically involving alcohol or prescribed drugs. Patients took these drugs primarily in order to help them cope with anxiety.

A further conspicuous presenting feature involved a high rate of recent attendance in general practice or hospital clinics in order to "find someone who really believes me or understands my problem." Associated with these levels of attendance was an often-repeated inconclusive or negative clinical examination and laboratory testing for antibodies to HIV (see Table 17.2).

TABLE 17.2
Presenting Features

Feature	Patient Numbers			
	Het M (N = 6)	Het F (N = 2)	Bi (N = 3)	Hom (N = 8)
Misinterpreted somatic features (aches, pains, etc.)	6	2	3	7
Anxiety	6	2	3	8
Depression	5	2	2	5
Obsessive-compulsive	6	2	3	8
Suicidal	3	2	1	4
High clinic attendance/non-reassured	6	2	2	5
Previous negative HIV antibody tests*	5 (1.4)	2 (2.5)	2 (2)	4 (1.7)

*Numbers in brackets refer to mean number of tests taken in those tested.

TABLE 17.3
Background Features

Feature	Patient Numbers			
	Het M (N = 6)	Het F (N = 2)	Bi (N = 3)	Hom (N = 8)
Sexual adjustment difficulties	3	1	3	8
Covert sexual activity	6	2	2	7
Sex-related guilt	6	2	2	5
Bargaining toward "low-risk" future	6	2	3	8
Low level of HIV-related sex activity risk	6	2	2	8
Previous STD history	0	0	2	3
Previous psychiatric/psychological history	4	2	0	4
Social isolation /high relationship dependence	4	2	1	6
Genuine intercurrent non-STD disease	1	1	1	1

BACKGROUND FEATURES

Background features resulting from the assessment protocol are presented in Table 17.3.

There were striking consistencies in the difficulties patients had experienced in coming to terms with their sexuality from their adolescense onward. These difficulties included issues of self-acceptance of homosexuality; and problems in the expression of sexual desire or attachment, often associated with constricting religious or familial imperatives on sexual expression. This was usually associated with a subsequent history of covert sexual expression and a high level of guilt associated with this. For example, in heterosexual subjects, anxiety-provoking sexual activity may have taken place outside or prior to marriage or a stable emotional relationship without being divulged, and it thus engendered considerable guilt over broken fidelity. In the context of homosexuality and bisexuality, in only two cases was a male patient able to express his homosexuality openly, all other subjects remaining "closeted" for fear of the reactions of others or because of self-esteem difficulties associated with being homosexual. While sexual expression in this latter group did not necessarily result in a high level of sexual guilt, in only one case was there a history of resulting sexual activity that was judged to be at high risk for acquisition of HIV. A central issue in difficulties of sexual adjustment relating to all subjects concerned a history of "venereophobia," in which sexual activity was much constrained by the fear of acquiring STDs. This typically resulted in a history of low-risk sexual expression, particularly in recent years; for example, intermittent episodes of mutual masturbation only. Five patients had a history of prior STD, all of which had occurred six or more years prior to intervention for their current concerns.

Interestingly, the fears associated with possible HIV infection had led to a significant tendency toward sexual bargaining—a propensity toward those sexual activities or relationships associated with a considerably reduced likelihood of future HIV infection. Thus, within the heterosexual group, there was a uniform expression of a desire for future HIV infection. Thus, within the heterosexual group, there was a uniform expression of a desire for future monogamy or celibacy, and, in most other subjects, there was an expressed desire for future celibacy, monogamy, or heterosexuality.

Ten subjects had a previous psychiatric disturbance for which they had been treated. The most common disorders reported were those related to anxiety or depressive disorders; one had a history of obsessive-compulsive disturbance; and, interestingly, four patients had a history of eating disorder (anorexia nervosa or bulimia). For some, the prior psychiatric or psychological intervention related to recurring concern over possible venereological infections such as herpes ("venereophobia"), and in others related to "mediahyped" public-health issues, such as breast cancer and Legionnaires' disease. Two subjects had diagnosable, intercurrent physical disease, knowledge of which did nothing to lessen the obsessive disorders associated with their fear of HIV. Two other subjects had nonspecific viral illness not related to HIV infection as determined on repeated antibody screening. Clinical investigation suggested that in both cases the viral infection was probably an influenza-type illness.

The other background feature measured in the sample was that of social isolation or high dependence in existing stable relationships. Thirteen of the subjects studied had stable relationships characterized by high levels of dependence in a context of general social (and sexual) isolation or withdrawal.

DISCUSSION

Bisexual and Heterosexual Worried-Well Subjects

Five out of eight heterosexual subjects, and one of the three bisexual subjects, were married, and a triggering stimulus to their obsessive fears of HIV had been guilt associated with covert sexual activity outside of this marital relationship. Similarly, five of the eight experienced significant difficulties during their adolescent sexual adjustment, and, in most cases, patients had prior psychiatric or psychological involvement of a formal nature. Within this group, there was also a high level of social isolation in later years, even in the context of marriage. Two subjects within the bisexual group had STDs in the years prior to the recognition of the HIV pandemic. Interestingly, the mean age of bisexual and heterosexual worried-well persons is 39 years, which contrasts significantly with the average of 30 years in the homosexual worried-well population.

Homosexual Worried-Well Subjects

The consistent clinical picture emerging from the analysis of this group is of a younger homosexual man who has experienced significant difficulties in coming to terms with his sexual orientation; and who has been involved in covert, low-risk sexual activity resulting in a minimal prior history of STD infection. There is a consistent high level of social isolation in this group, also coinciding with significant sexual guilt. Identification of self with high-risk HIV infection had led to the appearance of significant anxiety and obsessive disorders in the context of depression, and in some cases suicidal ideation. This, in turn, appears to reinforce previous levels of social isolation and withdrawal. Further, there is association with a medium to high level of attendance for confirmatory assessment of clinical and laboratory features prompted by a high level of somatic distress.

OVERVIEW

The presentation of subjects in the worried-well study closely resembles that of subjects revealed in the context of prior epidemics, notably STDs such as syphilis. "Syphilophobia" was first recorded in the medical literature in 1586, almost exactly 400 years ago (Macalpine, 1957). Since the emergence of the AIDS epidemic and the increasing media coverage of the syndrome and its causative agent, HIV, large numbers of psychologically vulnerable persons appear to have adopted the epidemic as a vehicle for the expression of their sexual or psychological/psychiatric vulnerability (Miller, 1987; Nicholas, Glover, Parr, Leonard, & Miller, 1987).

It is important to note that there are considerable overlaps in the phenomenology of both heterosexual and homosexual groups, and it seems likely that we will experience more difficulties in future patient management in both low- and high-risk social groups. It is clear that persons with demonstrated psychiatric/ psychological history and vulnerability, involved in covert and usually low-risk sexual activity, suffering significant sexual guilt and consequent practical non-identification with high-risk groups present a discrete clinical phenomenon. A low level of self-esteem often results, and somatic symptoms of anxiety and depression will often be misinterpreted as evidence of infection, resulting in high rates of obsessive-compulsive disorder and depression.

If one uses the background criteria as yardsticks by which to measure psychological vulnerability newly presented from all risk groups, it is conceivable that the potential for psychosocial morbidity will be recognized and, hopefully, minimized before these disorders progress to levels of functional incapacity. Criteria for the identification of vulnerable persons in this regard a presented in Table 17.4.

TABLE 17.4
Worried-well Checklist of Presenting and Background Features

Presenting features:

Acute, high-level anxiety with multiple anxiety-related somatic features

Intervention-resistant ideas/beliefs that such symptoms relate to HIV infection

Frustration and depression at inability of doctors to successfully "diagnose" HIV infection/disease

Repeated (involuntary) dwelling on thoughts/images of HIV infection, disease, and decay

Prominent fears that HIV infection has been passed on to loved ones, children, etc.

Obsessive-compulsive features including bodily checking, washing, and repeated questioning of physicians

Conspicuous guilt over sexual and/or lifestyle activities seen as leading to "infection"

Expressed or covert suicidal ideation/planning, sometimes with a history of unsuccessful attempts

Background features:

History of covert and usually "low-risk" sexual expression, in context of guilt and stress

Venereophobia relating to sexual expression/history, usually involving no (serious) prior STDs

Difficulties in post-adolescent sexual adjustment

Previous psychiatric/psychological history (e.g., depression, obsessive disorders, adjustment disorders, hypochondriasis, eating disorder), or high level of physician attendance

Previous multiple negative HIV antibody tests

High dependency in close relationships and relative social isolation/poor social "networking" or support

Poor family support and/or family non-awareness of sexuality

Bargaining toward future monogamy, celibacy, or low-risk sexual expression

HYPOCHONDRIASIS

In attempting to formally achieve a reliable diagnostic measure with which to characterize this form of presentation, the clinician is forced to consider the chronology of presenting phenomena. This means asking the question, "Which comes first—the obsession or the depression?" As clinical experience with this study group indicates, the obsessional state has, in some cases, lifted

TABLE 17.5
DSM III Diagnostic Criteria for Hypochondriasis

A. The predominant disturbance is an unrealistic interpretation of physical signs or sensations as abnormal, leading to preoccupation with the fear or belief of having a serious disease.

B. Thorough physical evaluation does not support the diagnosis of any physical disorder that can account for the physical signs or sensations or for the individual's unrealistic interpretation of them.

C. The unrealistic fear or belief of having a disease persists, despite medical reassurance, and causes impairment in social or occupational functioning.

D. The disturbance is not due to any other mental disorder, such as schizophrenia, affective disorder, or somatization disorder.

with the prescription of antidepressants (Miller, 1987). However, this is not universally the case, and a depressive state cannot, therefore, always be assumed to be the primary disorder, particularly where associated features of obsessive-compulsive disorders are prominent (American Psychiatric Association, 1980).

Similarly, while most of those studied give ample evidence of anxiety disorders, it is rare for patients to present without other complicating features. Anxiety disorder is usually an intercurrent phenomenon in this population (Salkovskis & Warwick, 1986).

Given the core features of these clinical presentations—a preoccupation with health, an insufficient medical pathology, selective attention to bodily changes/features, a negative construing of any bodily sensations or changes, and selective attention to and disbelief of medical information that contrasts with the patients' assumptions—a more enduring and relevant diagnosis appears to be that of hypochondriasis (APA, 1980). DSM III diagnostic criteria for hypochondriasis are presented in Table 17.5.

These criteria clearly have considerable relevance for the diagnosis of patients represented in this survey. In addition, however, this classification widens the range of treatment options open to the clinician. For example, Salkovskis and Warwick (1986) have presented promising suggestions for management of hypochondriacal patients using cognitive-behavioral approaches.

TREATMENT

Obsessive states are among the most difficult to treat in contemporary psychology (Carnwath & Miller, 1986). This subject population also emphasizes the difficulties involved in trying to prove the absence of disease. Patients will also present frequently with high-level anxiety, panic states, depression, and serious suicidal planning; and interventions that can intercept such plans and undermine the motivators of such levels of distress will be necessary to avoid significant psychosocial morbidity in the future.

Previous studies have highlighted the importance of identifying the exact nature of patient anxieties and any correlative symptoms (e.g., Wolcott, Fawzy, & Pasnau, 1985). For many patients, this information-gathering process will be of help in itself, at least temporarily, as it provides them with an opportunity to vent their anxieties in a way that they have not done before, particularly if their worries relate to covert sexual activities that they have not been able to divulge to stable sexual partners or associates. Such data gathering will also frequently indicate a poor coping response to stress in general; and it may well be that by highlighting methods of stress reduction or appropriate daily planning that minimizes exposure to stressful events or obsessive triggers, the patient will experience some relief, particularly from associated anxiety symptoms.

Along with the process of clinical indentification goes the equally important process of placing the patient's worries in the context of (a) information concerning his or her low level of risk of exposure to the virus through his reported sexual activity; and (b) his broader anxieties or concerns that form a context for this current presentation. It must be affirmed that the continual requests made for reassurance from medical staff actually perpetuate the problem by repeatedly distracting attention—the patient's and the physician's—from the *real* bases of their anxieties. Strict therapeutic contracting that involves limiting therapist/ physician contact with the patient, limiting time spent during consultations discussing HIV/AIDS symptoms and statistics, and developing a consistent and thorough examiniation of his or her background vulnerabilities, affirming realistic anxiety/distracting or confronting activities and prior successful coping strategies, may be the most promising course (Miller, Acton, & Hedge, 1988).

Various methods in the behavioral psychotherapy paradigm have been found to be successful in some cases, although, of course, with many of these patients, the current anxieties form just the latest manifestation of chronic neurotic conditions. Salkovskis and Warwick (1986) emphasize that the treatment of hypochondriacal states requires a minimum number of steps. First, engagement, in which the patient is educated about the meaning and the frequency of specific bodily changes. Second reattribution, in which alternative explanations for the reported bodily changes are constructed. Third, behavior modification, particularly those behaviors which maintain the cycles of obsessive and/or depressive response (e.g., by instituting a program of response prevention). Such approaches require familiarization with principles of cognitive treatment of hypochondriacal states. These include recognizing that the aim is to help the patient to identify what the problem is, not what it isn't; drawing a careful distinction between providing relevant information or irrelevant or repetitive information; and working on patients' beliefs, collaboratively, rather than discounting them. Recognition of these issues is particularly important for maintaining patient compliance throughout treatment and for future medical management (Frost, 1985).

Pharmacological interventions, particularly where depression is the underlying disorder, may be of value; although they, too, pose a dilemma. Those medications traditionally used for depressive or obsessive states usually produce marked side effects to therapeutic doses which tend to exacerbate patients' fears and hypochondriacal dispositions, given their somatic sensitivities. On the other hand, the severity of presentations often makes immediate pharmacological intervention seem necessary. Short-term anxiolitic prescriptions, beta-blockers, or low-dose neuroleptic prescriptions may be of use somatically, but do little to intercept obsessive content. Behavioral psychotherapy may assist where background vulnerability and relationship disturbances, arising from the fears of HIV disease, exist; and, in some cases, psychiatric admission will be required, particularly where suicidal risk is prominent (Miller, 1986a; 1986b).

The need for acute psychiatric admission protocols for this population is particularly evident, given the high level of suicidal planning and activity within the groups surveyed. Additionally, appropriately trained psychiatric staff acting in a liaison capacity with STD or GUM clinics must be available for early recognition and intervention.

CONCLUSION

This brief series of patients reveals consistent presenting and background psychological phenomena in the population of worried well, presenting in the context of the HIV pandemic. This group also conforms to the psychiatric classification of hypochondriasis, and these consistencies lead to a number of clinical options in a patient group with considerable management difficulties. The consistency in presenting and background features within this population enables early clinical identification of chronic psychosocial vulnerability and likely chronic management difficulty in those attending for HIV antibody testing, particularly following heightened media coverage of HIV/AIDS. Further, with the development of promising treatment packages for hypochondriasis, particularly from the cognitive/behavioral psychotherapy paradigm, the scope for affective clinical interventions complementing the traditional interventions for depression and obsessive disorders is becoming increasingly wide. Clearly, with identification of this important clinical group becoming more reliable, the need for sustained evaluation of such interventions is paramount.

ACKNOWLEDGMENTS

Portions of this study were first presented at the IIIrd International Conference on AIDS, Washington, D.C., June 1–5, 1987. The author thanks Drs. Barbara Hedge and Ulrike Schmidt (Academic Department of Psychiatry, The

Middlesex Hospital Medical School) for constructive comments on earlier drafts of this chapter.

REFERENCES

American Psychiatric Association. (1980). *Diagnostic and statistical manual of mental disorders* (3rd ed.). Washington, D.C.: Author.

Bhanji, S., & Mahoney, J. D. H. (1978). The value of a psychiatric service within the veneral diseases clinic. *British Journal of Venereal Disease, 54*, 266-268.

Carnwath, T., & Miller, D. (1986). *Behavioural psychotherapy in primary care: A practice manual.* London: Academic Press.

Catalan, J., Bradley, M., Gallwey, J., & Hawton, K. (1981). Sexual dysfunction and psychiatric morbidity in patients attending a clinic for sexually transmitted disease. *British Journal of Psychiatry, 138*, 292-296.

Christ, G. H., & Wiener, L. S. (1985). Psychosocial issues in AIDS. In V. T. DeVita, S. Hellman, & S. A. Rosenberg (Eds.), *AIDS: Etiology, diagnosis, treatment and prevention* (pp. 275-298). Philadelphia: J. B. Lippincott.

Des Jarlais, D. C., & Friedman, S. R. (1987). HIV infection among intravenous drug abusers: Epidemiology and risk reduction. *AIDS, 1*, 67-76.

Dilley, J. W., Ochitill, H. N., Perl, M., & Volberding, P. A. (1985). Findings in psychiatric consultations with patients with acquired immune deficiency syndrome. *American Journal of Psychiatry, 142*, 82-86.

Fitzpatrick, R., Frost, D., & Ikkos, G. (1986). Survey of psychological disturbance in patients attending a sexually transmitted diseases clinic. *Genitourinary Medicine, 62*, 111-115.

Forstein, M. (1984). The worried well. In S. Nichols & D. Ostrow (Eds.), *Psychiatric implications for acquired immune deficiency syndrome.* Washington, DC: American Psychiatric Press.

Friend, J. (1727). *The history of physick* (2nd ed., Part 2). London: Walthoe.

Frost, D. P. (1985). Recognition of hypochondriasis in a clinic for sexually transmitted disease. *Genitourinary Medicine, 61*, 133-137.

Glover, L., & Miller, D. (1987). AIDS: Counselling and support, (1) Hospital and statutory services. In M. Adler (Ed.), *Diseases in the homosexual male* (pp. 163-174). London: John Wiley.

Goldberg, D. (1978). *Manual of the General Health Questionnaire.* Windsor, Canada: NFER Nelson.

Goldberg, D., Cooper, B., Eastwood, M., Kedward, H., & Shepherd, M. (1970). A standardised psychiatric interview for use in community surveys. *British Journal of Preventative and Social Medicine, 24*, 18-23.

Green, J. (1986). Counselling HTLV-III seropositives. In D. Miller, J. Weber, & J. Green (Eds.), *The management of AIDS patients* (pp. 151-168). London: Macmillan Press.

Ikkos, G. (1987). *Psychiatric aspects of sexually transmitted diseases: A review.* Unpublished manuscript.

Ikkos, G., Fitzpatrick, R., Frost, D., & Nazeer, S. (1987). Psychological disturbance and illness behaviour in a clinic for sexually transmitted diseases. *British Journal of Medical Psychology, 60*, 121-126.

Jeffries, D. (1986). Virology. In D. Miller, J. Weber, & J. Green (Eds.), *The management of AIDS patients* (pp. 53-63). London: Macmillan Press.

Kernoff, P., & Miller, R. (1986). AIDS-related problems in the management of hemophilia. In D. Miller, J. Weber, & J. Green (Eds.), *The management of AIDS patients* (pp. 81-92). London: Macmillan Press.

Kite, E., & Grimble, A. (1963). Psychiatric aspects of venereal disease. *British Journal of Venereal Diseases, 39,* 173-180.

Macalpine, I. (1957). Syphilophobia: A psychiatric study. *British Journal of Venereal Disease, 33,* 92-99.

Mayou, R. (1975). Psychological morbidity in a clinic for sexually transmitted disease. *British Journal of Venereal Disease, 51,* 57-60.

Miller, D. (1986a). Psychology, AIDS, ARC and PGL. In D. Miller, J. Weber, and J. Green (Eds.), *The management of AIDS patients* (pp. 131-150). London: Macmillan Press.

Miller, D. (1986b). The worried well. In D. Miller, J. Weber, & J. Green (Eds.), *The management of AIDS patients* (pp. 169-173). London: Macmillan Press.

Miller, D. (1987, June 1-6). *Predictors of chronic psychosocial disturbance arising from the threat of HIV infection: Lessons from heterosexual, bisexual and homosexual worried-well patients.* Poster presented at IIIrd International Conference on AIDS. Washington, D.C.

Miller, D., Acton, T.M.G., & Hedge, B. (1988). The worried well: Their identification and management. *Journal of the Royal College of Physicians of London, 22* (3), 158-165.

Miller, D., Green, J., Farmer, R., & Carroll, G. (1985). A "pseudo-AIDS" syndrome following from a fear of AIDS. *British Journal of Psychiatry, 146,* 550-551.

Miller, D., Green, J., & McCreaner, A. (1986). Organising a counselling service for problems related to acquired immune deficiency syndrome (AIDS). *Genitourinary Medicine, 68,* 116-122.

Nicholas, H., Glover, L., Parr, D., Leonard, P., & Miller, D. (1987, June 1-6). *The effect of a government AIDS media campaign on a general population: Antibody test requests and reasons.* Paper presented at IIIrd International Conference on AIDS. Washington, D.C.

Oates, J. K., & Gomez, J. (1984). Venereophobia. *British Journal of Hospital Medicine, 32,* 435-436.

Pedder, J. R., & Goldberg, D. P. (1970). A survey by questionnaire of psychiatric disturbance in patients attending a venereal diseases clinic. *British Journal of Venereal Diseases, 46,* 58-61.

Salkovskis, P. M., & Warwick, H. M. C. (1986). Morbid preoccupations, health anxiety and resurrance: A cognitive-behavioural approach to hypochondriasis. *Behaviour Research and Therapy, 23,* 597-602.

Temoshok, L., Mandel, J. S., & Moulton, J. M. (1986, May 13). *A longitudinal psychosocial study of AIDS and ARC in San Francisco: Preliminary results.* Paper presented at annual meeting of American Psychiatric Association, Washington, D.C.

Wolcott, D. L., Fawzy, F. I., & Pasnau, R. O. (1985). Acquired immune deficiency syndrome (AIDS) and consultation-liaison psychiatry. *General Hospital Psychiatry, 7,* 280-292.

Author Index

Printed and bound by CPI Group (UK) Ltd, Croydon, CR0 4YY
17/10/2024
01775685-0008

Subject Index